DICTIONARY OF HEALTH INFORMATION TECHNOLOGY AND SECURITY

Dr. David Edward Marcinko, MBA, CFP©

Certified Medical Planner©

Editor-in-Chief

Hope Rachel Hetico, RN, MSHA, CPHQ

Certified Medical Planner©

Managing Editor

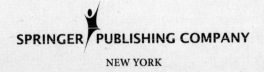

SPRINGER PUBLISHING COMPANY

NEW YORK

Springer Publishing Company, LLC
11 West 42nd Street
New York, NY 10036
www.springerpub.com

Acquisitions Editor: Sheri W. Sussman
Production Editor: Carol Cain
Cover design: Mimi Flow
Composition: Apex Publishing, LLC

07 08 09 10/ 5 4 3 2 1

Library of Congress Cataloging-in-Publication Data

Dictionary of health information technology and security / David Edward Marcinko, editor-in-chief, Hope Rachel Hetico, managing editor.
   p. ; cm.
  Includes bibliographical references.
  ISBN-13: 978-0-8261-4995-4 (alk. paper)
  ISBN-10: 0-8261-4995-2 (alk. paper)
  1. Medical informatics—Dictionaries. 2. Medicine—Information technology—Dictionaries. 3. Medical informatics—Security measures—Dictionaries. I. Marcinko, David E. (David Edward) II. Hetico, Hope R.
[DNLM: 1. Informatics—Dictionary—English. 2. Medical Informatics—Dictionary—English. 3. Computer Communication Networks—Dictionary English. 4. Computer Security—Dictionary—English. W 13 D557165 2007]

R858.D53 2007
610.3—dc22   2007005879

Printed in the United States of America by RR Donnelley.

The *Dictionary of Health Information Technology and Security* is dedicated to Edward Anthony Marcinko Sr., and Edward Anthony Marcinko Jr., of Fell's Point, Maryland. They constantly reminded us to present concepts as simply as possible, as we endeavored to create a comprehensive Dictionary relevant to the entire health care industrial complex.

Contents

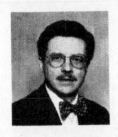

Dr. David Edward Marcinko, MBA, CFP©, CMP©, is a health care technology futurist, economist, lexicographer, and board certified surgical fellow from Temple University in Philadelphia. A prolific writer, he edited five practice-management books, three medical texts in two languages, six financial planning books, three CD-ROMs, a quarterly periodical and a four volume comprehensive dictionary series (www.HealthDictionarySeries.com) for physicians, hospitals, financial advisors, accountants, attorneys, and health care business consultants. Internationally recognized for his work, he provides litigation support and expert witness testimony in State and Federal Court, with hundreds of clinical publications archived in the Library of Congress and the Library of Medicine at the National Institute of Health. His thought leadership essays have been cited in journals such as: *Managed Care Executives, Healthcare Informatics, Medical Interface, Plastic Surgery Products, Teaching and Learning in Medicine, Orthodontics Today, Chiropractic Products, Podiatry Today, Investment Advisor Magazine, Registered Representative, Financial Advisor Magazine, CFP© Biz (Journal of Financial Planning), Journal of the American Medical Association (JAMA.ama-assn.org), The Business Journal for Physicians* and *Physician's* Money Digest; by professional organizations such as the Medical Group Management Association (MGMA), American College of Medical Practice Executives (ACMPE), American College of Physician Executives (ACPE), American College of Emergency Room Physicians (ACEP), Health Care Management Associates (HMA), and PhysiciansPractice.com; and by academic institutions such as the Northern University College of Business, Creighton University, UCLA School of Medicine, Medical College of Wisconsin, Washington University School of Medicine, University of North Texas Health Science Center, University of Pennsylvania Medical and Dental Libraries, Southern Illinois College of Medicine, University at Buffalo Health Sciences Library, University of Michigan Dental Library, University of Medicine and Dentistry of New Jersey, Emory University School of Medicine, Georgetown University, and the Goizueta School of Business at Emory University, among others.

Dr. Marcinko received his undergraduate degree from Loyola University (Baltimore), completed his internship and residency training at Atlanta Hospital and Medical Center, received fellowship confirmation in Las Vegas, earned his business degree from the Keller Graduate School of Management (Chicago), and earned his financial planning diploma from Oglethorpe University (Atlanta). He is a former licensee of the Certified Financial Planner© Board of Standards (Denver) and holds the Certified Medical Planner© (CMP©) designation. He held general securities (Series #7), uniform securities state law (Series #63), and registered investment advisory representative (Series #65) licenses from the National Association of Securities Dealers (NASD). He was a Certified Physician in Healthcare Quality (CPHQ); a certified American Board of Quality Assurance and Utilization Review Physician (ABQAURP); and is a member of the American Society of Health Economists (ASHE) and the International Health Economics Association (iHEA); a member of the American Health Information Management Association (AHIMA) and the Healthcare Information and Management Systems Society (HIMSS); a member of the Microsoft Professional Accountant's Network (MPAN); a registered member of the U.S. Microsoft Partner's Program (MPP); a member of the Microsoft Health User's Group (MS-HUG); a Sun Executive Boardroom program member sponsored by CEO Jonathan Schwartz; a member of the Healthcare Informatics Executive Panel and member of SUNSHINE [Solutions for Healthcare Information, Networking, and Education], an international community for health care IT innovation created by HIMSS and Sun Microsystems, Inc. (NASD-SUNW). He is also a life, disability, health, property-casualty, annuity, and insurance professional for the State of Georgia.

After a brief stint as a visiting instructor in finance and health care administration at several business schools in the Southeast, he was appointed Academic Provost of iMBA Inc., to lead the firm's adult online learning (heutagogy) initiatives as an educator, interactive Web site engineer, Office-Live™ and Windows Vista™ operating system beta-tester for the Microsoft Corporation of Redmond, Washington (NASD-MSFT), and interim Chief Visionary Officer for a B2B telecommunication firm that failed in its bid for venture capital, but flourished in the private sector. Dr. Marcinko also has numerous other editorial and reviewing roles to his credit. His most recent offering from Springer Publishing Company is *The Business of Medical Practice* (Advanced Profit Maximization Techniques for Savvy Doctors [second edition]). A favorite on the lecture circuit often quoted in the media, he speaks frequently to medical and financial societies throughout the country in an entertaining and witty fashion.

Currently, Dr. Marcinko is Chief Executive Officer for the Institute of Medical Business Advisors, Inc. (www.MedicalBusinessAdvisors.com). The firm is headquartered in Atlanta, has offices in five states and Europe, and works with a diverse list of individual and corporate clients. It sponsors the professional Certified Medical Planner© charter designation program (www.CertifiedMedicalPlanner.com). As a national educational resource center and referral alliance, the iMBA Institute and its network of independent professionals provide solutions and managerial peace-of-mind to medical professionals, emerging health care organizations and their consulting business advisors and financial fiduciary consultants.

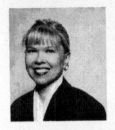

Hope Rachel Hetico, RN, MSHA, CPHQ, CMP©, received her nursing degree (RN) from Valparaiso University and Master's of Science Degree in Health Care Administration (MSHA) from the University of St. Francis, in Joliette, Illinois. She is the editor of a dozen major textbooks and a nationally known expert in managed medical care, medical reimbursement, case management, health insurance, security and risk management, utilization review, HIPAA, NACQA, OSHA, HIPAA, HEDIS, and JCAHO rules and regulations.

Initially, a devotee of pedagogy, Ms. Hetico became an apostle of adult learning using the andragogic principles of *i*MBA for corporate, professional, and practitioner audiences. She continually recruits and hosts a think-tank of talented thought–leadership visionaries, essayists, and experts for the *i*MBA Lexicon Query Social Network© and collaborative Web site (www.HealthDictionarySeries.com). With this documented history of identifying innovations in education and accelerating their adoption by the medical and financial services industries, she is frequently quoted in the health care business media and brings a decade of entrepreneurship and creative leadership skills to the *i*MBA National Network© of independent advisors.

Prior to joining the Institute of Medical Business Advisors as Chief Operating Officer, Ms. Hetico was a hospital executive, financial advisor, insurance agent, Certified Professional in Healthcare Quality (CPHQ), and distinguished visiting instructor of Healthcare Administration for the University of Phoenix, Graduate School of Business and Management. She was also national corporate Director for Medical Quality Improvement at Apria Healthcare, a public company in Costa Mesa, California [NYSE-AHG].

Currently an IT ontologist, Senior Linguistic Docent© for *i*MBA, and devotee of health information technology and heutagogy, Ms. Hetico is also Managing Editor for *Healthcare Organizations: Financial Management Strategies* (www.HealthCareFinancials.com), an interpretive reference guide with quarterly print updates dedicated to advancing corporate financial management strategies for hospitals, clinics, and related entities. She is charged with its leadership in the exploding health care institutional marketplace, while continuing to nurture its rapidly growing list of institutional and individual subscriber clients.

Preface

There is no privacy…get over it.

—*Scott McNealy*
Former CEO, Sun Microsystems, Inc.

This year marks the 25th anniversary of the IBM 5150, the first personal computer to be taken seriously as a business tool, rather than a hobby. The IBM PC was by no means the first personal computer on the market. IBM tried in 1975 with a $9,000 behemoth that never took off. Commodore, TRS, and Apple had been in the home computer business since 1977. They all found favor with home enthusiasts but failed to break into the corporate boardroom. After the 5150's debut on August 12, 1981, Apple took out an ad in the *Wall Street Journal* congratulating the company on finally noticing the PC market. A famous headline proclaimed, "Welcome, IBM. Seriously."

Yet, the emergence of serious health care information technology (HIT) and security, as a distinct field, may be traced back for more than 40 years when the vision for an electronic health record (EHR) was born. At a time which predated the PC, HIT experts believed EHRs would be adopted within a few years. The reality is that little happened until 1991, when the Institute of Medicine's report on computer-based patient records encouraged investing in new products. Unfortunately, few physicians took advantage of them because of expense and a lack of standardization for enterprise wide compatibility.

In fact, according to The Center for Studying Health System Change, the proportion of doctors with access to HIT doubled between 2002 and 2006.[1] Yet, according to George Washington University and the Massachusetts General Hospital, less than 24% of office-based physicians take advantage of HIT, and only 9% use more advanced systems that can help reduce costs and medical errors.[2] Few health care facilities comply with federal laws to protect patient privacy, while more patients refuse to sign release forms for medical information. Such trends bode ill for a national electronic health data exchange as neither mainframes, nor mini-computers, or open-source codes like UNIX or Linux provide the pricing and confidentiality demanded by the mission-critical health care industry. Moreover, although hardware accelerators seemed to represent the next evolution in health care computing performance following vector chips of the 1970s, RISC-based machines of the 1980s, and clusters of the 1990s; it is the WANs, networking mobility, and programmable blogs, vlogs virtual machines and collaboration philosophy of the 2000s, that promise to provide the needed cross-vendor capability to make true health care connectivity a reality.

Today, HIT is again at the top of the list for all physicians and health care organizations as the Vista© OS and the Microsoft-Intel© platforms offer substantially more functionality and reduced complexity for technophobic physicians than ever before. And, this time, all signs indicate that considerable progress will be made in the near future.

So, what has caused this paradigm change? In two words: financing and security.

The reality is that regulations-induced spending, including the Patriot Act and the Health Insurance Portability and Accountability Act (HIPAA), have placed more demands on health care technology budgets than ever before. Attention to HIT intensified when President George W. Bush called for widespread adoption of EHRs within the next decade.[3] In addition to digitizing the clinical information, patients, providers, and policymakers are looking ahead to securely sharing information electronically among all health organizations. The initiative was met with skepticism when a laptop computer was stolen by two teenagers containing unencrypted SSN information on 26.5 million retired veterans, 50,000 active-duty military, and 38,000 names last year. And, according to Trend-Micro, bot-infestations also occurred at government agencies such as the U.S. Department of Defense, the U.S. Navy, the Pittsburgh Supercomputing Center, and the Argonne National Laboratory, among others; costing U.S. consumers more than $8 billion because of computer-related crimes during the past two years.[4]

Enter the Trustworthy Computing initiative of the Microsoft Corporation as a hallmark feature of its Vista© for Health care Operating system as an optimizer of the most demanding health care enterprise workloads; including transaction processing, data mining, practice intelligence, enterprise resource planning applications, and high-scale performance computing.

Naturally, health data would also become available to compare mortality rates for surgeons at individual hospitals; for insurers to pay-for-performance; for consumers to compare prices on various health insurance products; and for patients with Consumer Directed Health Plans (CDHPs) to price shop for physicians, tests, and procedures. Such a connected and collaborative health system would also enable patients and doctors to access EHRs, prescription records, radiology and electro-cardiac images, and to facilitate access management within the decade. But, with huge projected costs, the disruptive potential of such an electronic health system is great; and so is its disruptive jargon if IT terms are not codified and understood in some ontological way. Thus, a robust solution for mission critical health care operations and EHRs now seems finally on the horizon as new HIT security concepts are commonplace in health care administration; along with its innovative jargon.

Still not convinced of linguistic HIT importance? Just consider the tortuous and contorted term, Regional Health Information Organization, or RHIO, which may be defined as a: *centralized, decentralized or hybrid architecture facilitating the coordinated interchange of electronic health information among autonomous databases representing various users, applications, workstations, main frames and stakeholder where each controls its interactions by means of an export schema to specify shared components, and an import schema to specify non-local information that a component wishes to manipulate.* Or, the simple term, electronic health record (EHR), which has more than 27 definitions, redundancies, restrictions, components, and tortuous derivations listed in the Health Information Management Systems Society (HIMSS) compendium, for 2006.

Nevertheless, HIT is more than verbal chicanery; it is an integral component of the protean health care industrial complex. Its language is a diverse and broad-based construct, covering many other industries: mathematics, engineering, and computer science; medicine, law, and nursing; as vernacular expressions from the street are co-mingled. Even seemingly "non-health technology" terms used by hackers, enthusiasts, and professional IT administrators are common because of their centrality to the health enterprise system. The discipline is not contained in a single space however, and its language needs to be codified to avoid confusion. But, the field is rapidly changing in a political environment seemingly flushed with cash. More terms have reached the health care information technology marketplace in the last few years than in all previous decades.

For example, terms such as fat-servers, thin-blades, cracker, dongle, deadly embrace, mashup, cinnamon bun, IMers, ICRers, CMing, war chalking, and Black Hating did not exist just a decade ago. Eponyms, standards, and laws such as the Clinger-Cohen Act, Moore's Law, Sar-Box, RICO, HIPAA, SONET, Huffman Code, SNOMED, MP3 protocols, GNU, IRC, HL7, and the Parkerian Hexad, were similarly absent; as were slang expressions such as viruses, trojans, worms, back-doors, lossy compression, pharming, phishing, vishing, or buffing. Latin phrases such as *ad-hoc, de-facto, de-jour,* and *qui-tam* no longer seem like a linguistic novelty.

And so, the *Dictionary of Health Information Technology and Security* was conceived as an essential tool for doctors, nurses, and clinicians; CTOs, CIOs, CMOs, CKOs, CSOs, CTSs, medical executives, and health care administrators; lawyers, management, and medical business consultants; HMOs, PPOs, and MCOs, as well as medical, dental, business, and health care administration graduate students and patients.

With more than 5,000 definitions, explanations, terms, and plurals; 3,000 whimsical abbreviations, morphemes, lexemes, code-names, slang terms, and acronyms; and a 2,000-item oeuvre of resources, readings, and nomenclature derivatives, the *Dictionary* is really a 3-in-1 reference. It contains more than 10,000 entries that cover the IT language of every health care industry sector: (i) layman, purchaser, and benefits manager; (ii) physician, provider, and health care facility; and (iii) payer, intermediary, and consulting professional. We highlight new terminology and current definitions, influential companies, products, people, programs, and applications; and we include a list of confusing acronyms and alphabetical abbreviations. The *Dictionary* also contains rich HIT offerings of the past that are still in colloquial use today. These backward-compatible definitions are contemporaneously expanded where appropriate with simple examples, illustrations, and cross-references to research various other definitions, or to pursue relevant and related terms.

Of course, by its very nature the *Dictionary of Health Information Technology and Security* is ripe for periodic updates by engaged readers working in the fluctuating health information technology and security milieu. It will be periodically updated and edited to reflect the changing lexicon of terms, as older words are retired and newer ones are continually created. Accordingly, if you have any comments, suggestions, or would like to contribute substantive unlisted abbreviations, acronyms, eponyms, or definitions to a future edition, or to nominate an expert, please contact us directly at the Institute, or though our Web site blog. We are flexible, market responsive, and committed to making this encyclopedic tool a valuable resource of the future.

David Edward Marcinko
Hope Rachel Hetico

NOTES

Preface

1. Marietti, C. (2006). Standing orders. *Healthcare Informatics,* 23(12), 8.
2. Claburn, T., Greenemeier, L., & McGee, M. (2006, October 16). The bots. *Information Week,* 32,43.
3. Executive Order (2006, August). Promoting quality and efficient health care in federal government administered or sponsored health care programs.
4. Kolbasuk, M. (2006, October 18). Targeted treatment? *Information Week,* 32, 32.

Foreword

Whither the *Dictionary of Health Information Technology and Security*?

A simple query that demands a cogent answer!

There is a myth that all stakeholders in the health care space understand the meaning of basic information technology jargon. In truth, the vernacular of contemporary medical information systems is unique, and often misused or misunderstood. It is sometimes altogether confounding. Terms such as, RSS, DRAM, ROM, USB, PDA, and DNS are common acronyms, but is their functionality truly understood?

Computer technology and online security is also changing, and with its rapid growth comes an internal lingo that demands still more attention from the health care sector. Legislation, such as the Health Insurance Portability and Accountability Act (HIPAA) of 1996, the Wired for Health Care Quality Act (WHCQA) of the Senate in 2005, the Health Information Technology Promotion Act (HITPA) of the House in 2006, and the National ePrescribing Patient Safety Initiative (NEPSI) of 2007 has brought to the profession a plethora of new phrases such as "electronic data interchange," "EDI translator," "ANSI X-12" and "X12 277 Claim Status Notification Transactions," and so forth. Hence, health care informatics is now being taught in medical, dental, graduate, and business schools as its importance is finally recognized.

Moreover, an emerging national Heath Information Technology (HIT) architecture—in the guise of terms, definitions, acronyms, abbreviations, and standards—often puts the nonexpert medical, nursing, public policy administrator, or paraprofessional in a position of maximum uncertainty and minimum productivity. Unfortunately, this opinion stems from the underappreciation of HIT as a prima facia resource that needs to be managed by others. The *Dictionary of Health Information Technology and Security* will therefore help define, clarify, and explain.

So too, embryonic corporate positions such as Chief Medical Information Officer (CMIO) or Chief Medical Technology Officer (CMTO) continue to grow as hospitals, clinics, and health systems become more committed to IT projects that demand technology savvy physician-executives. Many medical errors can be prevented and guesswork eliminated when the *Dictionary of Health Information Technology and Security* is used by informed cognoscenti as well as the masses. This book contains more than 10,000 entries and code names, with extensive bibliographic references that increase its utility as a useful tool and illustrated compendium.

Of course, authoritative linguistic sources such as the *Dictionary* serve a vast niche. Electronic Health Records (EHRs) and e-prescribing has languished, and more than 9 in 10 hospitals have not yet implemented Computerized Physician Order Entry systems (CPOEs).[1] And, HIT lags far behind other sectors in ease-of-use. As an educator, my task is to help students, late-adopters, and adult-learners understand key medical information concepts. This daunting task is aided by the *Dictionary* as my charges use it, become more conscientious in their studies, and recognize its value as a tool for virtually every health care worker.

My suggestion is to use the *Dictionary of Health Information Technology and Security* frequently. You will refer to it daily.

I also recommend the entire *Health Dictionary Series*© by Dr. David Edward Marcinko and his colleagues from the Institute of Medical Business Advisors, Inc.

Richard J. Mata MD, MS, MS-CIS
Certified Medical Planner© (Hon)
Chief Medical Information Officer (CMIO)
Ricktelmed Information Systems
Assistant Professor Texas State University

NOTE

Foreword

1. Healthcare Informatics and The Leapfrog Group. (2007, January). *Top Hospital List, 24*(1), 64, Skokie, IL.

Acknowledgments

The explosion of technology is transforming all aspects of health care from patient treatment, to clinical research, and to policy and administration. And, as this information drives innovation and the way it is delivered, medical professionals, patients, laymen, and stakeholders are increasingly challenged to use all available linguistic resources productively. When information access is appropriate and actionable, all concerned become more productive and quality of care improves.

The *Dictionary of Health Information Technology and Security* therefore serves a vital function as a printed search engine for members of the health care industrial complex to find, analyze, and understand terms, meanings, phrases, and HIT information in ways never before possible. Users find acronyms, slang, and peer-reviewed terms and derivations quickly and easily, and overall health policy and administration improves. Even basic computer science principles, operating systems, and programming language terms in AppleTalk©, JAVA, C, C+, HTML, JavaScript, VisualBasic, Unix, Linux, and others are included.

Creating the *Dictionary of Health Information Technology and Security* was a significant effort that involved all members of our firm. Major source materials include those publications, journals, and books listed as references, as well as personal communication with experts in the field. We draw from the experiences and insights of our students, colleagues, and clients from numerous health care organizations, clinics, universities, and medical practices. We are grateful to them for sharing their wisdom with us.

Over the past year, we also interfaced with public resources such as various state governments, the federal government, Federal Register (FR), the Centers for Medicare and Medicaid (CMS), Institute of Medicine (IOM), INFOSEC, the Healthcare Information and Management Systems Society (HIMSS), Microsoft Health User's Group (MSHUG), SUNSHINE [Sun Microsystems Inc., Solutions for Healthcare Information Exchange], American Health Information Management Association (AHIMA), American National Standards Institute's Healthcare Informatics Standards Board (ANSI-HISB), North Carolina Supercomputing Center (NCSC), and the U.S. Department of Health and Human Services (HHS), as well as numerous private professionals to discuss its contents. Although impossible to acknowledge every person that played a role in its production, there are several people we wish to thank for their moral support and extraordinary input.

Among these are: Paras Chaudhari from the Syracuse University School of Information Studies; the late Russell Coile, Jr., Senior Vice President, Superior Consultant Co, Southfield, MI (SUPC-NASD); Ahmad Hashem, MD, PhD, former Global Healthcare Productivity Manager, Microsoft Healthcare Industry Solutions Group, Microsoft Corporation, Redmond, WA; Richard D. Helppie, former Managing Director of Affiliated Computer Services, Inc. (NYSE: ACS) and Founder of Superior Consultant Corporation (NASD-SUPC); Parin Kothari, MBA, from the Syracuse University Whitman School of Business Management and Founder of ConsultBrown.org; Dr. Richard J. Mata, MS-MI, MS-CIS, San Antonio, TX; Dr. Brent A. Metfessel, MS, Senior Scientist-Institute for Clinic Systems Improvement, Bloomington, MN; Carol S. Miller, BSN, MBA, Program Manager-Science Applications, International Corporation-Health Solutions Business Unit, Falls Church, VA; Dr. William P. Scherer, MS, Boca Raton, FL; and Ted Nardin, CEO, and assistant editor Alana Stein of Springer Publishing Company, LLC., New York, who directed the publishing cycle from conception to release.

Instructions for Use

- **Alphabetization.** In compiling a dictionary of this size, we have had to be selective and take full responsibility for what is included herein and what is not. We believe it reflects state-of-the-art HIT lexicology but are cognizant that new terms and jargon are being invented and used every day. The quickest way to identify a word not found in any book, therefore, is to do a Web search. But take care, the definition may not be correct or peer reviewed. Entries in this dictionary are alphabetized by letter rather than by word, so that multiple-word terms are treated as a single word. Alpha-numeric definitions and unusual terminology are listed phonetically. Charts, graphs, tables, equations, lists, and other visual items are included to enhance reading understanding and interest.
- **Copyright, Trade, Product, and Service Mark Disclaimer.** Companies, products, programs and applications mentioned in this dictionary do not constitute endorsements. All trade marks, copyright, and service marks that may or may not be listed are acknowledged as belonging to their respective companies and owners. We make no attempt to determine or report their legal status. These include, but are not limited to:
  - IBM®, DB2®, Domino, eServer, iSeries, Lotus®, Lotus Discovery Server, Lotus Knowledge Discovery System, Lotus Workflow, LotusScript®, Lotus Notes®, pSeries, QuickPlace, Rational, Sametime®, Tivoli, VisualAge, WebSphere®, xSeries, and zSeries are trademarks of International Business Machines Corporation.
  - Intel® and Pentium® are trademarks of Intel Corporation.
  - Java® is a trademark of Sun Microsystems.
  - Linux® is a trademark of Linus Torvalds.
  - Macintosh, iPod, and Mac OS are trademarks of Apple Computer, Inc.
  - Microsoft®, FoxPro®, PowerPoint, SharePoint®, Visual Basic®, Visual FoxPro®, Visual Studio®, Windows®, and Windows NT® are trademarks of Microsoft Corporation.
  - Novell®, DirXML, GroupWise®, iFolder, NetMail, NetWare®, Suse®, Ximian, and ZENworks® are trademarks of Novell, Inc.
  - Oracle® is a trademark of Oracle Corporation.
  - Palm® and Palm Computing® are trademarks of Palm, Inc.
  - Certified Medical Planner© (CMP©), Health Dictionary Series© (HDS©), HealthcareFinancials©, and Medical Investment Policy Statement© (MIPS©) are copyrighted terms owned by *i*MBA, Inc©.

- **Cross-References, Synonyms, and Variations.** Contrasting or related terms, as well as synonyms and variations, may be included in the *Dictionary* to enhance reader understanding. Once an entry has been fully defined by another term, a synergistic term may also be suggested (e.g., health maintenance organization; managed care organization or health services organization). Colloquial slang terms are listed when appropriate, along with more than 200 notable *movers and shakers* in public and private IT and security (e.g., Adelman, Belovin, Berners-Lee, Cerf, Diffie, Gosling, Hellman, Kolodner, Noonan, Ranum, Rivest, Roberts, Schneier, Shamir, Whitfield, and Zimmerman). These visionaries were among the first wave of independent researchers to begin proselytizing about the serous commercial software vulnerabilities, and by extension, the Internet and HIT.

- **Definitions.** Because many academic and real-world words have distinctly different meanings and iterations depending on their context, it is left up to the reader to determine their relevant purpose. And, although health information technology and security may be sparsely included elsewhere in nontechnical terms, or as a brief glossary or appendix in a specific text, it may be difficult to quickly return to a portion of the book containing the desired terms. Therefore, the *Dictionary* offers an expanded presentation of terms and definitions from many perspectives and sources. Yet, it is realized that one person's definitional diatribe may be another's parsimony. Moreover, the various meanings of a term have been listed in the *Dictionary* by bullets or functional subheadings for convenience. Older mature terms still in use are also noted (e.g., CMS, micro-computer and CP/M) as well as contemporaneous new items (war-dialer, phracker, phreaker, sploits, Wi-Fi, Internet2), in order to help better appreciate the growing spectrum of IT and security relationships within the health care industry. Eponyms and HIT legislative acts are included; and Latin phrases with some foreign and slang terms are defined as they become part of the global health care IT and online security language.

- **Disciplines.** The meaning of various words and phrases are given multiple utility according to their field of use, and there are fewer fields immersed in the cross-pollination of concepts than health care IT and security. Accordingly, professional definitions from the disciplines of mathematics, engineering, statistics, technology, ethics, security, software programming, computing, networking, and electronics; as well as health policy, administration, and managed care are all included as they integrate with our core focus on health care information technology, computer networks, the Internet, and online security.

- **Endorsement Disclaimer.** Products, applications, programs, or companies mentioned in this *Dictionary* are mentioned for illustrative purposes only and are not an endorsement for any particular firm or device. For further information about any company or product name, consult the manufacturer's literature.

- **Italics.** Italic type may be used to highlight the fact that a word has a special meaning to the HIT industry (e.g., *modifier, Medicare + Choice, International Classification of Diseases, Tenth Edition Clinical Modification*). It is also used for the titles of publications, books, and journals referenced in the *Dictionary*.

- **Linguistic Disclaimer.** All definitions, abbreviations, eponyms, acronyms, variations and synonyms, and information listed in the *Dictionary* are intended for general understanding, and do not represent the thoughts, ideas, or opinions of the Institute of Medical Business Advisors, Inc©. Great care has been taken to confirm information accuracy, but we offer no warranties, expressed or implied, regarding currency and are not responsible for errors, omissions, or for any consequences from the application of this information. Furthermore, some terms are not complete because many are written in simplest form. The Internet space, computer HIT industry, security sectors, and their leaders are evolving rapidly, and all information should be considered time-sensitive.

- **Notice of Liability.** Every effort has been made to ensure that the *Dictionary* contains accurate and current information. It was reviewed by educators, physicians, and IT practitioners in the field to ensure current, accurate technical content, and every attempt was made to capture the scope of health technology practice in use, today. However, the publisher, editors, and *i*MBA Inc., shall not be held responsible for any loss or damage suffered by readers as a result of the information contained herein. The right of the coeditors to be associated with this work has been asserted in accordance with the Copyright, Designs, and Patents Act of 1988.

- **Unusual Definitions.** Unique trade or industry terms from Internet culture, new media, digital audio and photography, code-names, numerics, emoticons, and humor that play an active role in the field of HIT and security are included in the *Dictionary* along with a brief explanation, as needed (e.g., lossless, The L0pht, *Cult of the Dead Cow,* etc.). For related health insurance and managed care terms; health economics, finance, legal policy, and administration meanings, please review our three companion works in the comprehensive *Health Dictionary Series©* by *i*MBA Inc.

- **Use.** Beyond the immediate health care information technology and security space of professors, students, residents, interns fellows, medical practitioners, and health care entities, the *Dictionary* can be used as a handy quick reference source and supplement to sales literature for vendors, third-parties, clients, CIOs, CTOs, CSOs, CKOs, and purchasing agents, and to answer questions as well as inquiries about product specifications, functionality, or software as a service pricing. Fast, succinct, and technically accurate responses to such questions can sometimes mean the difference between closing and not closing a technology product sale; negotiating a favorable HIT or security contract, or reducing costs when purchasing a health-related information technology system or outsourced product and service. And, let us not forget about savvy consumers who will find the *Dictionary of Health Information Technology and Security*© a wealth of information in readily understood language. Astonishingly, the HIT system purchase decision itself is often made directly by the physician or layman without sufficient basic knowledge of security or technical acronyms, definitions, or IT policy explanations!

Terminology: A–Z

Acronyms, Abbreviations, and Eponyms

Abbreviations with multiple meanings are included in the *Dictionary* because the industry does not possess a body of standardized acronyms, eponyms, and abbreviations.

Bibliography

Collated printed readings, electronic references, and organizations from a variety of sources allow further research into specific subjects of interest, as well as an opportunity to perform critical comparisons not possible without other narrative periodicals or publications. Information on vendors and emerging and mature HIT servicing companies is also included.

- Print Media Textbooks
- Print Media Publications
- Print Media Journals
- Electronic Internet Media
- Associations and Organizations
- Committee on Improving the Patient Record in Response to Increasing Functional Requirements and Technological Advances

TERMINOLOGY: A–Z

e-Health is an emerging field in the intersection of medical informatics, public health and business, referring to health services and information delivered or enhanced through the Internet and related technologies. In a broader sense, the term characterizes not only a technical development, but also a state-of-mind, a way of thinking, an attitude, and a commitment for networked, global thinking, to improve health care worldwide by using information and communication technology.

Gunther Eysenbach,
Editor, Journal of Medical Internet Research, MD, MPH

A

A: Hyper Text Markup Language (HTML) computer anchor, or Web site or Web page location link.

ABELINE®: Internet2 high-performance computer network of Cisco Systems®, Nortel Networks®, and Qwest Communications®; backbone of the information superhighway Internet 2 concept.

ABELL, ROSEMARY: Board member and past president of the North Carolina Healthcare Information and Communications Alliance, Research Triangle Park, NC, and Director of National Healthcare Vertical Solutions, Keane Inc., Raleigh, NC.

ABEND: The sudden and abrupt end to a computer program or online session.

ABORT: To cancel a computer system or online session command; retry; fail.

ABS: Absolute value function for computer systems or online access.

ABSOLUTE ADDRESS: Fixed computer system memory location.

ABSOLUTE LINK: A direct hyperlink to a specific file on a network server.

ABSOLUTE URL: Web site address that contains all computer system machine contact information: full address, directory, and file.

ABSTRACT: Abbreviation, definition, information synopsis, or medical executive summary; hardcopy or electronic.

ABSTRACT MESSAGE: An electronic health or other message, within a message; data files, application errors, and so forth.

ABSTRACT SYNTAX: An electronic transmission description method of basic medical data or other information element types.

ABUSE: CPT errors to upgrade codes for additional medical reimbursement but without purposeful fraudulent intent.

The *Journal of Medical Internet Research* is the first international scientific peer-reviewed journal on all aspects of research, information, and communication in the health care field using Internet- and intranet-related technologies.

ACCELERATOR: Any device that speeds up a computer system application, program, or process.

ACCEPTABLE USE POLICY: Established computer networks and online guidelines for health care facility or medical data control and user protocol; access authorization.

ACCESS: To allow computer, server, or network use, manipulation, medical data or health information entry, or information and file inspection; communication between terminal and host; the ability or the means necessary to read, write, modify, or communicate, or to otherwise make use of any computer system resource.

ACCESS 2003®: MSFT database management software application with error checking, automatic property updating, object dependencies viewing, export and import data functionality, with links to lists on Microsoft Windows® SharePoint® Services sites, and so forth: expanded ability to import, export, and work with Extensible Markup Language (XML) data files.

ACCESS AUTHORIZATION: Information-use, policies, or procedures that establish the rules for granting or restricting access to a medical informatics or health systems user, terminal, transaction, program, or health process; acceptable use.

ACCESS AUTHORIZATION RECORDS: Establishes a procedure to assure that access and authorization to medical records are maintained; records should include who has access, the level of access, at what locations, and at what times.

ACCESS CODE: A number, password, or biometric identifier used to gain computer network entry.

ACCESS CONTROL (AC): Policy and procedures that allow or prevent computer, server, or network access; to triage files for read, write, and erase functionality; enable authorized use of a resource while preventing unauthorized use or use in an unauthorized manner; a method of restricting access to resources, allowing only privileged entities access; types of access control include, among others, mandatory access control, discretionary access control, time-of-day, classification, pretty-good protection, and subject-object separation; access code.

ACCESS CONTROL ENFORCEMENT (ACE): Subject user validation for requesting access to a particular process or computer network enforcing with a defined security policy that provides for enforcement mechanisms distributed throughout the health system; not only the correctness of the access control decision, but also the strength of the access control enforcement to determine the level of security obtained; checking identity and requested access against access control lists is a common access control enforcement mechanism; medical file encryption is an example of an access control enforcement mechanism; access control.

ACCESS CONTROL GRID (ACG): Spreadsheet, table, graph, or visual of an enterprise-wide health information management system.

ACCESS CONTROL LIST (ACL): A table that tells an OS which access rights each health user has in a particular information system, such as medical file directory, individual file or entry for each system user with access privileges such as the ability to read, write, or to execute a file (e.g., MSFT Windows NT/2000, Novell's NetWare, Digital's OpenVMS®, and Unix-based systems).

ACCESS CONTROL POLICY (ACP): Security rules and regulations for point-of-entry health data privacy and medical accountability; access control.

ACCESS CONTROL SYSTEM (ACS): Schematic of health information management system entry with restrictions and user rights; access control list.

ACCESS ESTABLISHMENT: A policy that sets the rules for determining the right of a person to have access to health information for job performance; the security policies, and the rules established therein, that determine an entity's initial right of medical data access to a terminal, transaction, program, or process; access control.

ACCESSION NUMBER: Cancer registry numerically ordered medical chart file or health information registration.

ACCESS LEVEL (AL): Authorization or security clearance level to use a computer, server, or network.

ACCESS LEVEL AUTHORIZATION (ALA): Establishes a procedure to determine the computer or network access level granted to individuals working on or near protected health information, medical data, or secure health data.

ACCESS MEASURES (AM): Ability to commence computer, server, or network use after security verification with passwords, identification numbers, fingerprint, voice, iris scan, or other biometric recognition systems.

ACCESS MODE: Method of computer, server, or network entry, with health information and medical data security protection mechanism; read, write, protect, create, delete, and so forth.

ACCESS MODIFICATION: The security policies and the rules that determine the type and reason for change or alteration to a health entity's established right of access to a terminal, transaction, program, or process.

ACCESS POINT (AP): Wireless LAN, MAN, or WAN receiver/transmitter that connects wired devices and networks; bridge link.

ACCESS RIGHTS (AR): Permission to use a computer, server, or network usually assigned by a health care department managing director, medical data or health information technology officer, CTO, CIO, CSO, or CKO.

ACCESS SECURITY: To allow computer or health care network entry using ID, password, secure socket layer (SSL) encryption, biometrics, and so forth; unique identification and password assignments are usually made to medical staff members for access to medical information on a need-to-know basis, and only upon written authority of the owner of the data; *need-to-know* is determined by the individual covered health care entity but generally can be categorized into the following areas:

- access by medical care providers to individual patient data, for use in patient care or specific hospital operations.
- access for research, planning, and quality improvement processes within the hospital.
- access by those employees in the health record department whose role includes record processing-maintenance.
- use of PKI (Private/Public Key Infrastructure) for public and private sectors, as needed, along with SSL technology and biometric encryption.
- individual IDs and passwords may not be shared with another user.
- passwords changed frequently, as designated by system design.
- users limited to one log-on at a time, as designated by individual platform design.
- multiple attempts to sign on with an improper access code result in a lock-out status of the individual until access privileges are restored by health information services.
- access of all users is monitored by identification and password assignments; warning notices displayed on each screen to inform staff of the confidential nature of the information and that their access is being monitored.
- maintenance of the access assignments completed with employee change in status (e.g., termination, change of position).
- employee's information.
- system employee choice of whether personal data will be accessible or restricted for view by medical staff only in the hospital system; the option of requesting restricted access on selected systems and not others will not be available.
- an employees' access to their own patient information must follow the process as defined in the release of information policies and procedures.
- pre-employment data will be retained only in the local employee health database.
- sensitive information (psychiatry, substance abuse, VIP, protected patients) is defined in the release of information policies and procedures.

ACCIDENTAL THREAT: Unintentional computer system assault or damage, as from physical properties, user mistake, or other nonmalicious source.

ACCOUNT: Health information electronic record keeping system for private medical data; patient specific file.

ACCOUNTABILITY: The health care information technology security objective that generates the requirement for actions of a medical entity to be traced uniquely to that entity; supports nonrepudiation, deterrence, fault isolation, intrusion detection and prevention, and after-action recovery and legal action; the property that ensures that the actions of an entity can be traced uniquely to that entity (ASTM E1762—95).

ACCOUNTABLE INFORMATION (AI): Keystroke, mirroring, or health data manipulation that evidences computer, server, or network entry or processing.

ACCOUNTING: Creating an historical record of who was authenticated, at what time, and how long they accessed a health or other computer system.

ACCOUNT LOCKOUT: Security system feature that prevents account access following several aborted attempts after a predetermined period.

ACCOUNT NAME: The user identifier on an e-mail account; username@host name.

ACCREDITED STANDARDS COMMITTEE (ASC): Organization that helps develop American National Standards (ANS) for computer and health information technology; accredited by ANSI for the development of American National Standards; ASC X12N develops medical electronic business exchange controls such as 835-Health Care Claim Payment/Advice and 837-Health Care Claim.

ACCURACY: Computer, server, or network misinformation or miscoding percentages or error rates; current medical data and information free form error.

ACKERMAN, MICHAEL, J., PHD: High Performance Computing and Communications Director, National Library of Medicine, Washington, D.C.

ACOUSTIC COUPLER: A modem device that changes a sequential train of pulses into sounds of a given frequency to be received by a traditional telephone.

ACQUIRE: To obtain a health data, medical information, or other file from a digital camera, video recorder, or scanner.

ACROBAT©: Software systems from Adobe Systems, Inc.® for creating and reading fixed portable document files (.pdf) functional on several different platforms.

ACTIVATION: To transfer Enterprise JavaBean® (EJB) information to more permanent storage or electronic memory.

ACTIVE CONTENT: Java®, JavaScript®, Active X®, or similar programs that are downloaded from a Web browser and executed in a single step, rather than as fixed HTML tag Web page content, which offers a static environment.

ACTIVE DESKTOP: The ability to use an Internet site Web page as a computer screen itself, rather than merely running a Microsoft program application.

ACTIVE INTRUSION: Intentional and unauthorized computer or network entry; manipulation, cracking, or hacking.

ACTIVE STAR TOPOLOGY NETWORK: Hub and spoke stellate computer network systems configuration that sends out signals, information, data, or other communications back to a centralized management station; repeatable network reciprocity.

ACTIVE THREAT: Potential intentional and unauthorized computer, server, or network entry; breach of security, manipulation, or software hacking.

ACTIVE WINDOW: The computer screen or window frame currently in use.

ACTIVE X©: MSFT Windows© object control used to enhance user interaction with a software application; a way to cope with user account control security.

ACTIVITY: The action for the creations of a product or service; application or file, and so forth.

ACTIVITY DATE: Charge-master data element of the most recent health care activity or medical data input.

ACTOR: The role one plays in a health information management system; title or position; or an application responsible for certain health information technology, medical, or other electronic tasks.

ADA: Computer program language of the 1970s that linked subprograms and compiled them separately prior to execution; Augusta Ada Byron.

ADAPTER: A simple circuit device that allows one computer system to work with another; for example, an I/O card.

ADD NOISE: Speckled texture to a digital image or GUI application; slang term.

ADD ON: A hardware unit that can be added to a computer to increase its capabilities, or a software application or utility program that enhances a primary program.

ADD/REMOVE UTILITY: Windows© or other similar utility program that demonstrates all computer installed programs; programs are best uninstalled from here.

ADDRESS: The unique identifier for a computer or the number of a storage or memory location; Internet Service Provider (ISP), file name, or e-mail identifier.

ADDRESS BOOK: A Web-browser e-mail address recording feature.

ADDRESS CLASS: One of four TCP/IP computer network types (A–D); the first three are used for Internet Protocol addressing.

ADDRESS MUNG(ING): To alter an e-mail address in the security attempt to prevent mass collection and spamming.

ADDRESS RESOLUTION: High-level Internet Protocol address conversion to its low level physical address.

ADDRESS RESOLUTION PROTOCOL (ARP): A method for mapping an Internet Protocol address to a physical machine address that is recognized in its local network.

ADELMAN, LEONARD, PHD: Professor of Computer Science and Director of the Laboratory for Molecular Science at USC; IT data security expert.

AD-HOC APPROACH: Common computer connectivity strategy to support many applications, vendors, hardware, and software and connections to disparate health information systems; a self-forming computer network; a query not determined when run against a health or other data base.

AD-HOC MODE: Peer-to-peer networking that does not have an access point when wireless; infrastructure mode; slang term.

ADMINISTRATIVE CODE SET (ACS): HIPAA code sets that indicate general medical business functions rather than specific health information; nonclinical or nonmedical code sets.

ADMINISTRATIVE CONTROLS: Procedures and policies that dictate health information system access, use, modification, and management of computerized resources.

ADMINISTRATIVE HEALTH CARE DATA: Nonclinical, nonmedical patient electronic data, files, and information, usually about third party payer, contact information, and reimbursement status.

ADMINISTRATIVE INFORMATION: Health care data used for purchasing, operations, financial, human resource, executive decision-making, and other managerial and business purposes; nonclinical IT information.

ADMINISTRATIVE RECORD: Nonclinical and nonmedical file of health care business or related data.

ADMINISTRATIVE SAFEGUARDS: Managerial actions, policies, and procedures to manage the selection, development, implementation, and maintenance of security measures to protect electronic protected health information or medical data, and to manage the conduct of a covered entity's workforce in relation to the protection of that information.

ADMINISTRATIVE SERVICES ONLY (ASO): The third party nonclinical administration of a health plan; occurs when a self-insured entity contracts with a Third Party Administrator (TPA) to administer a health plan.

ADMINISTRATIVE SIMPLIFICATION (AS): The use of electronic standard code sets for health information exchange; Title II, Subtitle F of HIPAA gives HHS the authority to mandate the use of standards for the electronic exchange of health care data; to specify what medical and administrative code sets should be used within those standards; to require the use of national identification systems for health care patients, providers, payers (or plans), and employers (or sponsors); and to specify the types of measures required to protect the security and privacy of personally identifiable health care and medical information (Table 1).

ADMINISTRATIVE SYSTEMS: Typical hospital information and computer technology systems that usually include the following functions:

Table 1: Administrative Simplification Compliance Act Regulations

Title	Description	Status
Model Compliance Extension Plan Federal Register Notice	ASCA required the Secretary to develop a model compliance extension plan for use by covered entities when requesting the one-year extension for implementing the HIPAA transactions and code sets.	Covered entities that did not submit an extension request by October 15, 2002 should come into compliance as soon as possible, and should be prepared to submit a corrective action plan in the event a complaint is filed against them.
Electronic Medicare Claims Submission 42 CFR Part 424 CMS-0008-F	This final rule implements the requirements for electronic submission of Medicare claims, submitted on or after October 16, 2003. In addition, this rule also implements the conditions upon which a waiver could be granted for these requirements. CMS will not process incoming non-HIPAA-compliant electronic Medicare claims submitted for payment beginning October 1, 2005.	Final rule estimated publication date: December 2006. Interim final rule published August 15, 2003 (PDF). Information on Medicare waiver for small providers billing on paper.
Exclusion from Medicare Proposed Rule	ASCA gives the Secretary discretion to exclude from the Medicare program any covered entities that are not compliant by October 2002 *and* have not submitted a compliance extension plan.	Schedule being developed.

(Continued)

Table 1: Continued

Final Rule on HIPAA Enforcement (Released February 16, 2006—Effective Date March 16, 2006)	
Part of Administrative Simplification	**Responsible for Enforcement**
Privacy	HHS Office for Civil Rights (OCR) Fact Sheet: How to File a Health Information Privacy Complaint Complaints, which must be submitted in writing within 180 days of an unauthorized disclosure, can be faxed or mailed to the appropriate OCR regional office, or sent via e-mail.
Transactions and Code Sets	Centers for Medicare and Medicaid Services (CMS)
	CMS and OCR will work together on outreach and enforcement and on issues that touch on the responsibilities of both organizations—such as application of security standards or exception determinations.
	CMS' Online Complaint Submission Form allows complaints to be submitted about covered entities' noncompliance with the HIPAA transaction standards. Complaints can also be submitted on a paper-based form available by download from the site (PDF).
Security	Centers for Medicare and Medicaid Services (CMS)
Identifiers	Centers for Medicare and Medicaid Services (CMS)

- admission scheduling and facility access management
- accounts payable and receivable
- patient and payer billing, internal finance, budgeting, and accounting
- patient demographic information for admission and other data items
- staffing and staff scheduling
- pharmacy inventory
- patient census
- facility maintenance

ADMINISTRATIVE USER ACCESS LEVEL: Computer access security level for nonclinical health care information.

ADMITTED TERM: Accepted definition for synonyms terms from an accredited health lexicon or other lexicology body.

ADOBE ACROBAT©: Popular Portable Document Format (PDF) exchange program from Adobe Systems®, Inc., which allows documents created on one computer platform to be displayed and printed without loss of rich text-enhancing features.

ADOBE SYSTEMS®, INC.: A graphics and desktop publishing software company founded by Dr. John Warnock in 1982 to pioneer desktop publishing with fonts and applications; Photoshop©; Illustrator©; PageMaker©; Premier©; GoLive©; and so forth.

ADVANCED DIAGNOSTIC CARD (ADC): Card, file tape, disk, CD, or software program used to run automatic computer facilities diagnostic and security test systems.

ADVANCED ENCRYPTION STANDARD (AES): An encryption security standard that replaced the 40-bit WEP keys using 128, 192, or 256 bit keys; successor to Data Encryption Standard (DES) of the U.S. NIST.

ADVANCED MICRO DEVICES (AMD): A manufacturer of digital CPUs in Sunnyvale, CA; Intel© competitor with the K-6 Pentium competitor, as well as Athlon™ and Duron™ CPU products; released the Turion™ (Table 2) and MT-37 chips for gamers in 2005, among others:

ADVANCED ORGANIZATIONS TECHNOLOGY: All the electronic medical data interchange systems that allow computers, networks, servers, patient information kiosks, and automatic patient response and input information systems to be integrated as one unit.

ADVANCED RESEARCH PROJECTS AGENCY (ARPA): Governed under the Department of Defense; agency involved with the use of telemedicine and its development, and continuing research; responsible for establishing the network, which later became known as the Internet.

ADVANCED STREAMING FORMAT (ASF): Electronic communications file format for sound, video, graphics, and text transmissions; and so forth.

ADWARE: Internet programs that open pop-up windows while browsing or surfing the Internet; slang term.

AETNA'S AEXCEL NETWORK©: Proprietary analytic software and database system to evaluate medical and health providers' relative costs compared to other doctors providing similar services.

AGASSI, ANTOINE: Chairman, Governor's e-Health Advisory Council, Tennessee.

AGENT: A background computer utility program that reports results to the end user upon completion.

AGGREGATE: To gather, assemble, or collect separate health information or other sets of medical data from two or more sources.

Table 2: Turion™ 64 Mobile Technology

AMD Turion™ 64 Mobile Technology Family

AMD Turion™ 64 X2 Dual-Core Mobile Technology

For Thin and Light Notebooks (Socket S1)

TL-60 (64-bit, 2.0 GHz, Dedicated 1M L2 cache, 1600 MHz HyperTransport™ bus)

TL-56 (64-bit, 1.8 GHz, Dedicated 1M L2 cache, 1600 MHz HyperTransport bus)

TL-52 (64-bit, 1.6 GHz, Dedicated 1M L2 cache, 1600 MHz HyperTransport bus)

TL-50 (64-bit, 1.6 GHz, Dedicated 512k L2 cache, 1600 MHz HyperTransport bus)

AMD Turion™ 64 Mobile Technology

For Thin and Light Notebooks (Socket 754)

ML-44 (64-bit, 2.4 GHz, 1M L2 cache, 1600 MHz HyperTransport bus)

ML-42 (64-bit, 2.4 GHz, 512k L2 cache, 1600 MHz HyperTransport bus)

ML-40 (64-bit, 2.2 GHz, 1M L2 cache, 1600 MHz HyperTransport bus)

ML-37 (64-bit, 2.0 GHz, 1M L2 cache, 1600 MHz HyperTransport bus)

ML-34 (64-bit, 1.8 GHz, 1M L2 cache, 1600 MHz HyperTransport bus)

ML-32 (64-bit, 1.8 GHz, 512k L2 cache, 1600 MHz HyperTransport bus)

MT-40 (64-bit, 2.2 GHz, 1M L2 cache, 1600 MHz HyperTransport bus)

MT-37 (64-bit, 2.0 GHz, 1M L2 cache, 1600 MHz HyperTransport bus)

MT-34 (64-bit, 1.8 GHz, 1M L2 cache, 1600 MHz HyperTransport bus)

MT-32 (64-bit, 1.8 GHz, 512k L2 cache, 1600 MHz HyperTransport bus)

AMD Opteron™ Processor

1000 Models	2000 Models	Price	8000 Models
AMD Opteron 1218 SE	AMD Opteron 2220 SE		AMD Opteron 8220 SE
AMD Opteron 1218	AMD Opteron 2218		AMD Opteron 8218
AMD Opteron 1216	AMD Opteron 2216		AMD Opteron 8216
AMD Opteron 1214	AMD Opteron 2214		AMD Opteron 8214

(Continued)

Table 2: Turion™ 64 Mobile Technology *(Continued)*

AMD Opteron™ Processor

1000 Models	2000 Models	Price	8000 Models
AMD Opteron 1212	AMD Opteron 2212		Dual-Core AMD Opteron 8212
AMD Opteron 1210	AMD Opteron 2210		
	AMD Opteron 2216 HE		AMD Opteron 8216 HE
	AMD Opteron 2214 HE		AMD Opteron 8214 HE
	AMD Opteron 2212 HE		AMD Opteron 8212 HE
	AMD Opteron 2210 HE		
100 Models	200 Models		800 Models
Dual-Core AMD Opteron 185	Dual-Core Model 285		Dual-Core Model 885
Dual-Core AMD Opteron 180	Dual-Core Model 280		Dual-Core Model 880
Dual-Core AMD Opteron 175	Dual-Core Model 275		Dual-Core Model 875
Dual-Core AMD Opteron 170	Dual-Core Model 270		Dual-Core Model 870
Dual-Core AMD Opteron 165	Dual-Core Model 265		Dual-Core Model 865
	Model 256		Model 856
AMD Opteron 154	Model 254		Model 854
AMD Opteron 152	Model 252		Model 852
AMD Opteron 150	Model 250		Model 850
AMD Opteron 148	Model 248		
AMD Opteron 146	Model 246		
AMD Opteron 144			
	Dual-Core Model 275 HE		Dual-Core Model 875 HE
	Dual-Core Model 270 HE		Dual-Core Model 870 HE

(Continued)

Table 2: Continued

1000 Models	2000 Models	Price	8000 Models
	Dual-Core Model 270 HE		Dual-Core Model 870 HE
	Dual-Core Model 265 HE		Dual-Core Model 865 HE
	Dual-Core Model 260 HE		Dual-Core Model 860 HE
	Model 250 HE		Model 850 HE
	Model 248 HE		Model 848 HE
	Model 246 HE		

AMD Athlon™ 64 Processor Family

AMD Athlon™ 64 FX Processor

Athlon 64 FX-62 (64-bit, 2.8 GHz, Dedicated 2 MB L2 cache, 2000 MHz Hyper-Transport bus, AM2 only)

AMD Athlon™ 64 X2 Dual-Core Processor

Athlon 64 X2 5200+ (64-bit, 2.6 GHz, Dedicated 2 MB L2 cache, 2000 MHz HyperTransport™ bus, AM2 only)

Athlon 64 X2 5000+ (64-bit, Energy Efficient, 2.6 GHz, Dedicated 1 MB L2 cache, 2000 MHz HyperTransport bus, AM2 only)

Athlon 64 X2 5000+ (64-bit, 2.6 GHz, Dedicated 1 MB L2 cache, 2000 MHz Hyper-Transport bus, AM2 only)

Athlon 64 X2 4600+ (64-bit, Energy Efficient, 2.4 GHz, Dedicated 1 MB L2 cache, 2000 MHz HyperTransport bus)

Athlon 64 X2 4600+ (64-bit, 2.4 GHz, Dedicated 1 MB L2 cache, 2000 MHz Hyper-Transport bus, AM2 and 939)

Athlon 64 X2 4200+ (64-bit, Energy Efficient, 2.2 GHz, Dedicated 1 MB L2 cache, 2000 MHz HyperTransport bus)

Athlon 64 X2 4200+ (64-bit, 2.2 GHz, Dedicated 1 MB L2 cache, 2000 MHz Hyper-Transport bus, AM2 and 939)

Athlon 64 X2 3800+ (64-bit, Energy Efficient Small Form Factor, 2.0 GHz, Dedicated 1 MB L2 cache, 2000 MHz HyperTransport bus)

Athlon 64 X2 3800+ (64-bit, Energy Efficient, 2.0 GHz, Dedicated 1 MB L2 cache, 2000 MHz HyperTransport bus)

(Continued)

Table 2: Turion™ 64 Mobile Technology *(Continued)*

Athlon 64 X2 3800+ (64-bit, 2.0 GHz, Dedicated 1 MB L2 cache, 2000 MHz Hyper-Transport bus, AM2 only)

AMD Athlon™ 64 Processor

Athlon 64 3800+ (64-bit, 2.4 GHz, 512 KB L2 cache, 2000 MHz HyperTransport bus, AM2 and 939)

Athlon 64 3500+ (64-bit, 2.2 GHz, 512 KB L2 cache, 2000 MHz HyperTransport bus, AM2 and 939)

Athlon 64 3500+ (64-bit, Energy Efficient Small Form Factor, 2.2 GHz, 512 KB L2 cache, 2000 MHz HyperTransport bus)

Athlon 64 3200+ (64-bit, 2.0 GHz, 512 KB L2 cache, 2000 MHz HyperTransport bus, AM2 and 939)

Mobile AMD Athlon™ 64 Processor

For Full-Size Notebooks

4000+ (64-bit, 2.6 GHz, 1M L2 cache, 1600 MHz HyperTransport bus)

3700+ (64-bit, 2.4 GHz, 1M L2 cache, 1600 MHz HyperTransport bus)

3400+ (64-bit, 2.2 GHz, 1M L2 cache, 1600 MHz HyperTransport bus)

3200+ (64-bit, 2.0 GHz, 1M L2 cache, 1600 MHz HyperTransport bus)

3000+ (64-bit, 1.8 GHz, 1M L2 cache, 1600 MHz HyperTransport bus)

AMD Sempron™ Processor Family

AMD Sempron™ Processor

Sempron 3400+ (64-bit, Energy Efficient Small Form Factor, 1.8 GHz, 256 KB L2 cache, 1600 MHz HyperTransport bus, AM2)

Sempron 3200+ (64-bit, Energy Efficient Small Form Factor, 1.8 GHz, 128 KB L2 cache, 1600 MHz HyperTransport bus, AM2)

Sempron 3000+ (64-bit, Energy Efficient Small Form Factor, 1.6 GHz, 256 KB L2 cache, 1600 MHz HyperTransport bus, AM2)

Sempron 3800+ (64-bit, 2.2 GHz, 256 KB L2 cache, 1600 MHz HyperTransport bus, AM2)

Sempron 3600+ (64-bit, 2.0 GHz, 256 KB L2 cache, 1600 MHz HyperTransport bus, AM2)

(Continued)

Table 2: Continued

Sempron 3500+ (64-bit, 2.0 GHz, 128 KB L2 cache, 1600 MHz HyperTransport bus, AM2)

Sempron 3400+ (64-bit, 1.8 GHz, 256 KB L2 cache, 1600 MHz HyperTransport bus, AM2)

Sempron 3400+ (64-bit, 2.0 GHz, 256 KB L2 cache, 1600 MHz HyperTransport bus, 754-pin)

Sempron 3200+ (64-bit, 1.8 GHz, 128 KB L2 cache, 1600 MHz HyperTransport bus, AM2)

Sempron 3000+ (64-bit, 1.6 GHz, 256 KB L2 cache, 1600 MHz HyperTransport bus, AM2)

Sempron 3000+ (64-bit, 1.8 GHz, 128 KB L2 cache, 1600 MHz HyperTransport bus, 754-pin)

Mobile AMD Sempron™ Processor Family

Mobile AMD Sempron™ Processor for Thin and Light Notebooks (Socket S1)

3600+ (64-bit, 2.0 GHz, 256k L2 cache, 1600 MHz HyperTransport bus)

3500+ (64-bit, 1.8 GHz, 512k L2 cache, 1600 MHz HyperTransport bus)

3400+ (64-bit, 1.8 GHz, 256k L2 cache, 1600 MHz HyperTransport bus)

3200+ (64-bit, 1.6 GHz, 512k L2 cache, 1600 MHz HyperTransport bus)

Mobile AMD Sempron™ Processor for Thin & Light Notebooks (Socket 754)

3400+ (2.0 GHz, 256k L2 cache, 1600 MHz HyperTransport bus)

3300+ (2.0 GHz, 128k L2 cache, 1600 MHz HyperTransport bus)

3100+ (1.8 GHz, 256k L2 cache, 1600 MHz HyperTransport bus)

3000+ (1.8 GHz, 128k L2 cache, 1600 MHz HyperTransport bus)

Mobile AMD Sempron™ Processor for Full-Size Notebooks (Socket 754)

3600+ (2.2 GHz, 128k L2 cache, 1600 MHz HyperTransport bus)

3400+ (2.0 GHz, 256k L2 cache, 1600 MHz HyperTransport bus)

3300+ (2.0 GHz, 128k L2 cache, 1600 MHz HyperTransport bus)

3100+ (1.8 GHz, 256k L2 cache, 1600 MHz HyperTransport bus)

3000+ (1.8 GHz, 128k L2 cache, 1600 MHz HyperTransport bus)

AGGREGATE DATA: The clinical and nonclinical information extracted from a patient record and anonymously combined with other records for analysis, statistical, or other studies.

AGORA: MSFT Windows Live Marketplace© Internet application; code name.

AHLTA: The U.S. military's medical data and electronic health record (EHR) initiative.

AIRPORT: A wireless short-distance connectivity docket or port for Apple Macintosh Computers®; conformed to 802.11 Wi-Fi standards in 1999 with access point and router.

AIRPORT EXPRESS®: Media Hub and Bridge introduced in 2004 by Apple Inc., to combine an AirPort Extreme® computer base station with a digital media hub; connected to a home stereo by analog or digital audio outputs, its "AirTunes" feature allowed Apple's iTunes jukebox software to stream music wirelessly from a Mac or Windows PC to a home stereo; AirTunes supports protected AAC titles purchased from Apple's music store.

AIRPORT EXTREME®: Airport computer connectivity docket from Apple Inc. that was released in 2003 and increased speed with an 802.11g standard; its base stations included a USB port for attaching a printer; some units included an analog dial-up modem.

AIRSNORT: A wireless computer hacking or network cracking utility tool; slang term.

AJAX: Asynchronous JavaScript® and XML; a development technique for creating interactive Web sites and applications; the intent is to make Web pages feel more responsive by exchanging small amounts of data with the server behind the scenes, so that the entire Web page does not have to be reloaded each time the user makes a change; meant to increase the Web page's interactivity, speed, and so forth; term coined and developed by Jesse James Garett in 2005; MSFT OfficeLive© and SharePoint© Groove, or the Zimbra© suite.

ALARM: Any communication or computer systems device that can sense an abnormal condition within the system and provide, either locally or remotely, a signal indicating the presence of the abnormality; a signal may be in any desired form ranging from a simple contact closure (or opening) to a time-phased automatic shutdown and restart cycle.

ALERT: A hardware or software generated health information management system warning; an active alert calls for an immediate alarm and response/reaction.

ALGEBRAIC CRYPTOGRAPHY: Security measure to encode text and protect privacy of health information using a code of prearranged numbers and mathematic equations.

ALGORITHM: Incremental stepwise procedure or software code for repeating a computer function or operation; clinical or critical medical path method for diagnostic/treatment protocols; cookbook medicine as for acute pulmonary edema.

ALIAS: An alternative name field or file link or application initiation; phony authentication or assumed name (Macintosh and UNIX).

ALIAS DOMAIN NAME (ADN): An e-mail protocol, within another e-mail protocol, for security or enterprise-wise identification purposes.

ALIAS POLICY: Health information management confidentiality policies and procedures required by patients or responsible persons for blinded e-mail information usually created by using an open-source majordomo mailing list.

ALL PROGRAMS MENU: Computer program storage placement area for Windows©.

ALPHABET FILING SYSTEM: Health information management recording system by which a patient's last name is used as the first component of an identifier, followed by first and middle names.

ALPHANUMERIC: Any combination of numbers, letters, or other symbols used for computer security codes, passwords, and so forth; a medical records filing system that uses the first two letters of a patient's last name followed by several numbers as an identifier.

ALPHA TEST: The initial examination of newly developed computer hardware, software, or peripheral devices; secondary stress or beta testing is more robust.

ALTAIR: Micro Instruments and Telemetry Systems, and MSFT Basic© driven hobbyist microcomputer, of 1975; 8080 Intel®-based CPU with BASIC code written by W. Gates and P. Allen; first home computer designed by engineer H. Edward Roberts, MD of Cochran, Georgia.

ALTA VISTA©: An Internet search engine from Digital Equipment Corporation®, now HP.

ALTERNATIVE BACKUP SITES: Off-site locations that are used for transferring computer operations in the event of an emergency.

ALWAYS ON: Continuous Internet connection; potential hacker access and security flaw.

AMAZON®: One of the first prominent and leading e-retail merchants; Seattle, WA.

AMENDMENT: HIPAA data privacy rule allowing the alterations of information while retaining the original.

AMERICAN DENTAL ASSOCIATION (ADA): The professional organization for dentists that maintains a hardcopy dental claim form and the associated claim submission specifications, and also maintains the Current Dental Terminology (CDT) medical code set; the ADA and the Dental Content Committee (DeCC), which it hosts, have formal consultative roles under HIPAA.

AMERICAN HEALTH INFORMATION MANAGEMENT ASSOCIATION (AHIMA): A large trade association of health information and medical data management professionals.

AMERICAN MEDICAL ASSOCIATION (AMA): A professional organization for allopathic physicians; the secretariat of the NUCC and maintains the Current Procedural Terminology (CPT) medical code set.

AMERICAN MEDICAL INFORMATICS ASSOCIATION (AMIA): An organization that promotes the use of electronic medical management and health care informatics for clinical and administrative endeavors.

AMERICAN MEGATRENDS, INC. (AMI): An early and leading supplier of BIOS software for motherboards, Norcross, GA.

AMERICAN NATIONAL STANDARDS (ANS): Policies and information technology regulations developed and approved by organizations accredited by ANSI.

AMERICAN NATIONAL STANDARDS INSTITUTE (ANSI): An organization that accredits various standards-setting committees and monitors their compliance with the open rule-making process that they must follow to qualify for ANSI accreditation; HIPAA prescribes standards mandated by ANSI accredited bodies; Part II, 45 CFR 160.103.

AMERICAN SOCIETY FOR TESTING AND MATERIALS (ASTM): Organization that develops health information standards and information for the medical profession (Health Committee E-31).

AMERICAN TELEMEDICINE ASSOCIATION (ATA): Established in 1993 as a leading resource and advocate promoting access to medical care for patients and health professionals via telecommunications technology; membership open to individuals, companies, and other organizations with an interest in promoting the deployment of telemedicine throughout the world.

AMERICA ONLINE© (AOL): A large commercial online Internet access service provider based in Dulles, VA; merged with Time-Warner in 2000.

AMIGA©: A now bankrupt maker of computer systems such as the Commodore Business Machines© of the later 1980s and early 1990s using Motorola technology; still active in Europe.

AMOROSO, JOSEPH: Director (Client Chief Information Officer) for the First Consulting Group; health data administrator.

AMPERSAND: The "&" symbol for the word *and*.

AMPLIFICATION: To increase broadband signal strength; the formal use of heuristic techniques, artificial intelligence, or gut feelings; slang term.

AMPLIFIER: Electronic devices that strengthen a signal as it traverses a communications channel.

ANALOG: Continuously variable physical information quantities (wave forms and frequencies) in devices operating on such data; for example, telephone or mercury thermometer, and so forth.

ANALOG COMPUTER: A computing machine that uses continuous physical processes for computations.

ANALOG DATA: Continuous information stream of health or other electronic data value.

ANALOG SIGNAL: Continuous data transmission stream of various frequencies and wavelengths, voice, light, or laser signals; a wave shaped electrical symbol that continuously changes with respect to size and shape depending on the information source; nondigital.

ANALOG TO DIGITAL: Conversion of older analog signals to electronic digital format.

ANALYSIS SESSION: A medical or health care information data mining segment.

ANALYSIS TOOL: Computer, network, or Web-based application that provides real-time information on system activity, modifications, attacks, and failures.

ANALYTIC REPRESENTATION: Environmental simulations or mathematical models that require a decision.

ANCHOR: A marker for HTML Web page or Web site document positions.

ANIMATED CURSOR: Mouse pointer for frames, rather than single images, producing an animation loop.

ANNOYBOT: A malicious Internet Relay Chat (IRC) robot or obnoxious utility program; slang term.

ANONYMIZED DATA: Originally identifiable heath data or medical information that has been rendered anonymous or unidentifiable.

ANONYMOUS FTP: File transfer protocol that allows cloaked access to public computer networks or the Internet using passwords such as: "guest," "unknown," "password," or "anonymous"; anonymous e-mailer; anonymous re-mailer, anonymous post, and so forth.

ANSWER: Computer or network configured to return phone calls, e-mails, Voice Over Internet Protocol (VOIP) calls, or other electronic communications prompts.

ANTENNA: A Wi-Fi high-gain or radiation pattern radio signal receiver/transmitter for wireless computer networks; omni-directional, patch, directional, or PC card attachment, and so forth.

ANTI-ALIAS: To eliminate the stair-step appearance of curved and slanted computer screen lines by illuminating nearby pixels.

ANTI-TEARING: The prevention of health or other data loss when contact is interrupted during communications; for example, abrupt smart card withdrawal.

ANTI-VIRUS, VIRUS PROGRAM (AVVP): Software that removes anti-virus programs; one of the first AVVPs was written by Vessilen Bontchev in 1989; Dark Avenger variant.

ANTI-VIRUS SOFTWARE: A software package or subscription service used to thwart malicious computer or network attacks, such as: Symantec®, McAfee®, Trend Micro®, Panda Software®, Sunbelt Software®, Computer Associates®, AVG®, or MS-FF®, and so forth.

ANTI-WORM: A software patch, fix; glitch repairer; do-gooder virus; slang term.

APACHE: Open free source archetypical engine of the Internet and incubator for related UNIX innovations through its software foundation; Web HTTP server program launched in 1995 by the Apache Group®.

APP: Computer software application; slang term.

APPLE COMPUTER, INC.©: Maker of non-PC hardware, software OSX operating systems, PDAs, and peripherals; leader of the data wireless revolution in music, photos, podcasts, iPod video, and so forth; based in Cupertino, CA, and founded by Steve Jobs and Stephen Wozniak.

APPLE IPOD©: Portable digital music and video player; iPOD Shuffle©, Nano©, and Hi-Fi.

APPLE IPOD© HIFI: Computer as a home entertainment hub with wireless connections for CDs, DVDs, stereos, high-end television sets, iPhone®, iTV®, and iPOD® series machines for easy access to music, photos, movies, and various digital media forms from other computer systems.

APPLE MACINTOSH: Streamlined computer from the Xerox-PARC developer of the window, icon menu, and pointing device (WIMP) interface.

APPLET: A small software application such as a work processor, limited function spreadsheet, or utility program often written in the JAVA programming language.

APPLETALK©: Macintosh© computer network communication protocol.

APPLEWORKS®: Productivity suite from the former Claris Corporation®; applications for the iMac machine from Apple Computer Inc®.

APPLIANCE: A dedicated, single-task, electronic device; appliance server, and so forth.

APPLICATION: A software program that performs a task, or subscription Internet service that does the same or directs the specific function of a computer; for example, Google Writely© word processor and Spreadsheet or Microsoft Office©, and so forth.

APPLICATION ARCHITECTURE: Common computer program for systems integration, reuse, and deployment in light of changing health care regulatory, business, clinical, and technology requirements.

APPLICATION DATA CRITICAL ANALYSIS: Formal assessment of health information, medical or other data systems security.

APPLICATION LAYER: Higher seventh layer for the Open Systems Connection (OSC) models, which allow computer network access using remote files, file transfer protocols, directory services, and so forth.

APPLICATION LEVEL PROXY: A type of firewall security technology.

APPLICATION META DATA: Data dictionary of forms, applications, menus, and health or medical information, and other electronic reports.

APPLICATION PROGRAM: Language that links a computer or network to the end user in order to perform an applied task; medical information systems.

APPLICATION PROGRAM INTERFACE (API): A set of routines, protocols, and tools for building software applications provided by most operating environments such as MS-Windows© so that programmers can write applications; although designed for programmers, APIs are good for health industry end users because they guarantee programs have a similar interface; e-mail, telephony calling systems, JAVA, graphics, and DirectX® API.

APPLICATION SECURITY: The use of software, hardware, and procedural methods to protect computer and medical programs and applications from external threats; security measures may be built into applications so that a sound program security routine minimizes the likelihood that hackers will be able to manipulate applications and access, steal, modify, or delete sensitive data; once an afterthought in software design, health data and other security is becoming an increasingly important concern during development as applications become more frequently accessible over networks and are, as a result, vulnerable to a wide variety of threats.

APPLICATION SERVER: A program or computer system that controls back-end functions, databases, or browsers, and so forth.

APPLICATION SERVICE PROVIDER (ASP): An entity that allows health care or other clients to use applications held on an off-site third-party server, usually on a subscription or per-member, per-month basis; midway between onsite processing and outsourcing, this model allows the client to control the processing workflow while eliminating the need to purchase and maintain the application software; service aggregator that acts as a customer relationship manager and single point of contact for health client interactions; software application delivery model; a vendor that hosts and supports a Web application that users access via a secure Internet connection.

APPLICATION TRAINING (AT): The education of medical staff in the correct ways of applying health information technology and related equipment so that it can be used to its fullest (clinical) capacity, and providing them with experience in the application of taught procedures; for example when different features will be employed for different patients or uses, the range of assistance the machine can offer them, how to alter the relationship between the machine and the patient or sample for different purposes, different procedures to pursue for different disorders or uses, and so forth.

APPLICATION WINDOW: Computer screen window with a running application.

APPLIED (ARTIFICIAL) INTELLIGENCE (AI): The electronic exhibition and manipulation of the computer-like characteristics of human intelligence; thinking machine.

APPLY: To activate and save changes from an options list in Windows© 98.

APPOINTMENT SYSTEM: A scheduling resource management process or application that integrates health care and medical components, such as physicians, facilities, times, and their effective utilization; access management.

APTITUDE TEST: Psychometrics to determine general abilities and skill acquisition capabilities.

APTIVE GROUP FREQUENCY HOPPING (AGFH): Technique that allows Wi-Fi and Bluetooth© wireless connectivity and co-operation.

AQUA: The Apple Macintosh OS X® GUI visual interface.

ARCHETYPE: The attributes or features declaration for a named computer system content type.

ARCHIE: A public domain file finding Internet utility program; archive; archie-client; archie-server.

ARCHITECTURE: Computer and health information systems configuration of hardware, software and networks, and so forth; a term applied to both the process and the outcome of thinking out and specifying the overall structure, logical components, and the logical interrelationships of a computer, its operating system, and network; a framework for applications, networks, and computer programs.

ARCHIVE: To store seldom-used computer programs or systems applications offline or offsite; backup systems.

ARCHIVING: A technique of transferring health information created during operations into a more permanent form; vary from manual backups, through periodic transfer to audio cassettes, to real-tune storage onto WORM (Write Once Read Many) disks; memory sticks or optical disks, and so forth.

ARDEN SYNTAX: A medical and clinical decision support system configuration; encoded language.

ARITHMETIC LOGIC UNIT (ALU): CPU that performs mathematic operations; math co-processor.

ARMORED VIRUS: A self-protecting and difficult to disassemble, malicious computer code; Whale variant.

ARPANET: The distributed Advanced Research Projects Agency Network of the Department of Defense; Internet precursor.

ARP SPOOFING: Unauthorized wired computer network access and Internet routing table corruption in order to steal PHI or other sensitive data.

ARRAY: A set of unique and sequentially sequenced health or other data elements.

ARTICLE: A post, text, or paper on a BBS or Internet users group.

ARTIFACT: An unwanted computer signal or visual image.

ARTIFICIAL INTELLIGENCE (AI): The use of computer systems, algorithms, and clinical decisions support systems to mimic human thought; medical diagnosis and treatment, and so forth.

ASC X12N: HIPAA transmission standards, specifications and implementation guides from the Washington Publishing Company; or the National Council of Prescription Drug Programs.

ASCII: American Standard Code for Information Interchange, or a generic computer language for numbers and characters; file, characters; transfer, string, and so forth.

ASP.NET: Originally called ASP+, it is the next generation of Microsoft's Active Server Page©, a feature of their Internet Information Server; both ASP and ASP.NET allow a Web-site builder to dynamically build Web pages by inserting queries to a relational database in the Web page. ASP. NET is different than its predecessor in two major ways: it supports code written in compiled languages such as Visual Basic, Perl, and C++, and it features server controls that can separate the code from the content, allowing GUI editing of pages; Although ASP.NET is not backwards compatible with ASP, it is able to run side by side with ASP applications. ASP.NET files can be recognized by their .aspx extension.

ASSEMBLER: A software program that translates assembly computer language into machine computer language; source code reader; cache; listing; language, and so forth.

ASSEMBLY LANGUAGE: Hardware dependent and machine driven second generation computer instruction language of simple phrases.

ASSOCIATE: A computer priority command always initiated on boot-up.

ASSOCIATION FOR ELECTRONIC HEALTH CARE TRANSACTIONS (AFEHCT): A professional society that promotes the use of electronic connectivity in the health care industrial complex.

ASSOCIATION RULE ANALYSIS: Useful if/then rule extraction from a medical database.

ASSUMPTION CODING: CPT code assignment without associated clinical signs and symptoms.

ASSURANCE: Grounds for confidence that the HIPAA health care information security objectives (integrity, availability, confidentiality, and accountability) have been adequately met by a specific implementation; "adequately met" includes: (1) functionality that performs correctly, (2) sufficient protection against unintentional errors (by users or software), and (3) sufficient resistance to intentional penetration or bypass.

ASTERISK: An ultra-low-cost PBX; the character symbol "*".

ASYMMETRIC (ASYNCHRONOUS) COMMUNICATION: Nonimmediate or not instantaneous reply communications method unlike the telephone; such as e-mail.

ASYMMETRIC CRYPTOLOGY: The use of two different but mathematically related electronic keys for secure health data and medical information storage, transmission, and manipulation.

ASYMMETRIC DIGITAL SUBSCRIBER LINE (ADSL): Technique used to increase bandwidth over standard land-linked copper telephone wires; a pair of modems connected by a copper line that yields asymmetrical transmission of data.

ASYMMETRIC ENCRYPTION: Encryption and decryption performed using two different keys, one of which is referred to as the public key and one of which is referred to as the private key; also known as public-key encryption.

ASYMMETRIC KEY: One half of a key pair used in an asymmetric "public-key" encryption system with two important properties: (1) the key used for encryption is different from the one used for decryption, (2) neither key can feasibly be derived from the other.

ASYMMETRIC MULTIPROCESSING: Assigning separate microprocessors for different tasks.

ASYNCHRONOUS: Occurring at different and varying times; flow of electronic information using start and stop bit parities, for beginning and end points.

ASYNCHRONOUS COMMUNICATION: Two way dual communications with time delay fracture; as with online Certified Medical Planner© "live" distance learning; there is a lapse in time from when a message is sent and when it is received.

ASYNCHRONOUS TRANSFER MODE (ATM): Electronic delivery mode that usually supports the simultaneous transmission of data, voice, and video streaming; two-way high band with communications; method of data transmission where a start signal precedes individual characters and one or more stop signals follow it; because of this start/stop system, delays may occur between characters; denotes the complete system of protocols and equipment associated with cell-based communications networks, which have the ability to transmit voice, data, and video traffic simultaneously using a statistical multiplexing scheme; this switching is expected to bridge the gap between packet and circuit switching; uses packets referred to as cells that are designed to switch cells so rapidly that there is no perceptible delay.

ATHLON®: A popular Intel Pentium©-like CPU made by the AMD Corporation® in 1999; AMD-K7 code name.

ATOM: An XML-based file format that allows lists of information "feeds" to be synchronized between medical and other publishers, patients, and consumers, composed of entries synchronizing Web content such as Weblogs and news headlines to other Web sites and directly to patient consumers.

ATOMIC DATA: A basic or low detailed level of health information or medical data sets.

ATOMICITY: Computer or network actions that must either be completed or aborted; go or no-go; usually for security purposes.

ATOMIC LEVEL DATA: Health data or medical information captured at the point of clinical contact; all or none transaction.

AT SIGN (@): Used to separate a recipient name from the domain name in an Internet e-mail address.

ATTACHMENT: Files, programs, spreadsheets, data, or images, and so forth, included and sent along with an e-mail message.

ATTACK: Aggressive and usually unwanted attempts to enter a secured computer system without authorization; usually for malicious mischief.

ATTACK TREE: An inverted tree diagram that provides a visual image of the attacks that may occur against an asset.

ATTACK VECTOR: Viruses that attack a computer from a wired or wireless network; the source or transmission of infection.

ATTEMPTED SECURITY VIOLATION: Unsuccessful attack to gain unauthorized access to a computer, server, or network.

ATTENDING PHYSICIAN IDENTIFICATION: A unique national identification number assigned to medical providers.

ATTENUATE: Signal weakness degradation over time and distance, usually regenerated with hubs for base-band and amplifiers for broad-band.

ATTRIBUTE: A computer system file access classification that permits it to be retrieved or erased; usual attributes are read/write, read only, archive, and hidden, and so forth; software or code information that describes a specific characteristic, such as a health directory or patient file; a health data abstraction.

ATTRIBUTES: Health information management system elements and medical information contained in a relational database.

ATTRIBUTE TYPE: Rough computer systems suffix classifier for medical data attributes.

AUDIO TELECONFERENCING: Simultaneous dual voice communications between two parties at remote locations; two way communications between physician and patient at various locations.

AUDIT: The monitoring of health care IT security relevant events is a key element for after-the-fact detection of and recovery from security breaches; HIPAA review.

AUDIT CONTROL: Mechanisms to record and examine computer system activity in order to identify suspected PHI or medical data access activities, assess the security system, and respond to potential weaknesses; the mechanisms employed to record and examine computer system activity.

AUDIT TRAIL: Data collected and potentially used to facilitate a health security review (ISO 7498–2); log used for security violation detection, auditing, error correction, recovery, and deterrence.

AUTHENTICATE: Medical records or health care data confirmed by signature; to verify the identity of a computer, server, or network user, by password, or public or private key infrastructure (PKI), or other means such as biometric identification; ensuring the identity of a user, process, or device, often as a prerequisite to allowing access to resources in a computer system or network.

AUTHENTICATION: Assurance that a claimed electronic or human user identity is valid; authentication service provides the means to verify the identity of a patient.

AUTHENTICATION HEADER (AH): IPSec protocol for tunnel identification and security.

AUTHOR: Originator of a medical or health care record; doctor, health practitioner, or medical provider.

AUTHORIZATION: Enables specification and subsequent management of the allowed health information data actions for a given system or computer network; a document signed and dated by the individual who authorizes use and disclosure of protected health information for reasons other than treatment, payment, or health care operations; must contain a description of the protected health information, the names or class of persons permitted to make a disclosure, the names or class of persons to whom the covered entity may disclose, an expiration date or event, an explanation of the individual's right to revoke and how to revoke, and a statement about potential redisclosures.

AUTHORIZATION CODE: Security access key; usually an alphanumeric password.

AUTHORIZATION CONTROL: Access control rules for medical information or a health information management system, which can be centralized, hierarchical, or individual.

AUTHORIZATION RIGIDITY: Health information management system lacking discretionary access control judgment.

AUTHORIZE: To authenticate a computer user or obtain consent for protected health care information (PHI); the granting or denying of access rights to a user, program, or process.

AUTO AUTHENTICATION: An automated authentication process.

AUTO BAUD DETECT: The detection and simultaneous adjustments of electronic communication speeds.

AUTO CALL: Automated call placements to predetermined numbers.

AUTO CALL NUMBER: External phone on the data line of an auto call feature.

AUTO CODE: Extracting medical records or health data information and converting it into computerized CPT and ICD-9-CM codes; computer assisted alphanumerical medical billing.

AUTO DIAL: Automatic dialing of stored telephone numbers, or e-mail addresses.

AUTOEXEC.BAT: Command file executed upon computer boot, for DOS and Windows©.

AUTOMAGIC: As if by magic; slang term.

AUTOMATED CLEARING HOUSE (ACH): Electronic check processing between banks and financial institutions, and customers, hospitals, clinical, and medical practices.

AUTOMATED DATA COLLECTION: The direct transmission of physiological health information or medical data from monitoring devices to either a bedside display system or a computer-based patient record.

AUTOMATIC CAMP-ON: Music replacement feature when a dialed telephone number is busy.

AUTOMATIC FORMS PROCESSING TECHNOLOGY: The ability to electronically and securely enter and abstract online PHI or medical data.

AUTOMATIC LOG-OFF: The cessation of an electronic computer session that is terminated after a predetermined time of inactivity.

AUTOMATIC PATCH: Automated computer system debugging feature usually performed without end-user awareness.

AUTOMATIC PRIVATE INTERNET PROTOCOL ADDRESS (APIPA): The basic sequence of computer networking to locate a specific private Web site used only for internal networks and not into the Internet from a router.

AUTOMATIC QUEUING: Instantaneous telephone call ported to a holding track until the correct connection is available; auto-save; automatic alert; automatic e-mail responder, and so forth.

AUTONOMOUS SYSTEM: Computer system networks, switches, and routers that are controlled by a singular authority through a common IGP.

AUTONOMY: Self determination regarding medical care or health care information access.

AUTORESPONDER: The e-mail equivalent of instantaneous fax-on-demand.

AUXILIARY STORAGE: Secondary or additional computer storage capacity; magnetic tape back-up, external floppy disk, zip drive, hard disk, flash memory stick, optical or CD-ROM, and so forth.

AVAILABILITY: The health care information security objective that generates the requirement for protection against intentional or accidental attempts to (1) perform unauthorized deletion of medical data, or (2) otherwise cause a denial of service or data.

AVATAR: A special user who is given the authority to access all file directories and files under the root directory in a UNIX-based computer system; virtual reality environment.

AWARENESS TRAINING: To provide training for all levels of personnel including a review of the medical organization's policies and procedures for keeping protected health information confidential.

AWK: A computer language replaced by PERL for scanning text files and processing lines and strings of code.

AZYXXI: A clinical data repository system company created by physicians that allows doctors to retrieve and view patient data from a variety of sources, including legacy, access management laboratory, and radiology; purchased by the Microsoft Corporation in 2006.

B

B2B: Business-to-Business.

B2C: Business-to-Consumer (Client).

B2P: Business-to-Patient.

BABBAGE, CHARLES (1791–1871): Inventor of the mechanical computing machine known as the "Analytic Engine" and precursor to electronic computers.

BACKBONE: High-speed transmission pathway for an interconnected computer network; high volume trunk in a computer network; slang term.

BACKBONE NETWORK: A high-speed, high-capacity transmission facility created to interconnect lower speed distribution channels from smaller branches of the computer or telecommunication network; Lucent Systems®; Nortel®; Cisco Systems©.

BACK DOOR: A means of access to a computer program that bypasses security mechanisms, sometimes installed by a programmer so that the program can be accessed for troubleshooting or other purposes; however, attackers often use back doors that they detect or install themselves, as part of an exploit; in some cases, a worm is designed to take advantage of a back door created by an earlier attack; trapdoor; for example, the worm Nimda gained entrance through a back door left by Code Red; slang term.

BACK DOOR TROJANS AND BOTS: Currently, the biggest threat to health care and all PC users worldwide according to the MSFT Corporation®.

BACK DOOR WORM: Malicious code spread by TCP port inoculation; Bagel variant of 2004.

BACK END: All computer systems components not seen or interacted with by the end user.

BACKGROUND: Program or application that is executing without operator or end-user input; any noise, print, processing, or task, and so forth.

BACKGROUND MODE: Occurs when a computer continues with a task function while another application is still running; printing, transferring, surfing, or using functions.

BACK PROPAGATION ALGORITHM: Training protocol for medical neural networks that propagates software code errors from output to hidden input.

BACK-UP: To copy, store, or mirror all health data programs, applications, and software for storage purposes; onsite or remote hot and cold backup locations exist; separately removed medium include another hard-drive, Rev® or Zip® drive, flash disk, tape drive or floppy disk, online storage, CD or DVD, and so forth; medical, health, or other information recovery or restoration feature.

BACK-UP UTILITY: Program to perform basic computer backup functions such as PowerQuest Drive Image©, Norton Ghost©, Stomp Backup My PC©, and Dantz Retrospect Professional Version©.

BACKWARD COMPATIBLE: To function with prior computer versions of itself; for example, Windows Vista® is mostly backward compatible with Windows XP©; XP with MSDOS©, and so forth.

BACTERIA: Computer system virus capable of health systems or enterprise wide replication; bacterium.

BAD SECTOR: A segment of computer disk storage that can't be read or written due to a physical problem in the disk; usually are marked by the operating system and bypassed; if data are recorded in a sector that goes bad, file recovery software and occasionally special hardware may be needed to restore it.

BADWARE: A software program or application that adds spyware, adware, and other unauthorized programs without user disclosure; slang term; www.stopbadware.org.

BALANCED BUDGET ACT: Title IV in 1997 that included financial provisions for Medicaid, Medicare, Medicare+Choice, child care, Medical Savings Accounts, Health Savings Accounts, Medigap plans, rural health care, and military retirees with related health care economic IT initiatives.

BALL, MARION J.: Associate Vice President for Health Information Resources, University of Maryland, Baltimore.

BANDWIDTH: Electronic information carrying capacity, measured in Mbps or Kbps or wireless frequency spectrum; bandwidth-on-demand; bandwidth reservation, bandwidth testing and trading; allocation, broker, exchange, management, demand, reservation, and so forth.

BANG: UNIX system exclamation point; slang term.

BANGPATH: An e-mail address that includes an exclamation mark; slang term.

BANNER: Application or Internet-based Web page advertisement; computer monitor/screen sign, or paid marketing area.

BANYAN VINES: A computer network operating system that shares information with a central server source; A DOS, WINDOWS®, OS/2, OSX bridge program; slang term.

BAR CHART: Visual representation or graph of nominal or ordinal data.

BAR CODE: Electronic identification tag for smart cards and inventory control.

BAR CODING SYSTEMS: Final FDA ruling issued in February 2004 that required bar codes on most prescription and nonprescription medications used in hospitals and dispensed based on a physician's order; the bar code must contain at least the National Drug Code (NDC) number, which specifically identifies the drug; although hospitals are not required at this time to have a bar code reading system on the wards, this ruling has heightened the priority of implementing hospital-wide systems for patient-drug matching using bar codes; a usual procedure for bar coding is as follows:

- drug given to the nurse for patient administration;
- in the patient's room, the provider scans the bar code on the patient's identification badge to positively identify the patient;
- medication container is passed through the scanner to identify the drug;
- match patient to the drug order; if no match including drug, dosage, and time of administration, an alert is displayed in real-time to correct the error prior to administration.

BARNETT, OCTO G., MD: Professor of Medicine, Harvard Medical School, and Director, Laboratory of Computer Science, Massachusetts General Hospital, Boston, MA.

BARRETT, CRAIG, R.: Chairman of the Board, the Intel Corporation.

BASEBAND: Individual digital bidirectional data transmission; a telecommunication system in which information is carried in digital (and analog) form on a single unmultiplexed signal; Ethernet network.

BASHSHUR, RASHID L., MD: Editor-in-Chief Emeritus, *Telemedicine and e-Health Journal.*

BASIC: A popular high-level computer language.

BASIC INPUT/OUTPUT SYSTEM (BIOS): Fundamental PC controller for data-read, memory, storage, keyboards, printers, peripherals, displays, and so forth; determines functionality upon PC boot-up.

BASTION SERVER: A firewall configured to withstand and prevent unauthorized access or services. It is typically segmented from the rest of the intranet in its own subnet or perimeter network.

BATCH: A group of health care or paper medical claims from many sources; batch job.

BATCH PROCESSING: The one-time processing of computer tasks, such as running a group of health care or paper medical claims from many sources, usually with time delayed output; job processing; punch cards.

BATCH TRANSMISSION: Processing several computer transactions at once.

BAT FILE: Data file name ending in .bat for computer command lists.

BAUD: A unit of digital transmission that indicates the speed of information flow. The rate indicates the number of events able to be processed in one second and is expressed as bits per second (bps). The *baud* rate is the standard unit of measure for data transmission capability; typical older rates were 1200, 2400, 9600, and 14,400 baud; the signaling rate of a telephone line in the number of transitions made in a second; 1/300 sec = 300 baud.

BAUD RATE: Transmission speed, per symbol/second, of electronic data information.

BAUMANN, HERMAN: Executive Director of Strategic Development for the American Hospital Association (AHA).

BAYER MATRIX: CMOS or CCD color pixel imagery.

BBL: Be Back Later; slang expression.

BEACONING: Problem ablation process for a token ring computer network.

BEAM: Infrared wireless computer network connection.

BEAM WIDTH: Radio antenna coverage angle.

BEAN: JAVA© open source computer language from Sun Microsystems, Inc; JAVA Bean; slang term.

BEDSIDE WORKSTATION: Computer network client machine in a patient hospital, hospice, or home bedroom.

BEEP CODE: Series of audio BIOS alarms caused by faulty PC hardware and sounded when a computer is started or booted-up; for example, AMI® and Award BIOS® beep codes.

BEHRINGER VERSUS PRINCETON MEDICAL CENTER: Court decision that confirmed patient privacy and held health care organizations responsible for that privacy.

BELL OPERATING COMPANIES (BOC): Grouped under the seven regional BOCs, or RBOCs.

BELLOVIN, STEVEN M.: Researcher on computer networks and security and Professor of Computer Science at Columbia University.

BENCHMARK: A performance test of hardware or software or other computer system peripheral devices.

BENIGN VIRUS: A prank software code that does no real harm; good-times virus.

BEOS: BeBox® computer operating system developed by Be, Inc®.

BEOWULF: Clustered computer network running on the Linux® operating system.

BERNERS-LEE, TIMOTHY: Created the World Wide Web in 1989, while working at CERN, using clickable hypertext links (hot links) in academic documents; inventor of the Web.

BERNOULLI BOX: Nonvolatile cartridge for a removable floppy disk drive with large storage capacity.

BETA TEST: The secondary or final stress examination of newly developed computer hardware, software, or peripheral devices; site, and so forth.

BIBLIOGRAPHIC DATABASE: Indexed computer or printed source of citations of journal articles and other reports in the literature; typically include author, title, source, abstract, and related information; MEDLINE® and EMBASE®.

BIFF: A sound, light, or other alerting method for incoming new e-mail transmissions; slang term.

BIG IRON: Large and expensive main frame computers or hardware legacy systems; slang term.

BILINGUAL: A computer system running two or more operating systems or languages.

BILLED CLAIMS: The fees or billed charges for health care services provided that have been submitted by a medical practitioner or health care provider to a payer.

BILLING CODE OF 1992 (UB-92): A Federal code billing form that requires hospitals follow specific billing procedures; similar to the Centers for Medicare and Medicaid (HCFA) 1500 form, but reserved for the inpatient component of health services.

BILLING CYCLE: The exact date for which certain medical services are billed; paper or electronically.

BILLING FLOAT: Time delayed between medical services provision, and invoicing the third party or patient.

BINARY: The principle behind computers using two digit commands of 0 and 1.

BINARY CODE: The computer coding system of binary digits; number, notation, files, transfer, tree, and so forth.

BINARY OPTION: An option that has two outcomes; generally structured to pay a predetermined fixed amount when-in-the-money; or correct, or pay nothing when-out-the money; or incorrect; either or medical diagnostic dilemma.

BINARY PHASE SHIFT KEYING (BPSK): Radio-modulation technique for wireless computer transmissions.

BIND: To link or assign one computer routine or address to another; to attach a productive device driver to computer adapter.

BINHEX: A Macintosh computer utility format that converts binary computer files to ASCII text files.

BIOETHICS: The application of moral principles to health and health care data information and processing.

BIOINFORMATICS: The application of medical and biological science to the health information management field.

BIOLOGICAL INFORMATION TECHNOLOGY (BIOIT): Cross industry alliance of the Microsoft Corporation to enhance the ability to use and share digital health and biomedical data.

BIOMETRIC: Personal security identity characteristics, such as a signature, fingerprints, voice, iris or retinal scan, hand or foot vein geometry, facial characteristics, hair analysis, eye, blood vessel, or DNA.

BIOMETRIC IDENTIFICATION: Secure identification using biometrics that identifies a human from a measurement of a physical feature or repeatable action of the individual (for example, hand geometry, retinal scan, iris scan, fingerprint patterns, facial characteristics, DNA sequence characteristics, voice prints, and hand-written signature).

BIONIC: A machine or instrument patterned after human beings or nature.

BIOPASSWORD: Start-up health care IT security pioneer of keyboarding patterns to boost online security through neural network patterns.

BIOS: The first operating system code employed upon computer initiation or start-up (boot-up); basic input/output system; supports all peripheral technologies and internal services such as the real-time clock.

BIOS INT. 13 ROUTINE: A DOS interrupt that is used to activate disk functions, such as seek, read, write, and format.

BIOTERRORISM: Germ or biological warfare.

BIT(S): Binary (2 digits) term coined by John Tukey in 1949; either Yes/No, On/Off, Dot/Dash, or an O/I value; the small unit of electronic transmission information; bit rate; bit stream; bit stuffing, and so forth.

BIT DEPTH: The number of pixel determining bits for tone or color range.

BIT LOCK: A hard drive encryption tool such as the MSFT Vista® 265-bit algorithm BitLocker Drive Encryption© that secures files, folders, or data drives.

BIT MAP: Pixel image of many bits that only defines in terms of black and white rather than a grayscale image.

BIT NET: An Internet-like system linking universities.

BIT ORDER: Serial transmission order of electronic health or other information bits.

BIT PIPE: Online or Internet resources for case studies, case law, reports, white papers, journals, literature, Web or pod casts, and so forth; slang term.

BITS PER SECOND (BPS): The number of binary digits transmitted per second that particularly applies to older modems, which transmit at either 14.4 Kbps (14,400 bps) or 28.8 Kbps (28,000 bps); newer modems are capable of 33.6 Kbps and 56 Kbps, and in some cases, transmission speed may extend to 128 Kbps; T lines and cable modems are fastest.

BLACKBERRY: A handheld portable digital device with e-mail capacity and wireless connectivity; from Research in Motion® (RIM).

BLACKCOMB: One of the purported follow-ups to the MSTF Windows Vista© OS; Chicago, Cairo, Longhorn, Memphis, Whistler, and so forth; product code names.

BLACK HAT (BH): A malicious computer hacker, cracker, or criminal; Black Hatting is the act of compromising the security of a system; slang term.

BLACK HOLE: The "place in cyberspace" where e-mail, IM, IRC, text, video, audio, or other messages or electronic transmissions disappear; slang term.

BLACK LIST: A list of Web sites and e-mail addresses that will not be accepted for deliverance.

BLADE: Machine that takes health and other data processing to a computer network server allowing the operating system and applications to be accessed remotely.

BLADE SERVER: Thin computer system that work in groups with servers stacked like a library bookshelf with easy chassis replacement, access, and functionality.

BLANK CHARACTER: A space character such as a letter or digit that comprises one computer byte.

BLANKET AUTHORIZATION: Wholesale medical data release permission for PHI within a certain time period or other range.

BLASTER WORM: Malicious code launched against Windows 2000© and XP PCs that caused DoD attacks in August 2003.

BLENDED THREAT: Computer health network attack that seeks to maximize severity of damage and speed of contagion by combining methods, such as using worms, trojans, and viruses while taking advantage of vulnerabilities in computers or other physical systems.

BLOATWARE: Inefficient, massive, slow software codes, computer programs, or applications; slang term.

BLOCK: Physical unit of stored medical or other data on an output/input electronic device; physical medical record unit.

BLOCK ALGORITHM: Computerized data encryption of larger information segments.

BLOCKER: Usually a software utility program that prevents unwanted e-mail transmissions, or spam; slang term.

BLOG: A type of online public Web site where entries are made as in a diary, and displayed in reverse chronological order; Weblog; slang term coined by Peter Merholz.

BLOGGER: One who writes and reads blogs; slang term.

BLOG LINE: Internet online news reporter and feed reader.

BLOGOSPHERE: The Internet universe of all blog Web sites.

BLOG ROLL: Feature that links to other blogs to alert them that you are linking to them; social blog networking.

BLUE FIN: A vendor-neutral application programming interface to help health care IT departments achieve interoperability across SANs built from multiple vendors; a standard to increase the reliability and security of storage products while also making them easier to manage.

BLUE SCREEN OF DEATH (BSOD): MSFT Windows® inoperable error message that requires computer rebooting; slang term.

BLUETOOTH® DEVICE: Machines, such as a cell phone with headset, transmitting across communications channels 1 to 14, over time.

BLUETOOTH® TECHNOLOGY: Wireless mobile technology standard built into millions of mobile phones, headsets, portable computers, desktops, and notebooks; named after Harold Bluetooth, a tenth-century Viking king; health care telemetry and rural data transmissions; the Bluetooth Special Interest Group (BSIG) advocates measures aimed at pushing health care interoperability for wireless devices and other computers designed for use in the medical field; other wireless stands include: Wi-Fi, ZigBe®, IrDA, and RFID.

BLUMENFELD, BARRY, MD, MS: Associate Director for Clinical Informatics, Research and Development, Partners Healthcare System.

BOMB: Any electronic virus, worm, Trojan, or other malicious computer code with a preset activation date for release.

BOOK, ERIC, MD: CIO and CMO of Blue Shield of California, and payment pioneer for chronic medical conditions.

BOOKMARK: A Web browser feature that allows one to record or store Web addresses, pages, sites, URLS, and so forth, for quick access.

BOOLE, CHARLES (1815–1864): First mathematician to use formula for logical human reasoning; father of modern digital computer programming.

BOOLEAN LOGIC: Mathematical algorithm and algebraic rules that govern logical computer functions developed by George BOOLE in the nineteenth century (AND, OR, and NOT are primary features of Boolean logic); query.

BOOT(ING) (UP): Starting or initiation of a computer operating system to load into random access memory and start executing its first instructions by examining the BIOS, hardware, floppy, and hard drive, RAM, CPU, OS, and so forth.

BOOT DISK: A floppy disk that contains needed computer operating system start-up files.

BOOT DRIVE: The disk drive on which a computer's operating system is installed.

BOOT PARTITION: Separation of computer system operating systems information and data files.

BOOT PASSWORD: BIOS option to secure and protect a computer start-up procedure.

BOOT SECTOR: Reserved sector on a hard disk used to load an operating system; a master boot record is typically the first sector in the first partition that contains a program that reads the partition table and points to another small program that causes the computer to boot the operating system.

BOOT TIME: Time between seeing the Windows© Splash Screen until the completed Windows Desktop (or similar startup time on other operating systems).

BORDER: The moveable edge of a Windows©-based computer screen used to change its size.

BORDER GATEWAY PROTOCOL (BGP): Method to advertise the reach of autonomous systems networks.

BORLAND INTERNATIONAL: Company founded by Philippe Kahn in Scotts Valley, California that first released the program Turbo Pascal©, the utility Sidekick©; followed by various C+ compliers, Paradox© database, Quattro© spreadsheet, and more recently Delphi©, Kylix©, and Java© development tools and templates; now the Inprise Corporation.

BOSS SCREEN: A fake computer screen of a business application or program that is quickly popped up when the boss walks by a workplace cubicle; slang term.

BOT: A smaller software algorithm for a minimally intelligent agent that is programmed to scour the Web for inventory prices in a certain range, or for medical journal articles that mention a disease or condition, and so forth; slang term.

BOTLENECK: Overloaded computer network.

BOTNET: A zombie army of Internet computers drones that, although their owners/users are unaware, have been set up to forward spam messages; a collection of broad-banded PCs hijacked during virus and worm attacks and seeded with software that connects back to the remote hacker for instructions.

BOUNCE: To correctly shut down or reboot a computer, system, or network; e-mail that is returned to sender.

BOUND APPLICATIONS: Computer programs that still run under a DOS or O/S2 operating platforms.

BOURNE, STEPHEN, R., PhD: Computer scientist from Trinity College, Cambridge, UK, and developer of the command line UNIX interface shell, which bears his name; chief technology officer for Ventures, an investment capital consulting firm in El Dorado, CA.

BOURNE SHELL: UNIX computer language and command interpreter; Steven Bourne.

BOZO: Electronic newsgroup miscreant fool, or Internet nerd; slang term.

BOZO FILTER: Software program that screens Internet e-mail messages based on specific individualized criteria; slang term.

BOZO LIST: A blacklist of miscreant IMers, IRCers, fax spammers, or e-mailers; slang term.

BRACES: Curly brackets or symbols used in computer programming to mark the beginning or end of a contained area or phrase.

BRAILER, DAVID, MD, PhD: First and former national coordinator for Health Care Information Technology (HCIT) for the Department of Health and Human Services in Washington, D.C., and who resigned in April 2006. Now, the current Vice President of the American Health Information Community (AHIC), and physician pay-for-performance expert, Washington, D.C.; in September 2006 replaced Robert Kolodner, who was chief health informatics officer of the Veterans Health Administration.

BRAIN DUMP: A large mass of health or medical data that may or may not be secure, or easy to understand, decipher, or digest; raw information overload.

BRAITHWAITE, WILLIAM, MD: Senior advisor on health information policy, Department of Health and Human Services (DHHS), CMO, e-Health Initiative Foundation.

BRANCH: A deviation from normal computer sequential instructions or operations.

BRAND SPOOFING: E-mail fraud where the perpetrator sends out legitimate-looking e-mails that appear to come from well-known and trustworthy Web sites in an attempt to gather personal and financial information from the recipient; a speculative phishing venture.

BRAUN, PETER: Researcher form Harvard University who established the appropriateness of relative value CPT codes along with William Hsiao, MD.

BREACH OF CONFIDENTIALITY: A third-party chain-of-trust violation regarding PHI.

BREACH OF SECURITY: A violation of medical information data integrity and security; unwanted disclosure of PHI.

BRIA, WILLIAM F., II; MD: Clinical Information Systems and IT Medical Director for the University of Michigan, Medical Center in Ann Arbor, President of the Association of Medical Directors of Information Systems in Keene, NH.

BRICKS AND MORTAR: A tangible and physical business such as a hospital, clinic, or medical practice; nonvirtual; real.

BRIDGE: A program or device that connects two computers or simple networks of dissimilar type; identical protocol interface.

BRIGHTCOVE: An Internet TV distributor.

BRIGHTNESS: The perception of luminance by the human eye; although many use luminance and *brightness* interchangeably, they are not exact synonyms.

BRIGHTON, JOHN, MD: CIO of Aetna U.S. Healthcare, headquartered in Blue Bell, PA.

BRITTLE: Friable, insecure, or unstable software output, application, or program.

BROADBAND: The total number of capacity bands available in a frequency-modulated and high-speed unidirectional electronic data transmission; high-speed, high-capacity electronic transmission channel of coaxial or fiber cables, instead of traditional copper telephone land-lines, which may carry voice, data, and video Internet or download transmission, simultaneously; modem or network, and so forth.

BROADBAND CODE DIVISION MULTIPLE ACCESS (BCDMA): A form of wireless technology where digital health information and medical data is sent over communication networks.

BROADBAND NETWORK: High-speed ringed computers or computer network.

BROADBAND OVER POWER LINES (BPL): Radio-frequency energy used to carry high-speed broadband-like electronic data packets traveling on electric current power lines, assisted by amplification *repeaters* and coupled with wired or wireless transmission to PCs, servers, or networks for Internet access beyond traditional phone companies and DSL cable providers (e.g., GreyStone Power Corp®., and TXU Corp®); plugging into the net.

BROADCAST: Data packet delivery to all nodes of a networked computer system.

BROADCAST MONITORING: The hub access point of a wired computer network where wireless data packets and information can be intercepted.

BROADCAST STORM: To incapacitate electronic transmissions by exceeding bandwidth capacity.

BROKEN LINK: An Internet Web page address hyperlink that is not functional.

BROKEN PIPE: A computer systems or network communications failure.

BROUTER: A computing device that provided both computer bridging and routing network functions; slang term.

BROWNOUT: A short period of insufficient electricity or power; longer blackout.

BROWSE: To search or scour the Internet for information or pleasure.

BROWSER: Software interface that supports messages, visuals, hyperlinks, searches, and audio information transmissions on the World Wide Web (WWW); for example, Internet Explorer© 7, Netscape Navigator©, Firefox©, Safari©, Opera©, Mozilla©, Thunderbird©, or GreenBorder Pro© running IE7® inside a safe "sandbox" so that malicious software cannot penetrate an OS while surfing.

BROWSER CACHE: Hard disk sector that holds visited Web page content to speed and enhance the Internet browsing experience.

BROWSER HIJACKER: A software program design to alter a user's browser settings.

BROWSER SHIELD: Ability to detect malicious code on a Web site and rewrite it for health data safety while preserving information on the Web page.

BROWSERSHIELD©: MSFT Internet Explorer© security platform to intercept and remove on the fly, malicious code (embedded scripts) hidden on Web pages and showing users safe equivalents of those pages; patch release alternative developed by Helen Wang.

BROWSING: Search the World Wide Web for electronic networked information; surfing; slang term.

BROWZER: British ISP and Web browser void of Web history or cache search tracking features.

BRUTE FORCE BANDWIDTH: LAN, WAN, or MAN optimization with software application acceleration to increase network transmission speed; to move health and other data faster, securely, and efficiently led by F5 Networks; slang term; Cisco NetScaler©, Packeteer®; slang term.

BRUTE FORCE CRACKING: A trial and error method used by application programs to decode encrypted health or other data such as passwords or through exhaustive effort rather than intellectual strategies; considered to be an infallible, although time-consuming, approach; power hacking.

BS 7799 / ISO 17799 MODEL: A health care security standard that suggests a multistep approach to protect health care information:

- business continuity planning
- system access control
- system development and maintenance
- physical and environmental security
- compliance
- personnel security
- security organization
- computer and network management
- asset classification and control
- security policy and procedures

BS 7799 / ISO 17799 SECURITY STANDARD: The International Organization for Standardization (ISO) is the world's largest developer of standards. Although ISO's principal activity is the development of technical standards, ISO standards also have important economic and social repercussions. ISO standards make a positive difference, not just to engineers and manufacturers for whom they solve basic problems in production and distribution, but to society as a whole. ISO 17799 is a comprehensive set of controls comprising best practices in information security. It is established as the major standard for information security. Its British precursor was published in the early 1990s as a Department of Trade and Industry (DTI)

Code of Practice, and in 1995 it was further developed and published by the British Standard Institution (BSI) as BS 7799. It outlines the specifications for an information security management system (ISMS). Security awareness is very much an integral part of any BS 7799/ISO 17799-compliant ISMS. A recurring theme throughout the standard is that people in an organization must be made aware of the security policies, procedures, and control requirements that they are expected to uphold. This would be a task of a health organization's Security Officer and IT department. ISO 17799 addresses topics in terms of policies and general good practices. The document specifically identifies itself as "a starting point for developing organization specific guidance." It states that not all of the guidance and controls it contains may be applicable and that additional controls not contained may be required. It is not intended to give definitive details or "how-to's." ISO 17799 offers a 10-step approach addressing the following major topics:

1. Business continuity planning
2. System access control
3. Systems development and maintenance
4. Physical and environmental security
5. Compliance
6. Personnel security
7. Security organization
8. Computer and network management
9. Asset classification and control
10. Security policy

BSD: UNIX language variant developed at University of California, Berkeley.

BUCHOLZ, WERNER: Scientist who coined the term *byte*, during the early design phase for the IBM Stretch® computer system, in 1956.

BUCKET BRIGADE: Occurs when an attacker intercepts messages in a public key exchange and then retransmits them, substituting their own public key for the requested one, so that the two original parties still appear to be communicating with each other; man-in-the-middle or fire brigade attack; slang terms.

BUDDY LIST: Collection of e-mail, IM addresses, cell phone–numbers, or contact information, and so forth.

BUFFER: Temporary computer input/output storage area to compensate for transmission speed irregularities.

BUFFER OVERFLOW: Data overflow that occurs when a program tries to store more information in a buffer than it was intended to hold, and spills into adjacent buffers, corrupting or overwriting the valid data held in them; although it may occur accidentally through programming error, buffer overflow is an increasingly common type of security attack on health or other data integrity.

BUG: Colloquial term coined by Admiral Grace Hopper; erroneous computer code or programming mistake; coding error, slang term.

BUGGY VIRUS: Incompetent malicious software code (virus) that fails to deliver its payload; slang term.

BUILD: A version of a computer program or application that is still in testing; although a version number is usually given to a released product, a build number is sometimes used instead.

BULLETIN BOARD (SERVICE) SYSTEM (BBS): A networked computer system to receive and host calls, communicate or exchange files, music, medical, or other data; noncommercial dial-up service; circa 1980s with dial-up connections; newsgroups; computer service that allows users in an isolated location to access a central host computer through a computer in order to read and send electronic messages.

BUNDLE: To sell computer software, hardware, and peripheral components as a single combined package.

BURN: To store health or other digital data on a CD-ROM, DVD, EPROM, and so forth; to electrically write data.

BURNS, LOUIS: Intel© Digital Health Group Manager.

BURST MODE: High-speed computer channel transmission flow.

BUS: A common channel, hardware configuration, or common pathway between CPU and multiple electronic devices; there are several bus types such as USB, AGP, SCSI, FireWire, and PCI.

BUSINESS ASSOCIATE (BA): 45 CFR § 164.522 A health care organization or person that works on behalf of a covered entity, such as an independent consultant or contractor, but is not employed by the Covered Entity or a link in the Chain of Trust (COT); a person or entity who, on behalf of a covered entity or an organized health care arrangement, performs or assists in the performance of one of the following:

- a function or activity involving the use or disclosure of individually identifiable health information, including claims processing or administration, data analysis, processing or administration, utilization review, quality assurance, billing, benefit management, practice management, and repricing.
- provides legal, actuarial, accounting, consulting, data aggregation, management, administrative, accreditation, or financial services for such covered entity or organized health care arrangement.

BUSINESS ASSOCIATE AGREEMENT (BAA): HIPAA security contract for the Business Associate of a covered entity with the following terms and conditions:

a. Business Associate agrees to not use or disclose Protected Health Information other than as permitted or required by the Agreement or as Required by Law.

b. Business Associate agrees to use appropriate safeguards to prevent use or disclosure of the Protected Health Information other than as provided for by this Agreement.

c. Business Associate agrees to mitigate, to the extent practicable, any harmful effect that is known to Business Associate of a use or disclosure of Protected Health Information by Business Associate in violation of the requirements of this Agreement. [This provision may be included if it is appropriate for the Covered Entity to pass on its duty to mitigate damages to a Business Associate.]

d. Business Associate agrees to report to Covered Entity any use or disclosure of the Protected Health Information not provided for by this Agreement of which it becomes aware.

e. Business Associate agrees to ensure that any agent, including a subcontractor, to whom it provides Protected Health Information received from, or created or received by Business Associate on behalf of Covered Entity, agrees to the same restrictions and conditions that apply through this Agreement to Business Associate with respect to such information.

f. Business Associate agrees to provide access, at the request of Covered Entity, and in the time and manner [Insert negotiated terms], to Protected Health Information in a Designated Record Set, to Covered Entity or, as directed by Covered Entity, to an Individual in order to meet the requirements under 45 CFR § 164.524. [Not necessary if Business Associate does not have protected health information in a designated record set.]

g. Business Associate agrees to make any amendment(s) to Protected Health Information in a Designated Record Set that the Covered Entity directs or agrees to pursuant to 45 CFR § 164.526 at the request of Covered Entity or an Individual, and in the time and manner [Insert negotiated terms]. [Not necessary if Business Associate does not have protected health information in a designated record set.]

h. Business Associate agrees to make internal practices, books, and records, including policies and procedures and Protected Health Information, relating to the use and disclosure of Protected Health Information received from, or created or received by Business Associate on behalf of, Covered Entity available [to the Covered Entity, or] to the Secretary, in a time and manner [Insert negotiated terms] or designated by the Secretary, for purposes of the Secretary determining Covered Entity's compliance with the Privacy Rule.

i. Business Associate agrees to document such disclosures of Protected Health Information and information related to such disclosures as would be required for Covered Entity to respond to a request by an Individual for an accounting of disclosures of Protected Health Information in accordance with 45 CFR § 164.528.

j. Business Associate agrees to provide to Covered Entity or an Individual, in time and manner [Insert negotiated terms], information collected in accordance with Section [Insert Section Number in Contract Where Provision (i) Appears] of this Agreement, to permit Covered Entity to respond to a request by an Individual for an accounting of disclosures of Protected Health Information in accordance with 45 CFR § 164.528.

The Business Associate agreement is usually part of a contract made in the procurement process, but can be part of a Memorandum of Understanding (MOU), Grant Agreement (GA), or other document.

BUSINESS ASSOCIATE AGREEMENT USES AND DISCLOSURES: HIPAA styled general use and disclosure permission provisions for covered entities [(a) and (b) are alternative approaches] with the following terms and conditions:

a. Specify purposes:
   Except as otherwise limited in an agreement, Business Associates may use or disclose Protected Health Information on behalf of, or to provide services to, Covered Entity for the following purposes, if such use or disclosure of Protected Health Information would not violate the Privacy Rule if done by Covered Entity or the minimum necessary policies and procedures of the Covered Entity: [List Purposes].

b. Refer to underlying services agreement:
   Except as otherwise limited in an agreement, Business Associate may use or disclose Protected Health Information to perform functions, activities, or services for, or on behalf of, Covered Entity as specified in [Insert Name of Services Agreement], provided that such use or disclosure would not violate the Privacy Rule if done by Covered Entity or the minimum necessary policies and procedures of the Covered Entity.

c. Specific Use and Disclosure Provisions [only necessary if parties wish to allow Business Associate to engage in such activities].

i. Except as otherwise limited in an Agreement, Business Associate may use Protected Health Information for the proper management and administration of the Business Associate or to carry out the legal responsibilities of the Business Associate.

ii. Except as otherwise limited in an Agreement, Business Associate may disclose Protected Health Information for the proper management and administration of the Business Associate, provided that disclosures are Required by Law, or Business Associate obtains reasonable assurances from the person to whom the information is disclosed that it will remain confidential and used or further disclosed only as Required by Law or for the purpose for which it was disclosed to the person, and the person notifies the Business Associate of any instances of which it is aware in which the confidentiality of the information has been breached.

iii. Except as otherwise limited in an Agreement, Business Associate may use Protected Health Information to provide Data Aggregation services to Covered Entity as permitted by 42 CFR § 164.504(e)(2)(i)(B).

iv. Business Associate may use Protected Health Information to report violations of law to appropriate Federal and State authorities, consistent with § 164.502(j)(1).

BUSINESS ENTERPRISE SECURITY DEFENSE FEATURES: (of industry leaders):

- Microsoft®: built anti-malware into Vista OS
- Intel®: chip-partitioning technology
- EMC®: ID vendor Authentica
- Oracle®: enterprise vault and secure back-up products
- Cisco®: integrated network firewalls

BUSINESS INTELLIGENCE: The goal or end product of medical knowledge management.

BUSINESS RELATIONSHIP: An entity or one who assumes responsibility for another especially concerning HIPAA:

- a Third Party Administrator (TPA) is a Business Associate that performs claims administration and related business functions for a self-insured entity.
- a health care clearinghouse is a Business Associate that translates data to or from a standard format in behalf of a covered entity.
- a contract that extends the responsibility to protect health care data across a series of subcontractual relationships.

BUSINESS RESUMPTION: Returning a computer system or network to functionality usually after an unanticipated cessation of activities.

BUSINESS UNIT: Workforce member subject to HIPAA regulations and who is engaged in providing a specific product or service that involves Protected Health Information (PHI) on behalf of the Covered Entity (CE).

BUS NETWORK: A small and inexpensive Land Area Network (LAN) of connected computers and systems; topology, system, and so forth.

BUTTON: A computer tool bar navigation icon.

BYTE (BINARY TABLE): A term first coined by Werner Bucholz in 1956, to represent a series of eight 1 or 0 used to symbolize a specific computer character; a ninth bit may be used in the memory circuits as a *parity bit* for error checking; originally coined to mean the smallest addressable group of bits in a computer, which has not always been eight; SI octet prefix: bits, bytes, kilobytes, megabytes, gigabytes, terabytes, petabytes, exabytes, zettabytes, and yottabytes.

C

C: A programming language developed by Bell Laboratories and Dennis Ritchie in the 1970s for UNIX operating system computers; C+ and C++ are extensions of the language with similar general purpose languages, such as Pascal and ALGOL.

C++: Object-oriented version of the C computer programming language and adopted by companies such as Apple Computer Inc.® and Sun Microsystems, Inc.®.

C#: MSFT.NET framework language similar to Java with increased object-orientated operating system interface.

C2C: Client (Customer) to Client (Customer).

C2P: Client (Customer) to Patient (Provider).

CABLE INTERNET: An Internet access by way of wired coaxial TV service.

CABLE MODEM: Coaxial wire used to connect a computer and TV system for Internet or online service.

CABLE / PHONE OPERATOR: Companies, such as BellSouth©, AT&T©, and Verizon Communications©, that are massive broadband users.

CABLE TELEPHONY: Telephone service enabled by a TV coaxial wire company.

CABLE TELEVISION (CATV): A transmission system that distributes broadcast television signals and other services by means of a coaxial cable.

CACHE: Temporary computer memory storage space that speeds RAM data access; memory cache ("cache store" or "RAM cache") is a portion of memory made of high-speed static RAM (SRAM) rather than the slower and cheaper dynamic RAM (DRAM) which is used for main memory and is effective because most programs access the same data or instructions so that by keeping as much of this information as possible in SRAM, a computer can avoid slower DRAM; disk cache uses conventional main memory, and the most recently accessed data is stored in a memory buffer; when a program needs to access data from the disk, it first checks the disk cache. Disk caching dramatically improves the performance of applications because accessing data in RAM is faster than accessing it on a hard disk; cache memory, farm, card, and so forth.

CACHE POISON: Malicious deletion or alteration of IDNSs and IP addresses that is stored in caches farms and passed on to other serves thereby contaminating the entire network.

CADDY: CD or CVD plastic holder or carrier.

CAIRO: Aborted Windows© OS; code term.

CALIFORNIA DATA BASE SECURITY BREECH INFORMATION ACT (SB-1386): A state law requiring organizations that maintain personal information about individuals to inform those individuals if the security of their information is compromised, and stipulates that if there's a security breach of a database containing personal data, the responsible organization must notify each individual for whom it maintained information; went into effect July 1, 2003 and was created to help stem the increasing incidence of identity theft.

CALL BACK: To identify a caller or calling terminal, and then disconnect the call, dial back, and authenticate the original call.

CALL CENTER: A telephonic central point of access for health care triage.

CALL WAIT: Telephone call alert notification while in use.

CANCEL: To end a computer input command; terminate transmissions.

CANCELBOT: Computer utility program that automatically cancels prearranged messages, e-mails, or IMs, and so forth.

CANNED: A previously written or off the self software product, routine, or program.

CANON GROUP: An early group of leading health care informaticists who defined the need for medical IT terminology standardization.

CANONICAL: The process of conforming with some specification in order to ensure that health or other data is in an approved format; generating or converting canonical data from noncanonical data; a core, standard for foundation for related medical and health care IT concepts.

CAPACITY: The ability to perform a number of tasks, per unit time.

CARBON COPY: Remote-controlled software for Windows© and MS-DOS®.

CARD BUS: 32-bit data bus specification format for fast Ethernet transmissions.

CARDINAL: The number of rows in a data table or entries in an index.

CARD READER: Machine hardware able to read computer punch cards, smart cards, magnetic strips, memory or flash sticks, microchips, RFID tags, and so forth.

CARET: Hat or circumflex character "^" that indicates mathematical exponentially; or a proofreading insertion symbol.

CAREWARE: A shareware software program that suggests charitable donations.

CARNIVORE: A digital FBI sting operation, e-mail and cell phone or wire-tap program to reduce health care and other types of fraud or e-commerce evil doers; code name.

CARRIER: An FTC regulated telecommunications company.

CARR, KEVIN D., MD: Program Director and CMIO for the Waterbury Health Access Program in Connecticut.

CASCADE: Overlapping computer screen or menu windows.

CASCADE MENU: The arrangement of window screens under a pull-down menu command.

CASE SENSITIVE: To interpret the difference between upper (capital) and lower (small)-case letters.

CATHODE RAY TUBE: The monitor or other means of displaying digital or analog data in a computer system.

CAVITY: A type of stealth or covert computer virus that alters or overwrites a small section of an infected file; allowing it to live and propagate; slang term.

CD AUTHORING: Software to produce and burn CDs and DVDs; for example, Roxio Easy CD Creator©, Ahead Nero©, and Pinnacle InstantCD©.

CELEBRITY VIRUS: Malicious code named after notables such as Rod Stewart, Jethro Tull, or Jennifer Lopez that overwrites target programs, but retains and renames them for easy treatment; slang term.

CELERON©: Intel© value brand CPU; code name Covington.

CELL: Transmission packet used on fixed Asynchronous Transfer Mode (ATM) and similar telephone networks; an elementary unit of storage.

CELL®: Microprocessor chip released by IBM in 2006 with more computing power than traditional chips in handling some handheld health care applications; first appeared in thin "blade" server systems.

CENSOREWARE: Software utility program that restricts Internet site visits, transmissions, and files, and so forth; security measure; slang term.

CENTER FOR HEALTH INFORMATION MANAGEMENT (CHIM): Industry association or health information technology and research.

CENTERS FOR DISEASE CONTROL AND PREVENTION (CDCP): An organization in Atlanta, Georgia, that maintains several code sets included in the HIPAA standards, including the ICD-9-CM codes.

CENTERS FOR MEDICARE & MEDICAID SERVICES (CMS): The organization that historically maintained the UB-92 institutional EMC format specifications, the professional EMC NSF specifications, and specifications for various certifications and authorizations used by the Medicare and Medicaid programs. CMS also maintains the HCPCS medical code set and the Medicare Remittance Advice Remark Codes (MRARC) administrative code set.

CENTRAL PROCESSING UNIT (CPU): Integrated motherboard chip that directs all arithmetic, logic, graphic, audio and video, on-ground connectivity, and wireless computer operations; health IT professionals (particularly those involved with mainframes and minicomputers) often refer to the entire computer as a CPU, in which case "CPU" refers to the processor, memory (RAM), and I/O architecture (channels or buses); with speeds exceeding 10 GHz; Intel®, AMD®, Motorola®, and so forth.

CENTRINO®: Intel© mobile brand wireless CPU.

CERF, VINTON, PHD: Early designer of ARPANET while a graduate student at UCLA; known as father of the Internet and coauthor of the TCP/IP protocol that allowed independent networks to form one large network; currently the chief Internet strategist for MCI WorldCom, evangelist for Google, and developer of the Internet Planetary Network (IPN); partner of Robert Kahn, PhD.

CERTIFICATE AUTHORITY: A third-party encryption verification agency for personal identification in health data communications.

CERTIFICATE OF DESTRUCTION (COD): Third-party verification and proof of medical data destruction or the secure annihilation of PHI.

CERTIFICATE OF REVOCATION LIST: Schedule of Public Key Infrastructure (PKI) approvals decommissioned by a certification authority.

CERTIFICATION: The formal approval of software, hardware, and end users for a computer system; the technical evaluation performed as part of, and in support of, the accreditation process that establishes the extent to which a particular computer system or network design and implementation meet a prespecified set of security requirements; may be performed internally or by an external accrediting agency.

CERTIFIED MEDICAL PLANNER© (CMP©): Professional economics designation (Certified Medical Planner©) first charted for advisors in 2000 that integrates the personal financial planning process (taxation, insurance, investing, retirement, and estate planning) for physicians, with specific knowledge of contemporaneous health information technology and managed care principles, such as financial, managerial and medical cost accounting, fringe benefits analysis, risk management, human resources and access management, managed care medicine, health care informatics, and human labor outsourcing, with medical practice valuation techniques, succession planning, and most health care business concepts as accredited by the Institute of Medical Business Advisors, Inc., Atlanta, Georgia (www.Medical.BusinessAdvisors.com); a CMP© charter-holder or CMP© certificant (www.CertifiedMedicalPlanner.com).

CETERIS PARIBUS: latin phrase for: "all things being equal," which acknowledges uncontrollable possibilities in a controlled testing hypothesis situation.

CHAIKEN, BARRY, MD, MPH: Vice President, medical affairs, McKesson Corp., Alpharetta, GA.

CHAIN OF CUSTODY: A process that documents everyone who has had contact with or direct possession of the evidence.

CHAIN OF TRUST (COT): Suggestion that each and every covered entity and Business Associate share responsibility and accountability for confidential PHI.

CHAIN OF TRUST PARTNER AGREEMENT: Contract entered into by two business partners in which it is agreed to exchange data and that the first party will transmit information to the second party, where the data transmitted is agreed to be protected between the partners; sender and receiver depend upon each other to maintain the integrity and confidentiality of the transmitted information; multiple two-party contracts may be involved in moving information from the originator to the ultimate recipient; for example, a provider may contract with a clearing house to transmit claims to the clearing house; the clearing house, in turn, may contract with another clearing house or with a payer for the further transmittal of those same claims.

CHAMPUS: Civilian Health and Medical Program of the Uniformed Services, U.S.C. Title 10 Section 1072(4).

CHANNEL: Telecommunication electronic pathway located between receiving and transmitting computer devices; a radio frequency assignment designed depending on the frequency band being used and the geographic location of the sending and receiving sites.

CHANNEL HOP: To quickly switch from one chat room, newsgroup, or IRC site to another without interacting; channel surfing; slang term.

CHARACTER: A set of basic symbols or elements to express data or information.

CHARACTER SPACING: The amount of font space reserved for each electronic character, letter, number, or symbol.

CHARGE-COUPLED DEVICE: A light-sensitive device that converts light information into electronic information via sensors that collect light as a buildup of electrical charge; the signal that results from this conversion can be converted into computer code and then used to form an image; commonly used in television and digital cameras and radiology image scanners.

CHARGE MASTER: A comprehensive review of a physician, clinic, facility, medical provider, or hospital's charges to ensure Medicare billing compliance through complete and accurate HCPCS/CPT and UB-92 revenue code assignments for all items including supplies and pharmaceuticals.

CHART: The paper and pen physical and written medical record; also an electronic medical record; electronic health record, and so forth.

CHART DEPLETION POLICY: Formal regulations for deciding when a medical record may be removed from resident medical records over a specific time period.

CHARTING BY EXCEPTION: Health information management and medical records and medical documentation system that focuses and records abnormal medical and clinical events.

CHART ORDER POLICY: Regulations for detailed health data and information documentation listings to define location and order within the medical record.

CHART TRACKING: Identifies the exact location and placement of PHI or other medical records.

CHAT: Real time conferencing ability enhanced by Internet keyboarding.

CHAT MODE: A split screen real time Internet communication program.

CHAT ROOM: Real time ISP sector devoted to a single medical topic or other topical keyboarding discussion; electronic forum or BBS; informal IRC site.

CHECK BOX: An on/off toggle switch queue in a software dialog box.

CHECK DIGIT: End product of an operating system checksum process.

CHECKED: MSFT error detection or debugging code in isolated development products.

CHECKSUM: Summation or additions of digits and bits according to rules of parity in order to verify health or other data integrity and authenticity; error detection mechanism.

CHEESE WORM: Usually helpful computer security patches for the Linux system, Lion worm that repairs exploits; slang term.

CHEUNG, NT, MD: Executive Manager, Healthcare Informatics Division, Hospital Authority of Hong Kong.

CHICAGO: MSFT Windows 95© version; code name.

CHIEF INFORMATION OFFICER (CIO): A senior corporate position with strategic responsibility for health information management and medical data and information technology and integrity.

CHIEF KNOWLEDGE OFFICER (CKO): A senior corporate position with strategic responsibility for health knowledge and medical data management.

CHILDREN'S ONLINE PRIVACY PROTECTION ACT (COPPA): A federal act that requires operators of online services or Web sites directed at children under the age of 13 to obtain parental consent prior to the collection, use, disclosure, or display of a child's personal information.

CHIP: Increasing small and more powerful semiconductors, such as processed silicone, gallium, or germanium, used in computers for certain electronic characteristics, such as storage, circuitry, or logic elements; integrated circuit: Moore's Law of microprocessor density.

CHIP INTERFACE: A fast computer connection between main processor and co-processor, or other chips: Geneseo; code name; Hyper-transport, or AMD chip-to-chip interface.

CHKDSK, CHKDSK /F: A DOS utility program that looks for lost clusters on a hard disk and reports the current amount of free memory and disk space; it has been replaced by ScanDisk.

CHOCKLEY, NANCY: President and CEO, National Institute for Health Care Management Research and Education Foundation (NIHCMREF); Washington, D.C.

CHURCH, GEORGE, PHD: Professor of Computational Genetics, Harvard Medical School.

CHURCH-TURING THESIS: Hypothesis that no mechanical computing device can do anything fundamentally different than another mechanical machine.

CIH VIRUS: Malicious computer code that first appeared in 1998 and tried to overwrite a computer system's BIOS and render it unbootable; Chernobyl virus variant.

CINNAMON BUN: The "@" sign; slang term.

CIPHER LOCK: A combination lock that uses buttons that must be pushed in the proper sequence in order to open the door.

CIPHER TEXT: Unreadable medical information in a secure and encrypted format.

CIRCUIT LEVEL PROXY: A type of nonapplication specific firewall technology; for example, SOCKS.

CIRCUIT SWITCH: Connection between a dedicated circuit network path and a telephone system.

CIRCUIT SWITCHED NETWORK: A line switching and dial-up service network that temporarily links multiple channels between multiple points and permits the medical user to exclusive use of an open channel to exchange protected health information.

CIRCULARITY: The endless cycle that suggests a computer cannot finish a task unit it has already completed; circular impossible logic; loop.

CISCO SYSTEMS®, INC.: Founded in San Jose, CA in 1984 as a leading manufacturer of computer network equipment, routers, bridges, frames, switches, and management software; CEO John Chambers.

CITATION: The record of an article, book, or other report in a bibliographic health or other database that includes summary descriptive information, for example, authors, title, abstract, source, and indexing terms.

CITRON, JEFFREY: CEO of Vonage© Holdings, which offers Internet telephone services enhancing health communications.

CLAIM: Medical invoice for health care services rendered; a doctor's medical bill.

CLAIM ADJUSTMENT REASON CODE: The code set for the difference between an original medical provider charge and ultimate reimbursement; a national administrative code set that identifies the reasons for any differences or adjustments between the provider charge for a claim or service and the payer's payment for it; code set used in the X12 835 Claim Payment & Remittance Advice and the X12 837 Claim transactions and maintained by the Health Care Code Maintenance Committee (HCCMC).

CLAIMANT: One who submits a claim for payment of benefits for a suffered loss, according to the provisions of a health insurance policy.

CLAIM ATTACHMENT: The hardcopy or electronic record needed to pay a medical claim.

CLAIMS CLEARING HOUSE: Organizations that examine and format claims for reimbursement.

CLAIM STATUS CODE: A national administrative code set that identifies the status of health care claims; used in the X12 277 Claim Status Notification transactions, and maintained by the Health Care Code Maintenance Committee (HCCMC).

CLAIM STATUS CODE CATEGORY: National administrative code set category that indicates the general category of the status of health care claims; code set is used in the X12 277 Claim Status Notification transactions and is maintained by the Health Care Code Maintenance Committee.

CLANCY, CAROLYN, MD: Director, Agency for Healthcare Research and Quality (AHRQ); DHHS.

CLARINET®: Subscription-based United Press International newsgroup; with feeds from Reuters®, SportsTicker®, and Commerce Business Daily®, and so forth.

CLARK, TERRY MD: President and CEO of physician distance-learning Medantic Technology©, Inc., and former Fulbright Scholar, NIH consultant, and Commissioner for the Presidential Task Force to improve Health Care for American Veterans.

CLASS: Electronic objects that share a common attribute; higher level abstraction for identification and definition; object oriented program; or U.S. FCC approval scheme:

- Class A: Approved for industrial or business use; high radio frequency interference potential.
- Class B: Approved for residential areas; low radio frequency interference potential.

CLASSIFICATION: Protection of health data from unauthorized access by the designation of multiple levels of access authorization clearances to be required for access, dependent upon the sensitivity of the information.

CLASSIFICATION LEVEL: Security clearance and authorization degree.

CLASSIFICATION SYSTEM: Any method to organized related health information for retrieval, manipulation, and storage.

CLEAN BOOT: A computer systems startup without load.

CLEAN CLAIM: A claim that meets all insurer requirements and is submitted before the filing limit; electronic invoice or hardcopy.

CLEAR: Setting of a bit or computer/electronic device register to zero.

CLEARANCE: Security classification for health information or medical data access and manipulation.

CLEARING HOUSE: HIPAA medical invoice, health care data transaction exchange, and medical data implementation service center that meets or exceeds Federally-mandated standardized Electronic Data Interchange (EDI) transaction requirements.

CLEAR MEMORY: To start computer RAM registers to a blank condition.

CLEAR TEXT: Easily read and unsecured language; plain text.

CLEARY, SCOTT: Project Management, e-Health, Connecticut.

CLICK: To push or release a button on a computer mouse or keyboard to activate an input instruction.

CLICKABLE IMAGE: An URL embedded picture, drawing, photograph, or similar visual hyperlinked item.

CLICK AND DRAG: To electronically grasp a computer screen icon and move it to a new location to exercise a specific function.

CLICK FRAUD: Phony computer clicks that drive up a Web site's revenue, rather than to search for a real product or service, for advertising driven sites.

CLICK STREAM: Mouse click trail that specifies a particular computer operation; click through.

CLICK THROUGH: The act of linking to a third party in order to measure advertising effectiveness.

CLICK TO CALL: Internet advertising model that allows Internet surfers to speak with a human being on company shopping and search platforms; product ordering intersection of eBay®, Skype®, and Google®.

CLIENT: A dumb receiving computer terminal with access to a central server or host that performs specific tasks but does not house or share network information.

CLIENT REGISTRY: Area where a patient's medical data and PHI is housed and stored.

CLIENT SERVER: A smart mainframe computer or central server that houses and shares specific health data or other information with clients or dumb network terminals.

CLIENT SERVER SYSTEM: A "repository," or computers known as "servers," that store large amounts of medical information and perform limited health data processing; communications with servers and client workstations that perform data processing and often have Graphical User Interfaces (GUI) for ease of use; both customizability and resource use is high, depending on the desired sophistication; many medical and clinical information systems that process data directly related to patient care use this configuration.

CLIENT SIDE APPLICATION: A program that runs on a computer network rather than a server.

CLINGER-COHEN ACT: Public Law 104–106; Information Technology Management Reform Act (ITMRA) of 1996.

CLINICAL CODE SETS: The confidential electronic identifiers for medical health services; medical code sets.

CLINICAL CODING: The assignment of alphanumerical codes to medical diagnostic and procedural verbiage and statements.

CLINICAL CONTENT OBJECT WORK GROUP (CCOWG): HL7 standard for shared clinical applications.

CLINICAL DATA: Protected Health Information (PHI) from patient, physician, laboratory, clinic, hospital, and/or payer, and so forth; identifiable patient medical information.

CLINICAL DATA INFORMATION SYSTEMS: Automatic and securely connected system of integrated computers, central servers, and the Internet that transmits Protected Health Information (PHI) from patient, physician, laboratory, clinic, hospital, and/or payer, and so forth.

CLINICAL DATA REPOSITORY (CDR): Electronic storehouse of encrypted patient medical information; clinical data storage.

CLINICAL GUIDELINES: Suggested and personalized medical protocols or treatment algorithm.

CLINICAL INFORMATICS (CI): The management of medical and clinical data; the use of computers, networks, and IT for patient care and health administration.

CLINICAL INFORMATION: All the related medical information about a patient; Protected Health Information (PHI) from patients, providers, laboratories, clinics, hospitals, and/or payers or other stakeholders, and so forth.

CLINICAL INFORMATION SYSTEM (CIS): A computer network system that supports patient care; relating exclusively to the information regarding the care of a patient, rather than administrative data, this hospital-based information system is designed to collect and organize data.

CLINICAL INFORMATION SYSTEM NETWORK: Computer information technology health system that encompasses a wide range of features, functions, and modules and may include the following:

- pharmacy information systems with bar coding and drug interaction checking.
- computerized physician (provider) order entry (CPOE) for clinicians to directly order tests and treatments online.

- departmental systems such as laboratory information systems, radiology systems, and intensive care clinical computing.
- electronic medical record systems (EMR) that allow physician orders, free text clinical notes, decision support, radiology images, and other areas to be nearly fully computerized, allowing a "paperless" medical institution.

CLINICAL INTEGRATION (CI): The confidential, sure and correct union of patient electronic medical information with all appropriate health care parties or decision makers: physicians, facilities, laboratories, and payers.

CLINICAL MESSAGING: Real-time or asynchronous clinical or medical data and/or PHI electronic exchanges; clinical instant messaging; CMing; slang term.

CLINICAL (CRITICAL) PATHWAY (CP): Formalized and mandated medical protocol or treatment algorithm; critical pathway.

CLINICAL PORTAL: A network centered HIM access computer device.

CLINICAL TERMS, VERSION 3 (CTV3): The UK National Health Services "read codes" used to facilitate medical information interchange; U.S. SNOMED counterpart.

CLINICAL WORKSTATION: A single point of clinical data access or electronic interface.

CLIP ART: Previously prepared graphic images used for desktop publishing, writing, and so forth.

CLIP BOARD: Windows© feature used to store electronic information; any temporary electronic storage cache.

CLIPPER: A general governmental cryptology security chip.

CLIPPER CHIP: Data protection chip proposed by the government and National Security Agency in 1993 to secure vital and individualized health and other information, but defunct by 1996; now used as a slang term for the invasion of privacy.

CLOCK: An evenly spaced computer impulse generator, in MHz, where 1 MHz = 1,000,000 cycles per second (CPS).

CLOCK SPEED: Microprocessor performance velocity and benchmark expressed in megahertz units; MHz.

CLONE: An IBM compatible personal computer made by a manufacturer other than IBM, which exited the PC business in 2005, to China-based Lenovo®, under the leadership of William Amelio, formerly of Dell, China; Compaq Computer, and so forth.

CLOSE: To exit a computer program and clear it from memory.

CLOSED CARD SYSTEM: Smart card central processor computer chip system, operating in a single environment such as hospital access management.

CLOSED INFORMATION SYSTEM: A type of electronic mailing list that allows only members of that mailing list to send messages to it; distinguished from 'open' or 'moderated.'

CLUSTER: 1024 bytes hard disk storage space; hard disk allocation unit or some number of disk sectors that are treated as a unit; smallest unit of storage that the operating system can manage.

CLUSTER COMPUTING: A series of networked connected computers.

CLUSTER VIRUS: A singular malicious computer code that attacks files but gives the appearance of mass infestation.

CMOS: Complementary MOS or the most widely used type of integrated circuit for digital processors and memories.

CMOS MEMORY: A small, battery-backed memory bank in a computer that holds configuration settings.

COASTER: A free CD or DVD give-away as a product/service promotional item; slang term.

COAXIAL CABLE: Transmission lines made of two cores; an inner white conductor encased in insulation, and an outer black conductor with PCV insulation; a single or dual transmission wire covered by an insulating layer, a shielding layer, and an outer jacket; because it contains a high bandwidth, it may be a broadband carrier with the ability to transmit data, voice, and video.

COBOL: Common Business Oriented Language was the first widely used high-level programming language for health care and other business applications, such as payroll, accounting, and other business applications; written over the past 35 years, they are still in use and it is possible that there are more existing lines of programming code in COBOL than in any other programming language; generally perceived as out-of-date and viewed as legacy applications; developed by Grace Hopper as a simple linguistically based computer language program that revolutionized the business computer.

COBWEB SITE: An old URL; dated Web site; slang term.

COCOA APP: Software written specifically for a Mac OS X; slang term.

CODE: A way of dealing with electronic data for a physical computing machine; method for systemically dealing with medical data or other information; computer program.

CODED DATA: Health information or medical data aggregated in a standardized way for comparison.

CODE EDITOR: Software that evaluates medical claims and compares it with clinical records that may affect reimbursement.

CODE LOOKUP: An electronic file with recoded medical codes and health care indexes.

CODE OF FEDERAL REGULATIONS (CFR): Governmental collection of federal regulations and guidelines published in the *Federal Register*.

CODER: One who converts a written diagnosis or medical treatment into a number-letter alphanumeric code for payment and reimbursement; biller.

CODER-DECODER (CODEC): A device that converts a digital signal to an analog signal at one end of transmission, and back again to a digital signal at the opposing end.

CODE RED WORM: Malicious software that infected the White House Web site in 2001 and capable of fast replication, hibernation, and re-infection; slang term.

CODE SET (CS): 45 CFR 162.103 Any HIPAA encryption or de-encryption electronic algorithms used for HIPAA medical information transactions; data elements such as tables of terms, medical concepts, medical diagnostic codes, or medical procedure codes; both the codes and the descriptions (Table 3).

CODE SET MAINTAINING ORGANIZATION: The association that creates and maintains HIPAA electronic code sets for secure health data transmissions; Part II, 45 CFR 162.103.

CODING: The transference of disease, injury, and medical treatment descriptions and narratives into designated and approved alphanumeric form.

CODING CLINIC: American Hospital Association quarterly publication on ICD-9-CM coding issues approved by the CMS.

CODING CONVENTION: The typeface, font, indentation, and punctuation marks used to determine how *ICD-9-CM Codes* are interpreted.

CODING CREEP: A slang term for elevated (increased-acuity) coding, in order to increase medical payments and reimbursement.

Table 3: Code Set Standards (NPRM)

Diseases, injuries, impairments, etc.: ICD-9-CM
Procedures: ICD-9-CM, CPT, CDT, HCPCS
Drugs—Most administrative transactions: HCPCS Pharmacy transactions: NDC
Devices: HCPCS
Standards for Unique Health Identifiers
(DHHS Indications Thus Far)
Provider Identifier: National Provider ID (NPI)
Health Plan Identifier: PAYERID
Employer Identifier: EIN
Individual Identifier: (Still under consideration)

CODING SPECIALIST: One who is an expert at assigning alphanumeric to diagnostic or medical procedures.

COGAN, JOHN, PHD: Senior Fellow of the Hoover Institution, Stanford University.

COHORT DATA: Patients grouped together and described by common characteristics such as age, sex, disease state, medications, complications, insurance coverage, and so forth.

COLD BACKUP: A database backup when the database is offline and thus not accessible for updating; offline backup.

COLD BOOT: Computer start-up from a powered-down, or off, state; a *hard boot*.

COLD SITE: An alternative backup site that provides the basic computing infrastructure, such as wiring and ventilation, but very little equipment.

COLLABORACARE CONSORTIUM: A partnership of electronic, DME, and other vendors that help provide regional health information organizations, provider communities, and health insurance plans with prepackaged, integrated components of payer/provider information exchange and medical EDI.

COLLABORATIVE NETWORK: A computer network or single-issue social Web site internally run, policed, and self-censored; wiki; collaborative filter; collaborative censor.

COLLABORATIVE STORAGE DATA SET: American Joint Commission on Cancer neoplasm staging standard; user derived database.

COLLECTION: The medical and/or electronic billing process.

COLLEGE OF HEALTH INFORMATION MANAGEMENT FOR EXECUTIVES (CHIME): Educational and certifying branch of the Center for Healthcare Information Management (CHIME), an industry association for health information technology and research; useful for CIOs and CTOs.

COLLEN MORRIS F: Director Emeritus and Healthcare Information Technology Consultant, Division of Research, Kaiser Permanente Medical Care Program, Oakland, California.

COLLISION: Malfunction of two computer network nodes attempting shared access at the same time.

COLLISION DETECTION: Ability to detect Ethernet traffic and avoid a nodal collision on a shared computer network.

COLOR MODEL: The dimensional coordinate system used to describe colors numerically, such as Red, Green, Blue (RGB); Hue, Lightness, Saturation (HLS); and Cyan, Magenta, Yellow, Black, and Lightness (CMYBL).

COLOR SATURATION: The sum of ink in a given area of an electronic image; because of dot gain and press conditions, there is no color saturation value above 300.

COLOR SPACE: A particular electronic color variant with a specific range of colors as its chief characteristic.

COMBINATION HALFTONE: An image that is comprised of elements of half tones and line art.

COM1/COM2/COM3: The first two serial communication ports on a PC.

COMMAND: Application option in a pull-down menu; computer system input.

COMMAND BUTTON: Dialog box Windows© icon for a preselected program, application, or input command.

COMMAND.COM: A computer program command that accesses and executes user/operator input; is used with DOS; Bourne, Korn, and C shells with UNIX operating systems.

COMMAND INTERPRETER: Software that can access and execute user input; the term.

COMMAND PROMPT: The place to input instruction for a DOS command; C:\ or A:\, or UNIX %.

COMM CLOSET: Physical location or storage area for computer and networking equipment; communication closet; wiring closet; slang terms.

COMMENT: Public opinion on proposed or potential HIPAA related regulations provided in response to an NPRM, Notice of Intent, or other federal regulatory notice; ignored computer program information seen only by the user.

COMMON CARRIER: A telecommunications company, charging published and nondiscriminatory rates and regulated by the government, that offers communications relay services to the general public by means of shared circuits.

COMMON FRAMEWORK: Includes all the technical documents and specifications, testing interfaces, and code, as well as a companion set of privacy and security policies and model contractual language to help medical or other organizations interested in information exchange to move quickly toward the necessary legal agreements for private and secure health information and data sharing.

COMMON GATEWAY INTERFACE (CGI): A Web server standard to pass a user's request to an application program and to receive data back to forward to the user.

COMMON SERVICES: Software shared across several applications.

COMMUNICATION ARCHITECTURE: The software and hardware capacity that facilitates electronic computer interactivity.

COMMUNICATION MULTIPLEXER: An instrument that permits health data from multiple, lower speed communication lines to share a single higher speed communication path.

COMMUNICATIONS BUS: Health Information Access Layer segment that allows standard messages and protocols.

COMMUNITY HEALTH INFORMATION NETWORK (CHIN): A connected electronic entity committed to securely share private patient health information among entities such as medical providers, clinics, laboratories, hospitals, outpatient centers, hospice, and other health care facilities; Community Health Management Information Systems (CHMIS), Enterprise Information Networks (EINs), Regional Health Information Networks (RHINs), and Health Information Networks (HINs).

COMPACT DISC (CD): Optical drive that can read or write data by burning tiny bumps into the surface; speed is in numbers such as 64X, 32X, or 24X; reading speed is higher than writing speed; developed by Philips Electronics®.

COMPACT DISC—READ ONLY MEMORY (CD-ROM): A computer drive that can read CD-R and CD-RW discs.

COMPACT DISC—RECORDABLE (CD-R): An optical disc that contains up to 650 megabytes of data and cannot be changed once recorded.

COMPACT DISC—REWRITEABLE (CD-RW): An optical disc that can be used to record data, erase it, and re-record again.

COMPACT FLASH: Nonvolatile flash storage; memory stick; thumb stick, and so forth.

COMPACT FLASH CARD: Smart card, memory stick, or processor chip that uses nonvolatile memory like that from the Macromedia Corporation©, now Adobe Systems©, Inc.

COMPAQ© COMPUTER: A first IBM PC clone manufacturer that acquired DEC and has since been acquired by HP.

COMPARTMENTED INTRANET: Internal computer network analogous to the watertight doors on a ship; supports the enforcement of health organizational policies and the limitation of damage in the event of a security breach as illustrated in Figure 1.

COMPATIBILITY: The ability of two pieces of hardware (a personal computer and a printer, for example) to work together; standards, published specifications of procedures, equipment interfaces, and data; for computer systems to work together; formats are essential to decreasing and possibly eventually extinguishing incompatibility; IBM PC clone to MacBook©.

COMPILED LANGUAGE: Computer code that runs very fast as an executable file.

COMPILER: Software language translator program for machine instructions.

COMPLEMENTARY CODE KEYING (CCK): Wi-Fi high-speed transmission technique; while a Baker sequence is its slower analog.

COMPLETE TRUST DOMAIN: The MSFT Windows NT© large complex network multiple account resource that communicates two-way trustworthy computing.

COMPLEX INSTRUCTION SET COMPUTER (CISC): Efficient microprocessors capable of high speeds and many transactions.

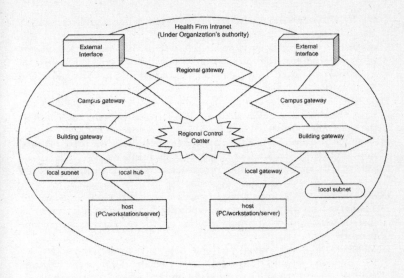

Figure 1: Compartmented health entity intranet.

COMPLIANCE: Conformity to HIPAA medical data security policies and standards as well as the data security procedures developed to meet user needs; improper conduct includes, but is not limited to a lack of discretion or unauthorized disclosure of any health information concerning a specific patient.

COMPLIANCE DATE: The date by which a covered health care entity must comply with a standard, implementation specification, requirement, or modification specified by the CMS, HHS, FRC, or other agency.

COMPLIANT: Year 2000, or Y2-K compatible hardware, software, or electronic computer peripheral devices; security moniker for trust.

COMPONENT: Self-contained application that is part of an object-oriented computer program; block of GUI applications.

COMPONENT CODE: Post-comprehensive code nomenclature that cannot be charged to Medicare when a comprehensive code is also charged.

COMPONENT CODING: Standardized medical report code regardless of physician specialty.

COMPONENT WARE: All the individual partitions, hardware, and software programs with protected patient information that support the health care industrial complex; clinical, laboratory, drug, facility, providers, payer, and third-party intermediary.

COM PORT: Serial port for connecting a cable to an IBM PC-compatible computer, usually, but not exclusively for data communications; referred to by the operating system as COM1, COM2, COM3, and so forth.

COMPRESS: To transform health or other data to minimize the space required for storage or transmission or to download more efficiently.

COMPRESSED FILE: Software utility program used to condense, transport, and archive programs with the file extension .zip.

COMPRESSED VIDEO: Video images that have been processed to reduce the amount of bandwidth adequate for capturing the necessary information so that medical images and health information can be sent over a telephone network.

COMPRESSION: Concentrated electronic data used to enhance and speed transmission or reduce storage capacity; especially useful for radiology, X-ray, MRI, and CT and PET scan images, and broadband transmissions.

COMPRESSION RATIO: The ratio of the number of bits in an original medical image to the number in a compressed version of that image; for example, a compression ratio of 3:1 would signify a compressed image with a third of the number of bits of the original image.

COMPRESSION SOFTWARE: A program that physically reduces the data size of an image or file achieved by deleting like elements of information for the purposes of compression, then restoring those elements upon decompression.

COMPU SERVE©: An early online information server based in Columbus, Ohio; subsidiary of AOL since 1998.

COMPUTED RADIOGRAPHY (CR): A system of creating digital radiographic images that utilizes a storage phosphor plate (instead of film) in a cassette; once the plate is exposed, a laser beam scans it to produce the digital data, which are then translated to an image.

COMPUTER: A machine and related system connection that contains an input/output device, storage capability, arithmetic and logic units, and a control unit, and used to accept, manipulate, and output data. The personal computer (PC) is the most important type of machine introduced by IBM® in 1981 and cloned by Compaq Computer Corporation® in 1983; IBM exited the product line to Lenovo® in 2005; PCs built by Apple Inc., such as the Macintosh (Mac), are graphically intense and usually used by schools, gamers, and artists; most health information technologists and technologies use the IBM-compatible platform (clone); desktop, laptop, notebook, handheld, pen, or PDA; categorized by class, generation, or mode of processing.

COMPUTER ABUSE: Illegal and unethical acts committed with a computer.

COMPUTER-BASED PATIENT RECORD (CBPR): The electronic capture, storage, processing, transmission, presentation, and security functionality of clinical patient medical information; electronic medical records; electronic patient chart.

COMPUTER-BASED PATIENT RECORD INSTITUTE (CBPRI): Nonprofit organization founded in 1992 to promote, focus, evaluate, standardize, and create policy on the use of electronic medical records (EMRs); past chairmen include Dr. Paul C. Tang and Dr. W. Ed Hammond.

COMPUTER CONFERENCING: Communications within groups through computers, or the use of shared computer files, remote terminal equipment, and telecommunications channels for two-way communication.

COMPUTER CRIME: Illegal acts committed with a computer; especially financial; medical fraud and coding abuse.

COMPUTERIZED PHYSICIAN ORDER ENTRY SYSTEMS (CPOES): Automatic medical provider electronic medical chart-ordering system that usually includes seven features:

- *Medication analysis system:* A medication analysis program usually accompanies the order entry system; in such cases, either after order entry or interactively, the system checks for potential problems such as drug–drug interactions, duplicate orders, drug allergies and hypersensitivities, and dosage miscalculations; sophisticated systems may also check for drug interactions with comorbidities (e.g., psychiatric drugs that may increase blood pressure in a depressed patient with hypertension), drug–lab interactions (e.g., labs pointing to renal impairment, which may adversely affect drug levels), and suggestions to use drugs with the same therapeutic effect but lower cost; physicians have the option to decline the alerts and continue with the order; alerts frequently override providers and provide feedback that can lead to modification of the alert paradigms; encouraging feedback increases the robustness of the CPOE system and facilitates continuous quality improvement.
- *Order clarity:* The verification of illegible signatures and orders as well as preventing possible errors in order translation; affirming orders takes professional time, and resources are spent duplicating the data; thus, real cost savings can be realized through the elimination of these processes.
- *Increased work efficiency:* Instantaneous electronic transmittal of orders to radiology, laboratory, pharmacy, consulting services, or other departments replaces corresponding manual tasks.

- *Point of care utilization:* Guidelines that are accessible through hand-held devices or bedside terminals offer the advantage of decision support during the patient encounter; the Institute for Clinical Systems Improvement (ICSI), for example, has guidelines installed on a 3Com™ Palm Pilot® for the purposes of walk-through during or around the time of the patient encounter; for other guidelines, software exists that allows a provider to interactively access guidelines through selection of appropriate pathways on the online decision tree.
- *Benchmarking and performance tracking:* The comparison of input data to evidence-based clinical guidelines allows the possibility of performance analysis compared to norms or benchmarks; rule must not be too rigid because in specific instances it may be appropriate to vary from guideline algorithms.
- *Online alerts:* In similar fashion to medication alerts from CPOE, guideline-based alerts show a medical provider where a clinical decision may conflict with evidence-based guidelines; provider is allowed to override the alert if he or she feels the clinical situation warrants special decision-making.
- *Regulatory reporting:* An increase in guideline compliance can support improvements in regulatory reporting, such as to JCAHO and CMS for acute myocardial infarction and heart failure treatment appropriateness, as an example.

COMPUTER NETWORK: Assemblage of electronically connected computers and peripheral devices to share medical or protected patient health information.

COMPUTER OUTPUT TO MICROFILM: The long term storage of computer files on microfilm, or *microfiche.*

COMPUTER PRIESTHOOD: Electronic machine expert; slang term.

COMPUTER SECURITY: Administrative and user hardware, software, Internet-based, and peripheral procedures used to protect patient medical and private health information.

COMPUTER SECURITY METHODS: Integrity safeguards implemented within health care information technology architecture using the networking, hardware, software, server, and firmware of the technology itself; includes (1) the hardware, firmware, and software that implements security functionality; and (2) the design, implementation, and verification techniques used to ensure that system assurance requirements are satisfied:

- patients, visitors, or employees;
- attempting to obtain another password or security code;

- using or attempting to use another's password or security code or allowing the use of one's code by another;
- unauthorized modification of information or database structure;
- unauthorized access, whether internally or from a remote location;
- unauthorized release of patient information.

COMPUTER TELEPHONY: The union of telephone and computer technologies to place calls within the public system; VOIP.

COMPUTER TRESPASS: Using a computer system without permission.

COMPUTER VIRUS: A software code snippet to control or damage computer information.

CONCENTRATOR: A computing network device that divides electronic data into two or lower bandwidth channels in order to speed transmission; hub and/or router.

CONCEPT VIRUS: Computer system code with no malicious or destructive payload; as in the JAVA StrangeBrew variant of 1998.

CONCURRENT CODING: CPT coding and billing while the patient is still in the hospital.

CONFERENCE: Real-time computer network communications; multiple private or public messages found on a system, usually specific to a particular topic and sometimes moderated by a host who leads the discussion; also called 'Folder,' 'SIG' (Special Interest Group), or 'Echo'; much like the newsgroups on the Internet.

CONFIDENTIAL: The property that health or other information is not made available or disclosed to unauthorized individuals, entities, or processes (ISO 7498–2); to keep medical data and protected health information (PHI) private.

CONFIDENTIAL HEALTH INFORMATION (CHI): Protected Health Information (PHI) that is prohibited from free-use and secured from unauthorized dissemination or use; patient specific medical data.

CONFIDENTIALITY: The health care information technology security objective that generates a requirement for protection from intentional or accidental attempts to perform unauthorized computer, server, or network data-reads; includes data in storage, during processing, and while in transit.

CONFIG.SYS: A DOS and early Windows© computer boot-up file with contents and peripheral attachment information.

CONFIGURATION MANAGEMENT (CM): Historical log of computer or network manipulations such as software and hardware installations, file or program additions or deletions, security changes, vendor numbers and codes, and so forth.

CONFIGURE: All the components that comprise a computer system or network and its peripheral devices.

CONFORMANCE: Dynamic and static option conditions for implementation in a standard.

CONGESTION: An overloaded computer system network, Internet, extranet, intranet, and so forth.

CONNECTIVITY: The potential for a computer, server, peripheral components, or network to establish links and communicate with like configured machines; Internet; wireless medical data transmission connectivity standards include: Bluetooth©, USB, Wi-Fi, Z-Wave©, and ZigBe©; the ability to send and receive information between two locations, devices, or business services.

CONNELLY, PAUL: Chief Information and Security Officer for Hospital Corporation of America (HCA).

CONSENT: A document signed and dated by the individual that a covered entity obtains prior to using or disclosing protected health information to carry out treatment, payment, or health care operations; consent is not required under the HIPAA privacy rule; § 164.506 for uses or disclosures to carry out treatment, payment, or health care operations.

CONSENT REQUIREMENT: A plain language document that will:

- inform individuals and patients that protected health information may be used and disclosed to carry out treatment, payment, or health care operations;
- refer the individual or patient to the notice required by §164.520 for a more complete description of such uses and disclosures and state that the individual has the right to review the notice prior to signing the consent;
- if the covered health care entity has reserved the right to change its privacy practices that are described in the notice in accordance with § 164.520 (b)(1)(v)(C), state that the terms of its notice may change and describe how the individual may obtain a revised notice;
- state that:
  - the individual or patient has a right to request that the covered entity restrict how protected health information is used or disclosed to carry out treatment, payment, or health care operations;
  - the covered entity is not required to agree to requested restrictions; and
  - if the covered entity agrees to a requested restriction, the restriction is binding on the covered entity;
- state that the individual has the right to revoke the consent in writing, except to the extent that the covered entity has taken action in reliance thereon; and
- be signed by the individual or patient and dated.

CONSOLE: Input/output device situated between computer operator and machine; main keyboard.

CONSOLIDATED HEALTH INFORMATICS (CHI): e-Government initiative with the goal of adopting vocabulary and messaging standards to facilitate communication of clinical information across the federal health enterprise.

CONSULTATION REPORT: The formal findings of a participating physician.

CONSULTATIVE COMMITTEE ON INTERNATIONAL TELEPHONE AND TELEGRAPH: Currently, the International Telecommunications Union Consultative Committee for Telecommunications (ITU-T); an international agency responsible for developing standards for telecommunications, as well as FAX and video/audio/imaging coder-decoder (CODEC) devices.

CONSUMER-DRIVEN (DIRECTED) HEALTH PLAN (CDHP): Health care re-insurance plan predicated on high deductibles, low premiums, and patient responsibility.

CONTACT: Electrical connection between surfaces that allows conduction or current flow.

CONTENT PROVIDER: A firm that provides online medical or other information over the Internet; NIH, iMBA, Inc., AOL, MSN, Library of Congress, and so forth.

CONTENT SPOOF: A type of security intrusion to present a faked or modified Web site to the user as if it were legitimate with the intent, typically, to defraud victims or to misrepresent a health or other organization, physician, or individual; trust exploitation between a health care organization and payers, patients, providers, TPAs, and so forth.

CONTENT STANDARD: HIPAA specifications for both data element and coding of secure transmissions.

CONTEXT-BASED ACCESS: An access control based on the context of a health transaction (as opposed to being based on attributes of the initiator or target); the "external" factors might include time of day, location of the user, and strength of user authentication.

CONTIGUOUS: Adjacent or touching; contrast with fragmentation.

CONTINGENCY PLAN: A plan for responding to a health system information technology emergency that includes performing backups, preparing critical facilities that can be used to facilitate continuity of operations in the event of an emergency, and recovering from a disaster; updated regularly.

CONTINUITY OF SIGNATURE CAPABILITY: Rule that the public verification of a signature shall not compromise the ability of the signer to apply additional secure signatures at a later date (ASTM E 1762–95).

CONTINUOUS SPEECH RECOGNITION: The translation of human voice into electronic written language; usually in real-time.

CONTRACT CODER: An interim CPT coder.

CONTROL ACCESS (CA): Authorized administration and clearance for individual computer, server, or network use and security.

CONTROL KEY: An alternate meaning to another activated keyboard computer input key.

CONTROLLED MEDICAL TERMINOLOGY: Health care concepts expressed as a particular lexicon of vocabulary.

CONTROLLER: Electronic circuit board or system to run a peripheral computer device.

CONTROL MENU: Windows© menu used to manipulate various interfaces or operating system features.

CONTROL PANEL: Windows repository for tools and applications, such as add/delete hardware, add/remove programs, display, system, and user accounts.

CONTROL PROGRAM FOR MICROPROCESSORS (CP/M): Older operating system for microprocessors such as the Zilog Z80© computer of the 1970s; predates DOS and created by Gary Kildall of Intergalactic Digital Research©; also the creator of BIOS (Basic Input/Output System); Quick and Dirty Operating System.

CONTROL RESOURCE: Application of an access control computer mechanism for health or other security; control rights.

CONTROL UNIT: Input/output device that directs computer operations, interprets code, and initiates commands to execute functions.

CONVENTIONAL MEMORY: Random Access Memory (RAM) used by MS-DOS© to run real-mode application.

CONVERSATION MODE: Transmission method that requires a computerized response.

CONVERSION: Changes to a source code or computer database; utility that changes file format.

COOKIE: Software information sent from Web sites via Internet browser to a personal computer hard drive for storage; cached information; authorize or unauthorized Web site visit electronic log; slang term; text-file that is stored in a user's browser to retain Web pages, sites, passwords, CCs, and so forth; slang term.

COOKIE FILTER: Software computer utility program that reduces or prevents information relay using cookies.

COOKIE POISONING: The modification of a cookie (personal information in a Web user's computer) by an attacker to gain unauthorized information about the user for purposes such as identity theft; the attacker may use the information to open new accounts or to gain access to the user's existing accounts; slang term.

COPROCESSOR: A designated computer chip, such as a graphics or math coprocessor, to work in conjunction with the main CPU; Xilinx®, and AMD® Torrenza; code name.

COPY: To duplicate and store health data, medical, or other information.

COPY PROTECT: To secure any electronic storage media from unauthorized duplication.

CORBA: An open, vendor-independent architecture and infrastructure that computer applications use to work together over networks.

CORE DUO PROCESSOR: Mobile Intel® CPU with two execution cores optimized for multithreaded applications and multitasking; allows simultaneously running multiple applications such as games, number-crunching programs while downloading music, or running virus-scanning security programs in the background.

COREL® CORPORATION: Company that introduced an early electronic drawing program in 1989, CorelDraw®, based in Ottawa, Ontario, Canada; since acquired the WordPerfect® line business applications and Linux distributor.

CORE MEMORY: Volatile and older data storage mechanism from MIT.

CORRECT CODING INITIATIVE (CCI): Quarterly guidelines for the appropriateness of CPT codes and medical billing combinations for Medicare payment.

CORRECTION: HIPAA data privacy rule allowing the alterations of electronic medical information while not retaining the original.

COTHREN, ROBERT M., PHD: Chief Scientist, Health Solutions Northrop Grumman Corporation.

COUNTERMEASURE: An action, process, device, or system that can prevent, or mitigate the effects of threats to a computer, server, or network and can take the form of software, hardware, and modes of behavior, such as personal and application firewalls, anti-virus software, and pop-up, spy, or ad-ware blockers.

COUNTERSIGNATURE: The ability to prove the order of application of signatures; analogous to the normal business practice of signing a document that has already been signed by another party (ASTM E 1762 -95); part of a digital signature.

COUSINEAU, LEO, MD: Director of Medical Informatics for the Kevric Company, Silver Spring, MD.

COVERED ENTITY (CE): 42 CFR § 164.504(e)(2)(i)(B). Any organization that deals with protected health information (PHI), for example:

- a health care provider submits invoices, or bills, and is paid for health care services and transmits any health information in electronic form;
- an individual or group health plan provides, or pays the cost of medical care. Health plans include group health plans, health maintenance organizations (HMOs), health insurance issuers, Medicare, Medicaid, and governmental health care programs; and

- a health care clearinghouse processes nonstandard data elements of health information into standard elements, receiving data and translating it from one format into another. Billing services, hospitals, clinics, nursing homes physicians, podiatrists, and dentists are other examples of covered entities.

COVERED ENTITY CONTRACT OBLIGATIONS: HIPAA Provisions for Covered Entities to inform Business Associates of privacy practices and restrictions [provisions dependent on business arrangement]:

a. Covered Entity shall notify Business Associate of any limitation(s) in its notice of privacy practices of Covered Entity in accordance with 45 CFR § 164.520, to the extent that such limitation may affect Business Associate's use or disclosure of Protected Health Information.
b. Covered Entity shall notify Business Associate of any changes in, or revocation of, permission by Individual to use or disclose Protected Health Information, to the extent that such changes may affect Business Associate's use or disclosure of Protected Health Information.
c. Covered Entity shall notify Business Associate of any restriction to the use or disclosure of Protected Health Information that Covered Entity has agreed to in accordance with 45 CFR § 164.522, to the extent that such restriction may affect Business Associate's use or disclosure of Protected Health Information.

COVERED ENTITY CONTRACT PERMISSIBLE REQUESTS: Covered Entity shall not request Business Associate to use or disclose Protected Health Information in any manner that would not be permissible under the Privacy Rule if done by Covered Entity. [Include an exception if the Business Associate will use or disclose protected health information for, and the contract includes provisions for, data aggregation or management and administrative activities of Business Associate]: (sample)

Terms and Terminations:
a. Term. The Term of this Agreement shall be effective as of [Insert Effective Date], and shall terminate when all of the Protected Health Information provided by Covered Entity to Business Associate, or created or received by Business Associate on behalf of Covered Entity, is destroyed or returned to Covered Entity, or, if it is infeasible to return or destroy Protected Health Information, protections are extended to such information, in accordance with the termination provisions in this Section. [Term may differ.]

b. Termination for Cause. Upon Covered Entity's knowledge of a material breach by Business Associate, Covered Entity shall either:
   1. Provide an opportunity for Business Associate to cure the breach or end the violation and terminate this Agreement [and the _____ __ Agreement/ sections ____ of the _____ Agreement] if Business Associate does not cure the breach or end the violation within the time specified by Covered Entity;
   2. Immediately terminate this Agreement [and the _____ Agreement/ sections ____ of the _____ Agreement] if Business Associate has breached a material term of this Agreement and cure is not possible; or
   3. If neither termination nor cure is feasible, Covered Entity shall report the violation to the Secretary. [Bracketed language in this provision may be necessary if there is an underlying services agreement. Also, opportunity to cure is permitted, but not required by the Privacy Rule.]
c. Effect of Termination.
   1. Except as provided in paragraph (2) of this section, upon termination of this Agreement, for any reason, Business Associate shall return or destroy all Protected Health Information received from Covered Entity, or created or received by Business Associate on behalf of Covered Entity. This provision shall apply to Protected Health Information that is in the possession of subcontractors or agents of Business Associate. Business Associate shall retain no copies of the Protected Health Information.
   2. In the event that Business Associate determines that returning or destroying the Protected Health Information is infeasible, Business Associate shall provide to Covered Entity notification of the conditions that make return or destruction infeasible. Upon [Insert negotiated terms] that return or destruction of Protected Health Information is infeasible, Business Associate shall extend the protections of this Agreement to such Protected Health Information and limit further uses and disclosures of such Protected Health Information to those purposes that make the return or destruction infeasible, for so long as Business Associate maintains such Protected Health Information.

COVERED ENTITY CONTRACT REQUIREMENTS: According to Section 164.306(a) of the HIPAA security rules, a covered entity must:

- ensure the confidentiality, integrity, and availability of all electronic PHI that it creates, receives, maintains, or transmits;
- protect against any reasonably anticipated threats or hazards to the security or integrity of such information;

- protect against any reasonably anticipated uses or disclosures of such information that are not permitted or required under the privacy rule;
- ensure compliance with the security rule by its workforce.

COVERED FUNCTION: All the processes performed by a covered entity, according to HIPAA; those functions of a covered entity, the performance of which makes the entity a health care plan, health care provider, or health care clearinghouse.

CP/M: Control Program for Microprocessors; a 1980s OS from Digital Research Inc. ® and precursor to DOS.

CRACKER: An unauthorized attempt to access a computer or computer system; hacker; slang term.

CRAPLETT: A small useless JAVA® application program; slang term.

CRASH: Computer operating system or program abrupt inactivity prior to reboot; freeze; slang term.

CRAW(LER): A small computer program that searches for information on the Internet; spider; Web-crawler; bot; robot; slang terms. Crawlers; software used to index the World Wide Web.

CRAY RESEARCH, INC.: Supercomputer maker founded by Seymour Cray in 1977.

CREDIT CARD (CC): Smart card used to immediately access unsecured credit for consumption.

CREEPING FEATURES: The unsystematic and ambiguous improvement of software by adding often unrelated and unintegrated components; slang term.

CRIPPLE WARE: Intentionally incomplete software program distributed as an inducement to purchase the complete and more robust version; slang term.

CRITICAL PATHWAY (CP): Intensive critical care medical, business management, or electronic algorithm; clinical pathway; medical pathway; cookbook medicine.

CROSS MAP: A reference from one term or concept to another, in a different lexicon or space.

CROSS PLATFORM: Functionality across more than one platform, computer, or networked system.

CROSS SITE SCRIPTING (XSS): A security exploit in which the attacker inserts malicious coding into a hyper link that appears from a trustworthy source, but the embedded programming is submitted upon activation as part of the client's Web request allowing the attacker to steal health data or other information.

CROSS-SITE TRACING (XST): A sophisticated form of cross-site scripting that can bypass security countermeasures already put in place to protect against XSS allowing an intruder to obtain health or other secure data using simple client-side script.

CROSS TALK: Adjacent electronic signal data overflow with information and transmission distortion.

CROSS WALK: An electronic data map or database.

CROUNSE, WILLIAM, MD: Global health care industry director for the Microsoft Corporation.

CRUNCH MODE: Working toward an approaching deadline; burning the midnight oil; slang term.

CRYPTOGRAPHIC KEY MANAGEMENT: Security keys and codes administered when protective functions are implemented in various health care electronic services.

CRYPTOGRAPHY: The science and art of keeping health information and other data secret; transforming health information and medical data so that it is secure while transmitted or stored.

CRYPTOLOGY: Any method used to transform intelligible electronic information and transmissions, to an unintelligible format in order to preserve identity and maintain security and prevent unauthorized use.

C SHELL: Interactive UNIX format developed by William Joy, at the University of California, and cofounder of Sun Microsystems.

CTRL+ALT+DEL: Keystroke combination that opens the Windows XP© Task Manager to access its options such as closing, running, switching, and viewing applications.

CUE: Embedded software code that specifies an action.

CURRENT DENTAL TERMINOLOGY™ (CDT): Dental medicine and procedural code set owned by the American Dental Association.

CURRENT DIRECTORY: The default computer system directory; cd in DOS and WINDOWS© or pwd in UNIX.

CURRENT PROCEDURAL TERMINOLOGY™ (CPT): A standardized mechanism of reporting services using numeric codes as established and updated annually; first produced, owned, and copyrighted in 1961 by the American Medical Association; medical diagnosis or procedure descriptor using a five digit CPT code number.

CURRENT PROCEDURAL TERMINOLOGY™ (CPT) MODIFIER: Additional code descriptors used after a five-digit CPT code number to indicate the medical service was altered or extraordinary compared to the standard CPT code description for payment:

- 21: prolonged EM services
- 22: unusual procedure services
- 23: unusual anesthesia
- 24: unrelated EM same physician services done post-operatively
- 25: significant and separate EM services by same-day physician
- 26: professional component

- 27: multiple same-day, outpatient EM encounters
- 32: mandated services
- 47: anesthesia by surgeon
- 50: bilateral procedure
- 51: multiple procedures
- 52: reduced services
- 53: discontinued procedure
- 54: surgical care only
- 55: post-operative management only
- 56: preoperative management only
- 57: decision for surgery
- 58: staged related procedure, same physician, post-operative period
- 59: distinct procedure service
- 62: two surgeons
- 63: procedures on infants less than 4 kg.
- 66: surgical team
- 73: discontinued ASC procedure prior to anesthesia administration
- 74: discontinued ASC procedure after anesthesia administration
- 76: repeat procedure by same physician
- 77: repeat procedure by another physician
- 78: return to OP by same physician during post-operative period
- 79: unrelated procedure, same physician, post-operative period
- 80: assistant surgeon
- 81: minimum assistant surgeon
- 82: assistant surgeon when qualified resident surgeon absent
- 90: reference laboratory
- 91: repeat clinical diagnostic laboratory test
- 99: multiple modifiers

CURSOR: Blinking computer screen icon light or tag for typing input identification; cursor control rate, speed, and control.

CUSEEMEE®: Real-time videoconferencing computer program for Cornell University, Ithaca, NY; video medicine for Windows® PCs and Macs®.

CUT: To highlight and delete a computer text or image.

CUT AND PASTE: To highlight and move a computer text or image from one document to another; copy and paste.

CYBER CAFÉ: A business location where patrons socially browse the Internet.

CYBER CASH: Internet telephony protocol for sending secure cash substitutes over the World Wide Web (WWW); e-money.

CYBER EXTORTION: A form of online criminal activity in which the Web site, e-mail server, or computer infrastructure of an enterprise is subjected repeatedly to denial of service (DOS) attacks who then demand money in return for promising to stop the attacks.

CYBERNETICS: The study of computer information processing in a human-like fashion; cyber life, sex, speak, and so forth.

CYBERNETICS SYSTEM: Automatic internal feedback for medical data, health, or other information; cyber speak.

CYBERPUNK: A malicious online miscreant; cop, dog; slang term.

CYBERSPACE: Term coined by science fiction writer William Gibson in the 1984 book, *Neuromancer*. "A new universe, a parallel universe created and sustained by the world's computers and communication lines. The tablet become a page, become a screen, become a world, a virtual world; A common mental geography, built, in turn, by consensus and revolution, canon and experiment. Its corridors form wherever electricity runs with intelligence. The realm of pure information."

CYBERSPACE SHADOW: Model of a patient or health organization; medical files or PHI.

CYBER SQUATTER: Online copyright, service, and trademark infringement from people seeking profit from pay-per-click advertising.

CYBER TERRORIST(M): Attacks by a terrorist group using computer technology and the Internet to cripple or disable a nation's electronic health care system or infrastructure.

CYBRARIAN: A computer network query database and interactive search engine.

CYBURBIA: The community of computer system users in cyberspace; varying Internet cultures; slang term.

CYCLE: A set of health data or other events that is repeated.

CYCLE BILLING: The time period in which health or other accounts receivable invoices, premiums, or other medical bills are periodically repeated and sent.

CYCLE TIME: Turn around time from start-to-finish of the medical claims cash conversion cycle.

CYLINDER: All tracks that reside in the same location on every computer disk surface; on multiple-platter disks, it is the sum total of every track with the same track number on every surface; on a floppy disk, it is a cylinder comprises the top and corresponding bottom track.

CYRIX CORPORATION®: Founded in 1988 as manufacturer of x86-compatible CPU chips and now involved in health care IT.

D

DAEMON: A UNIX utility program that executes a background operation such as e-mail handling, when required; a program that is "an attendant power or spirit" and sits waiting for requests to come in and then forwards them to other processes as appropriate.

DAISY CHAIN: To connect computer devices in sequence.

DAMAGED RECORD POLICY: Standards, methods, and protocol used to recover damaged electronic or traditional paper-based medical records and/or other private heath data and information.

DANCING BALONEY: Small visually animated images and tiny moving objects that add excitement to an Internet Web page; slang term.

DATA: A series of meaningful electrical signals that may be manipulated, transmitted, and stored; a sequence of symbols to which meaning may be assigned; medical information; plural of *datum*.

DATA ACCESS: The degree to which health care data and medical information is securely made available.

DATA ACCURACY: The extent to which medical information and other health data is current, precise, and correct.

DATA ADMINISTRATOR: One who manages, controls, and modifies a medical or other secure database.

DATA AGGREGATION: Protected or other health information that is created or received by a Business Associate in its capacity as the Business Associate of a covered entity; the combining of such protected health information by the Business Associate with the protected health information received by the Business Associate in its capacity as a Business Associate of another covered entity, to permit data analyses that relate to the health care operations of the respective covered entities.

DATA AUDIT: A process to addresses HIPAA security requirements by preserving historical information and transactional details that would otherwise be overwritten; capture of all insertions, updates, and deletions to health data in real time, enabling physician-executives and office managers to monitor what was changed, who made the change, and when; should also support live, secure data feeds so the audit-trail database is always current, enabling effective querying and reporting.

DATA AUTHENTICATION: The corroboration that information has not been altered or destroyed in an unauthorized manner; examples include the use of a check sum, double keying, a medical message authentication code, or digital signature.

DATA BACK-UP: A retrievable, exact copy of health, medical, or other information; mirror image; the process of copying data to another media and storing it in a secure location.

DATA BACK-UP PLAN: A documented and routinely updated plan to create and maintain, for a specific period of time, retrievable exact copies of health or other information.

DATA BANK: Any electronic server or repository of medical, health, or other information; database.

DATABASE: A computerized storage repository or server for medical or other data, with library-like index for rapid search functionality and retrieval; data bank.

DATABASE ADMINISTRATOR: One who manipulates, secures, and manages a large computerized database for hospitals, HMOs, insurance companies, health systems, or other enterprise-wide conglomeration.

DATABASE LIFE CYCLE (DBLC): The useful life or timeline of medical information or health data.

DATA CACHING: Temporary storage of new health care or other write data or high-demand read data in solid state memory, for the purpose of accelerating performance; after the cached data is written to disk or determined to be of low demand, it is overwritten with newly cached data.

DATA CAPTURE: The process of securely recording health or medical information.

DATA COMMUNICATION: The transfer of information from one computer to another using the OSI standard (ISO #7498) seven decision layers; physical, link, network, transport, session, presentation, and application.

DATA COMPRESSION: To increase computer file storage space with the elimination of redundancy, empty field, gaps, or fragments; stuffit, zip file, Winzip®, pcx utilities, and so forth; any method to reduce sheer volume of health data by more efficient encoding practices, thereby reducing image processing, transmission times, bandwidth requirements, and storage space requirements; some compression techniques result in the loss of some information, which may or may not be clinically important.

DATA CONDITION: An electronic description of certain medical and PHI data and related information.

DATA CONTENT: All the HIPAA elements, privacy, and data code sets inherent to an electronic medical information transmission.

DATA CORRUPTION: The purposeful or accidental destruction of data file integrity.

DATA COUNCIL: Health and Human Service body that is responsible for the ASS provisions of HIPAA.

DATA CUBE: A health or other information scheme in tabular structure used for analysis.

DATA DEFINITION LANGUAGE (DDL): A relationship tabular database of health or medical information used as structured query.

DATA DESCRIPTOR: All the text defining a HIPAA code or code set.

DATA DICTIONARY: Centralized relational database or integrated repository of electronic health data or medical files.

DATA DIDLING: The unauthorized manipulation of computer or network files, programs, or data; slang term.

DATA ELEMENT: The smallest unit of HIPAA protected, approved health, or other information.

DATA ENCRYPTION: Clocking device, software program, or algorithm used to conceal and protect stored transmitted data; especially through the Internet; security measure.

DATA ENCRYPTION STANDARD (DES): An older health or medical data private key cryptology federal protocol for secure information exchange; replaced by AES.

DATA ENTRY: Any method to enter information into a computer system, such as keyboarding, voice, or scanning technology.

DATA EXCHANGE: The transmission of secure electronic health or other information over communication channels, such as the Internet or an intranet.

DATA FIELD: Limited health data or other information-listing area.

DATA FILE: The electronic files used by a computer or on its connected network; a photographic image .jpeg file; a MSFT WORD© file with .doc extension, and so forth.

DATA GRANULARITY: The degree of health, medical, or other information detail and specificity.

DATA INDEPENDENCE: Static application program that allows physical or logical architectural structural changes.

DATA INTEGRITY: Secured health data protected from malicious mischief that has not been altered in an unauthorized manner; covers data in storage, during processing, and while in transit; the property that information has not been altered or destroyed in an unauthorized manner (ASTM E1762–95); precision; correctness; accuracy and timeliness.

DATA INTERCHANGE STANDARD (DIS): X12 HIPAA health data transmission standard format.

DATA INTERCHANGE STANDARD ASSOCIATION (DISA): The organization that provides X12 HIPAA transmission standards and formats.

DATA LEAKAGE: Minute and almost undetectable amounts of computer file storage or program loss.

DATA LINK: The union of two or more pieces of separately recorded electronic health care information.

DATA LINK LAYERS: The ISO/OSI reference model or seven tiered standard for computer network communications: application, presentation, session, transport, network, data, and physical.

DATA MANAGEMENT: Usually a large subsector of a major database management system.

DATA MAP: The integration and matching of one set of health data codes to another set of codes; cross-walking.

DATA MARK: Data base warehouse derivation focused on a single topic; medical or other information database that is user-friendly.

DATA MIGRATION: Ability to transfer health, medical, or other data from a legacy big-iron and enterprise wide computer system to PCs or linked networks.

DATA MINING: The electronic analysis of large databases in search of cohort commonalities, patterns, and useful trends; medical data and health status outcome-analysis algorithms.

DATA MODEL: The electronic storage, architecture, or format required to assist a medical, health care, or other business entity.

DATA ORIGINATOR: One who generates medical, health, or other information; patient, provider, payer, CE, or health care facility.

DATA ORIGINATOR AUTHENTICATION: Verification of health care or electronic medical or other information for security purposes.

DATA ORIGIN AUTHENTICATION: The verification that the source of electronic data received is as claimed.

DATA OVERFLOW: Internal computer file offset time delay.

DATA PROJECT MANAGER (DPM): One responsible for health data for a predetermined period, with the following general security responsibilities:

a. Secure Areas: The clinical workstation, mobile, or stationary is accessed by authorized personnel only. Access is normally controlled using a network-operating system generated password. The password should be changed at given intervals. Some organizations use biometric devices, such as retinal scanners for authentication.

b. Equipment Security: A system of inventory and maintenance is used for all IT equipment, including warranties and maintenance contracts. Servers and mainframes are normally installed and maintained in secure cooled environments.

c. General Controls: In order to prevent unauthorized access, damage, and interference to business premises and information, the following measures should be put in place:

   • Provide all personnel with security training;
   • Require personnel to report access to a particular area of the health care system by anyone who does not have authorized access;
   • Document security policies and procedures;
   • Secure workstations and personnel security mechanisms to prevent loss, damage, or compromise of assets and interruption to business activities and to prevent compromise or theft of information and information-processing facilities;

- Require IT staff to keep a secure tracking of personnel equipment inventories and secure the workstations so that unauthorized duplication of information is not possible.

DATA RATE: Baud information transfer speed.

DATA RECOVERY: Restoration of physically damaged or corrupt health care or other data on a computer disk or tape; older disks and tapes can become corrupted due to hardware failure, bad software, and viruses, as well as from power failures that occur while the magnetic media is being written.

DATA REPOSITORY: The portion of any information system that accepts, files, and stores medical data and other information from various sources.

DATA RETRIEVAL: The extraction or accessibility of protected health care storage information.

DATA SECURITY: The authentication and access management control process used to protect health care information.

DATA SET: Medical, health, or other information elements suitable for a specific use.

DATA STORAGE: The retention of health care information pertaining to an individual in an electronic format.

DATA STREAM: The undifferentiated flow of medical, health, or other information across a computer network.

DATA SUBJECT: Patient whose protected electronic health information is stored, manipulated, transmitted, or retrieved.

DATA TAG: A formatted word in JAVA® scripting code that electronically transmits Web site page scripting information through query string standards.

DATA TERMINAL READY (DTR): Modem access availability to an incoming electronic transmission.

DATA USER: One with an authentic and secure need to use, store, alter, or retrieve protected electronic health, medical, or other information.

DATA VALIDATION: Any method to determine the accuracy and completeness of health or other data using checksum and check digits tests, key tests, format tests, and so forth.

DATA WAREHOUSE: A database, repository, data bank, or data mart.

DATUM: Any single medical, health, or other fact or bit of information.

DAUGHTER BOARD: A board within another circuit board; additional memory, accelerator card, and so forth; motherboard.

DBASE: Ashton-Tate® database that allowed custom built programmable solutions.

DBI: Logarithmic ratio to measure radio antenna gain relative to isotropic antenna gain.

DBM: Logarithmic ratio used to measure power levels relative to one milliwatt unit.

D-CODE: Electronic code set for dental procedures.

DEAD BOLT LOCK: A lock that extends a solid metal bar into the door frame for extra security.

DEAD LINK: A broken or nonfunctional HTML Web page address.

DEAD LOCK CONDITION: The stalemate that occurs when two elements in an electronic process are each waiting for the other to respond; for example, in a health network, if one doctor is working on file A and needs file B to continue, but another doctor is working on file B and needs file A to continue, each one waits for the other, both are temporarily locked-out.

DEADLY EMBRACE: The impasse that occurs when two data elements are each waiting for the other to respond and are temporarily locked out.

DEADSPOT: Geographic area void of cell phone, wi-fi, or other mobility signals; slang term.

DEAD START: To cold boot-up a computer system.

DEBAYER: To decode a computer image to a full color one.

DEBIT CARD: Smart bank card used to immediately draw cash from a secured checking or other current account; electronic check.

DEBRANTES, FRANÇOIS: National Health Coordinator for Bridges to Excellence.

DEBUG: To remove unwanted, erroneous, or broken coding errors from a software program; slang term.

DECAY: To reduce signal or electronic charge strength.

DECIBEL: Unit of loudness or signal strength measure (dB); 1/10 of a bell; Alexander Graham Bell.

DECISION-SUPPORT SYSTEM (DSS): Computer tools or applications to assist physicians in clinical decisions by providing evidence-based knowledge in the context of patient-specific data; examples include drug interaction alerts at the time medication is prescribed and reminders for specific guideline-based interventions during the care of patients with chronic disease; information should be presented in a patient-centric view of individual care and also in a population or aggregate view to support population management and quality improvement.

DECISION TREE: Hierarchical treatment or other algorithm or knowledge-based selection choice system; medical or electronic decision support system.

DECODE: The conversion of coded data or information back to its original form.

DECOMPRESS: To restore compressed data or information back to its original size; lossy.

DECRYPTION: To decode a secure or encrypted message, data, file, or program; opposite of encryption; changing an encrypted message back to its original form.

DEDICATED LINE: Always available, always-on, telephone line, data line, or data port, and so forth; a permanent telephone line reserved exclusively for one patient, accessible all hours of the day; usually offers better quality than standard telephone lines, but may not significantly augment the performance of data communications; a leased or private line.

DEDICATED SERVER: Computer used only as a network system server.

DE FACTO: A standard or widely used format or language.

DEFAULT: Basic computer selection choice without manual intervention.

DEFAULT DRIVE: A nonspecified computer disk drive.

DEFAULT ROUTE: Alternate network address for unlisted data packets.

DEFENSE-IN-DEPTH: Multilayered security countermeasures that provide several lines or hurdles of defense.

DEFINITION FILES: Files that contain updated antivirus information.

DEFORD, DREXEL: Former MS-HUG Past-Chairman and VP/CIO, Scripps Health Care Systems.

DEFRAG(GER): A computer software utility program that removes ambient data from a hard or floppy disk, or other storage device.

DEFRAG(MENT)(ATION): To reorganize the files of a computer disk into contiguous order, because the operating system stores new data in whatever free space is available and data files become scattered across the disk as they are updated; this causes the read/write head to move around all over the disk to read back the data; a defragmented disk can speed up back-up procedures and facilitate restoration of backed-up files.

DEGAUSS: The removal of potentially damaging magnetic fields from a computer system, file, or storage unit; gauss is a unit of measure for magnetic strength; Carl Friedrich Gauss.

DE-IDENTIFIED HEALTH INFORMATION: Protected health information that is no longer individually identifiable health information; a covered entity may determine that health information is not individually identifiable health information only if: (1) a person with appropriate knowledge of and experience with generally accepted statistical and scientific principles and methods for rendering information not individually identifiable determines that the risk is very small that the information could be used, alone or in combination with other available information, to identify an individual, and documents the methods and results of the analysis; or (2) the following identifiers of the individual, relatives, employers, or household members of the individual are removed:

1. Name;
2. Street address, city, county, precinct, zip code, and equivalent geocodes;

3. All elements of dates (except year) for dates directly related to an individual and all ages over 89;
4. Telephone number;
5. Fax number;
6. Electronic mail address;
7. Social Security number;
8. Medical record numbers;
9. Health plan ID numbers;
10. Account numbers;
11. Certificate/license numbers;
12. Vehicle identifiers and serial numbers, including license plate numbers;
13. Device identifiers and serial numbers;
14. Web addresses (URLs);
15. Internet IP addresses;
16. Biometric identifiers, including finger and voice prints;
17. Full face photographic images and any comparable images; and
18. Any other unique identifying number, characteristic, or code.

DE-IDENTIFY: To remove specific identity descriptors from health or other information; blind.

DEJANEWS©: A Usenet news-group search engine; Google© group.

DE JOUR: A standards organization for computer languages or file formats.

DEL: Computer keyboard delete button.

DELAY: Time lag between input and the appearance of selected data or output figures.

DELBANCO, SUZANNE, PHD: CEO, Leapfrog Group.

DELETE: To remove, erase, over-write, or destroy a computer file.

DELIBERATE THREAT: Potential willful and malicious security intrusion of a computer, server, or network.

DELIMITER: The beginning and end of a computer program or application.

DELINQUENT HEALTH RECORD: An incomplete health file or medical data chart.

DELL COMPUTER CORPORATION®: A leading direct manufacturer of personal computers with large health care division founded in 1984 by Michael Dell of Austin, TX.

DELPI©: PASCAL-like object orientated computer language.

DELURK: To remove a chat room visitor who reads and watches conversations without input or conversation.

DEMODULATION: Analog to digital conversion with a modem or similar unit; reverse of modulation.

DEMON DIALER: Automated phone or computer system that attempts a blast phone connection or wireless connection with multiple receiving devices; cell phones, PDAs, and so forth; war dialer usually for advertising purposes.

DENIAL OF SERVICE (DOS): The prevention of authorized access to resources or the delaying of time-critical operations; the first mass distributed DoS attack hit Amazon®, eBay®, Microsoft®, and Yahoo® in 2000.

DENIAL OF SERVICE ATTACK (DOSA): Purposeful computer network non-availability usually due to simultaneously shared resource overload; wireless bogus content flood in a wired computer network.

DENTAL CONTENT COMMITTEE: ADA committee responsibly for dental billing codes, sets, and administrative standards.

DENTAL INFORMATICS: The access, management, storage, and secure retrieval of dental information.

DEPARTMENT OF HEALTH AND HUMAN SERVICES (HHS): The federal government department that has overall responsibility for implementing HIPAA.

DERIVATIVE: Reused information at the computer system application level.

DESCRIPTION: 45 CFR 162.103 Text that defines a code set.

DESCRIPTIVE STATISTICS: Mathematic data presentation in the form of visual impressions and verbal descriptions.

DESCRIPTOR: The text defining a code in a code set; 45 CFR 162.103.

DESELECT: Computer command to work with another object.

DESIGNATED CODE SET: A medical code or administrative code set designated by HHS for use in one or more of the HIPAA standards.

DESIGNATED CONTENT COMMITTEE (DCC): An organization designated by HHS for oversight of the business data content of one or more of the HIPAA-mandated transaction standards.

DESIGNATED RECORD SET: Contains medical and billing records and any other records that a physician or medical practice utilizes for making decisions about a patient; a hospital, emerging health care organization, or other health care organization is to define which set of information comprises "protected health information" and which set does not. The patient has the right to know who in the lengthy data chain has seen their PHI. This sets up an audit challenge for the medical organization, especially if the accountability is programmed, and other examiners view the document without cause.

DESIGNATED STANDARD: HIPAA standard as assigned by the department of HHS.

DESKTOP: Computer used on or under a desk or other surface with rectangular base or tower model; usually only the monitor, keyboard, printer, and mouse are placed on the user's desk.

DESKTOP PUBLISHING: Computer programs and applications used to create documents, tables, graphs, and page layouts for electronic and print publishing; MSFT Publisher©, Adobe Indesign©, Serif Page Plus© PageMaker©, and QuarkXPress©, and so forth.

DESTINATION DISK: Computer source file used to copy onto another disk; floppy.

DESTRUCTION DUE TO DISASTER: A covered entity or hospital's attempt to safeguard health information records and other documents in structurally safe, fire-resistant, and water-resistant storage environments; general safeguarding will ensure that combustible and hazardous chemicals and materials are maintained in a supervised environment with minimal risk for damage to hospital property; at all times, the CE and hospital will meet building and fire codes and OSHA guidelines:

- *Flooding/Water Damage:* Health records are maintained in permanent storage in shelves raised from the floor to prevent flooding and water damage; should flooding or water damage occur, every attempt is to be made to remove health records from the area with removal beginning on the lower shelves first, working upwards; if records cannot be removed prior to water damage, the health information management specialist and the administrative team will meet to determine what recovery mechanisms are feasible based on age and type of records, insurance coverage, costs, long-term damage, and so forth; if salvage operations are recommended, the health information management specialist will contact a reputable salvage vendor (AHIMA recommendation).
- *Fire and Other Damage:* If records cannot be removed prior to fire or other damage, the health information management specialist and the administrative team will meet to determine what recovery mechanisms are feasible based on age and type of records, insurance coverage, costs, long-term damage, and so forth; if salvage operations are recommended, the health information management specialist will contact a reputable salvage vendor (AHIMA recommendation).

DESTRUCTIVE MEMORY: Computer recollection that loses content after being read.

DETECT AND CONTAIN: The ability to notice and respond to an IT security breach as an essential portion of an effective health information technology security capability; achieved by incorporating detection, analysis, and response components into the organization's intranet, as illustrated in Figure 2.

DETMER, DONALD E., MD: Professor of Surgery and Business Administration and Vice President for Health Information Sciences, University of Virginia, Charlottesville.

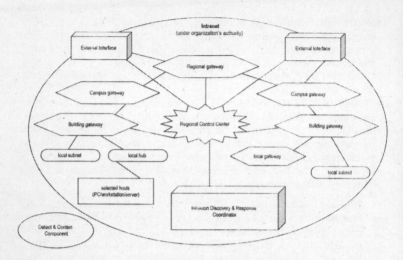

Figure 2: Health care IT security detection and containment.

/DEV: UNIX directory device link.

DEVICE: Any input/output computer system peripheral component.

DEVICE DRIVER: A software program that controls a peripheral computer device through the operating system.

DEVICE ID: Unique name given to computer hardware under plug-n-play architecture.

DEVICE LOCK: A steel cable and a lock used to secure a notebook computer.

DEVICE MANAGER: OS feature to view and alter software properties attached to a computer and related devices.

DEWEY, FORBES C., PHD: Director, Massachusetts Institute of Technology, Cambridge, MA.

DHHS RULE: Attempt to define medical data and PHI security standards as a set of scalable, technology-neutral requirements with implementation features that covered entities, providers, plans, and clearinghouses would have to include in their operations to ensure that electronically maintained or electronically transmitted health information pertaining to an individual patient remains safeguarded.

**DIAGNOSIS AND STATISTICAL MANUAL OF MENTAL DISORDERS, 4TH ED., REV.
(DSM-IV-R):** American Psychiatric Association manual of diagnostic criteria and terminology.

DIAGNOSIS (DIAGNOSTIC) CODE: The first ICD-9-CM diagnosis code describes the principal diagnosis; remaining codes are the ICD-9-CM diagnosis codes corresponding to additional conditions that coexisted at the time of hospital admission, or developed subsequently, and which had an effect on the treatment received or the length of stay.

DIAGNOSIS (DIAGNOSTIC) CREEP: Increased medical acuity coding of an illness, disease, injury, or treatment in order to increase reimbursement in a fee-for-service system; diagnostic upgrading; slang term.

DIAGNOSIS RELATED GROUPS (DRGS): (1) System of classifying patients on the basis of diagnoses for purposes of payment to hospitals. (2) A system for determining case mix, used for payment under Medicare's prospective payment system (PPS) and by some other payers; the DRG system classifies patients into groups based on the principal diagnosis, type of surgical procedure, presence or absence of significant co morbidities or complications, and other relevant criteria; DRGs are intended to categorize patients into groups that are clinically meaningful and homogeneous with respect to resource use; Medicare's PPS currently uses almost 500 mutually exclusive DRGs, each of which is assigned a relative weight that compares its costliness to the average for all DRGs.

DIAGNOSTIC: Software algorithm that tests hardware and peripheral computer components.

DIAGNOSTIC PROTOCOL: Medical pathways, algorithms, or diagnosis and treatment recommendations; cookbook medicine.

DIALOG BOX: Computer screen pop-up box that requests an input action.

DIALUP CONNECTION: Modem facilitated Internet or computer system connection through POTS; wired slow phone company Internet access; dialup access, loader, box, and so forth.

DIALUP LINE: A two-way cable used in traditional telephone networks.

DIALUP NETWORK: Process that allows a computer to be connected to a network or the Internet via a Web browser using a telephone dialup modem and land phone line.

DIAMOND, CAROL, MD: Chairman of the New York-based organization Connecting for Health.

DICHOTOMOUS DATA: Nominal health, medical, or other information units.

DIFFERENTIAL BINARY PHASE SHIFT KEYING (DBFSK): Wi-Fi modulation transmission technique.

DIFFIE, HELMAN: Public key data encryption method, protocol; VOIP security system standard.

DIFFIE, WHITFIELD, PHD: VP, Fellow, and CSO of Sun Microsystems, Inc.®, who discovered the concept of public key cryptography in 1975, now used in health data transmissions. He is a fellow of the Marconi Foundation and is recipient of awards from the IEEE, The Electronic Frontiers Foundation, NIST, NSA, the Franklin Institute, and ACM.

DIGERATI: Those knowledgeable about computers, software, hardware, peripheral components, and networks; digital elite; plural; slang term.

DIGG: An Internet news aggregator and medical–social bookmarking Web site.

DIGISPEAK: Online communications using acronyms for common phrases.

DIGIT: A single character numbering or binary system.

DIGITAL: Electronic and binary coded data; digital camera, computer, certificate, display, divide, fingerprint, modem, photography, recording, video, signature, standard speech, disk, mark, and so forth; technology that allows communications signals to be compressed for transmissions that are more efficient.

DIGITAL CAMCORDER: A digital camera/video-recorder.

DIGITAL CAMERA: Charged-Couple Device (CCD) with similar photographic/fax scanning technology; with ADC and DSP (Digital Signal Processor) capability, flash storage, and optical/digital zoom and focus features; no film camera; an image producing lens system made up of one or more light-sensitive integrated circuits, a myriad of light-sensitive elements, and circuits for timing, nonlinear amplification, and encoding color.

DIGITAL CERTIFICATE: An electronic ID card used in the RSA public key encryption health care system; X.509v3 or higher.

DIGITAL CONVERGENCE: The integration and use of computer communications, physicians, and patients.

DIGITAL DATA SYSTEM (DDS): A system for transmitting telephone traffic in digital format between major switching hubs that allows digital transmission of voice and data as a component of the analog plain old telephone system (POTS).

DIGITAL DICTATION: Vocal analog conversion to digital form, usually in real-time.

DIGITAL ENVELOPE: An encrypted message that uses public and private key methods.

DIGITAL EQUIPMENT CORPORATION® (DEC): Company later acquired by Compaq® in 1998, and then HP that produced the PDP8–11 computer line, VAX minicomputers, and Alpha microprocessors; founded by Ken Olson in 1956.

DIGITAL EXCHANGE (DAX): A computerized digital cross connection that permits specific channels from high-capacity lines to split out separately so that they may be directed elsewhere.

DIGITAL FILM: A memory card for an electronic camera; replacement for traditional camera film.

DIGITAL IMAGE: An image formed by independent pixels, each of which is characterized by a digitally represented luminance level; for example, a popular screen size for digital images was a 1024 by 1024 matrix of pixels x 8 bits, representing 256 luminance levels.

DIGITAL IMAGING AND COMMUNICATIONS IN MEDICINE (DICOM): Radiology broadband transmission imaging standards for X-rays, MRIs, CT, and PET scans, and so forth; health IT standard transmissions platform aimed at enabling different computing platforms to share image data without compatibility problems; a set of protocols describing how radiology images are identified and formatted that are vendor-independent and developed by the American College of Radiology and the National Electronic Manufacturers Association. The standard emphasizes point-to-point connection of digital medical imaging devices; DICOM 3.0 is the current version.

DIGITAL MEDIA HUB: A device that receives multimedia content streamed from a computer to a stereo or home theater system; usually residing in the same cabinet as the A/V equipment, it plugs into the A/V inputs of the receiver and connects to the home network via wired or wireless Ethernet; popular for audio collections, allowing files in MP3, AAC, and other formats to be organized on the computer using full-featured jukebox/player software such as iTunes® and WinAmp®.

DIGITAL RADIOLOGY: Medical digital imaging applied to X-rays, CT, PET scans, and related noninvasive and invasive technology; broadband intensive imaging telemedicine.

DIGITAL RESEARCH, INC. (DRI): Software company founded in 1976 by Gary Kildall to produce its CP/M computer operating system; a precursor of MS-DOS© and Windows©.

DIGITAL RIGHTS MANAGEMENT (DRM): The control and protection of digital intellectual, medical, health data, and related property.

DIGITAL SIGNAL: Discrete transmission of on/off electronic values; opposite of analog waves; public and private keys; an electrical signal in the form of discrete voltage pulses that transmit audio, video, and data as bits, which are either on or off, differing from analog signals, which are continuously varying; communications signals may be compressed using technology, allowing efficient and reliable transmission rotes.

DIGITAL SIGNATURE: Encrypted electronic authorization with verification and security protection; private and public key infrastructure; based upon cryptographic methods of originator authentication, computed by using a set of rules and a set of parameters so that the identity of the signer and the integrity of medical or other data can be verified.

DIGITAL SIGNATURE STANDARD (DSS): Encryption technology to ensure electronic medical data transmission integrity and authentication of both sender and receiver; date and time stamps; public and private key infrastructure.

DIGITAL SUBSCRIBER LINE (DSL): High-speed Internet connection.

DIGITAL TELECOMMUNICATIONS CHANNEL: Capable of transmitting high volume voice, data, or compressed video signals. DS1 and DS3 are also known as T1 and T3 carriers; early transmission rates were 64 Kbps for DS0, 1.544 Mbps for DS1, and 45 Mbps for DS3.

DIGITAL VERSATILE DISK (DVD): A technology that permits large amounts of data to be stored on an optical disk.

DIGITAL VERSATILE DISK—RECORDABLE (DVD-R): An optical disc technology that can record once up to 3.95 gigabytes of data on a single-sided disk and 7.9 GB on a double-sided disk.

DIGITAL VERSATILE DISK—REWRITEABLE (DVD-RAM): An optical disk technology that can record, erase, and rerecord data and has a capacity of 2.6 GB (single side) or 5.2 GB (double side).

DIGITAL VERSATILE DISK—REWRITEABLE (DVD+RW; DVD-RW): An optical disk technology that allows data to be recorded, erased, and re-recorded.

DIGITAL VIDEO DISK (DVD): Optical reader with writers exceeding X-48 speeds.

DIGITAL WATERMARK: Permanent and imperceptible images embedded into works by copyright owners.

DIGITIZE: To convert an electronic wave signal from analog to on/off values; the process by which analog, or continuous, information is transformed into digital, or discrete, information; because most computers are only capable of processing digital information and visual information is inherently in analog format, this process is essential in computer imaging applications.

DIJANGO: Open source Web application derivative language of the Python computer language; used to build Web applications with less code work.

DIMMED: A computer function that is not available for use.

DIP SWITCH: Dual-in-line package alternatives used to configure computer or networked hardware options.

DIRECT ACCESS: Data storage entry that is independent of physical computer locations.

DIRECT BROADCAST SATELLITE (DBS): A satellite designed with adequate power so that inexpensive earth stations, or downlinks, may by used for direct residential, health organization, or business reception.

DIRECT CAPTURE: A procedure by which medical image data are formed directly from the original source allowing a high quality image reproduction; images created from image files are identical to the original, regardless of the device used to capture them, such as a CT, PET scan, or an MRI.

DIRECT DATA ENTRY (DDE): The instantaneous and real time input of PHI from one computer source to another.

DIRECT DIGITAL IMAGING: Involves the capture of digital medical images so that they can be electronically transmitted for telemedicine purposes.

DIRECT MEMORY ACCESS (DMA): System that can control computer memory without using the Central Processing Unit (CPU).

DIRECT MEMORY ACCESS CONTROLLER: Independent system switch that can control computer memory without using the Central Processing Unit (CPU); enhancing speed.

DIRECTORY: A hard disk or electronic folder device for computer file name storage; an Internet search engine that organizes indices and topics.

DIRECTORY REPLICATION: To copy or mirror a set of master data directories; from export server to input server.

DIRECTORY WINDOW: The File Manager screen in Windows©.

DIRECT TREATMENT RELATIONSHIP: Synergy between an individual and a health care provider that is not an indirect treatment relationship.

DIRECT-X®: Windows multimedia application program interface that enables developers to access hardware without additional software specific code; optional sound and animation add-on functionality for Windows® multimedia presentations.

DISASTER PLAN: Various back-up methods used to recover lost data, or stay live and online in the event of system or network failure, regardless of source.

DISASTER RECOVERY: Outlines procedures for recovering any loss of health data in the event of fire, vandalism, natural disaster, or system failure.

DISASTER RECOVERY PLAN: A process to restore vital health and critical health care technology systems in the event of a medical practice, clinic, hospital, or health care business interruption from human, technical, or natural causes; focuses mainly on technology systems, encompassing critical hardware, operating and application software, and any tertiary elements required to support the operating environment; must support the process requirements to restore vital company data inside the defined business requirements; does not take into consideration the overall operating environment; an emergency mode operation plan is still necessary.

DISCLOSURE: Release of PHI outside a covered entity or business agreement space, under HIPAA; the release, transfer, provision of access to, or divulging of medical information outside the entity holding the information.

DISCLOSURE HISTORY: The methods in which CEs and BAs have dealt with PHI in the past.

DISCRETE SPEECH: Spoken language with pauses between words used for computer speech recognition software programs.

DISCRETIONARY ACCESS CONTROL (DAC): Limits computer or network access by restricting a subject's access to an object; generally used to limit a user's access to a file as it is the owner of the file who controls other users' accesses to the file.

DISH: An antenna shaped like a parabola that is the essential component of a satellite earth station, or downlink.

DISINFECTANT: A utility program that quickly erases all traces of how a computer system was used; removes user's tracks and e-fingerprints, sites visited, cookies, and so forth.

DISK: Fast rotating device, usually magnetic, used for the storage of electronic information, files, programs; floppy disk, hard disk, optical disk, Zip-disk, disk copy, crash, directory, farm, interface, jacket, memory, unit, and so forth.

DISK ARRAY: A computer optimized to be a single-purpose storage appliance that can hold 30–50 terabytes, or more, of health information spread over multiple large-capacity hard drives and all managed by a powerful central processing unit.

DISK BURN(ING): CDs optical storage method supported by Windows XP©; not DVDs.

DISK DEFRAGMENTER: A computer software utility program that removes ambient data from a hard or floppy disk, or other storage device and enhances performance and speed.

DISK DRIVE: The motor that rotates a data storage hard drive, as well as the read/write heads and all related mechanisms.

DISK DUPLEXING: Fault tolerant and redundant safe-guard storage device on two hard drives with separate channels and controls for security and safety; speedy.

DISKETTE: Magnetic electronic data memory and circular storage device (floppy) that is small, flexible, and transferable; first introduced in 1971 by Alan Shugart of IBM; sizes vary:

- 8.00 inch: A read-only format, which later became a read-write format.
- 5.25 inch: Common size for pre-1987 PCs, typically 360 K and 1.2 MB.
- 3.50 inch: Larger storage capacity than predecessors, from 400 K to 1.4 MB of data; most common sizes for PCs were 720 K DD and 1.44 MB HD; Macintosh supported disks of 400 K, 800 K, and 1.2 MB.

DISK FARM: A storage room full of computer disks.

DISK FORMAT: Data organization scheme on a floppy, hard, optical, flash, or other drive.

DISK FRAGMENT: A piece of a file written to a hard drive often in multiple fragments because there is no contiguous space available large enough to store the file.

DISK FRAGMENTATION: A condition where data is stored in noncontiguous areas on disk; as files are updated, new data are stored in available free space, which may or may not be contiguous; fragmented files cause extra head movement, which slows disk accesses; a defragmenter program such as Diskeeper® is used to rewrite and reorder the files.

DISK HEAD (READ/WRITE HEAD): A device that reads (senses) and writes (records) data on a magnetic disk (hard disk or floppy disk) or tape by discharging electrical impulses recorded as tiny magnetized spots of positive or negative polarity; when reading, the surface is moved past the read/write head, and the bits that are present induce an electrical current across the gap.

DISK INTENSIVE: Characterizing a process that requires reading from and writing to a computer disk.

DISKLESS PC: Computer terminal void of hard-drive functionality and used as an alternative to traditional thin client servers and blades; hybrid.

DISK MIRRORING: Fault tolerant storage technique that automatically or independently saves and copies vital electronic data on two physical disk drives on the same channel, for more security and safety than found in disk duplexing methods; copy.

DISK OPERATING SYSTEM (DOS): A series of IBM compatible programs that control computer and related components; operating system.

DISK PACK: Circular magnetic surfaces for electronic medical information, heath data, or other file storage.

DISK STRIP: Fault tolerant security storage technique that distributes data with-parity (AID 5) or nonparity (RAID 0) across three or more, or two physical disks, respectively.

DISK TRACK: The storage channel on a computer disk or tape; on magnetic disks (hard disks, floppy disks, and so forth) tracks are concentric (having a common center) circles.

DISK VOLUME: A physical storage unit, such as a hard disk, floppy disk, CD-ROM, and so forth.

DISPLAY CODES: User set parameters for the display of electronic search classification sets.

DISPOSABLE SMART CARD: Plastic card with magnetic strip holding a predetermined amount of electronic money storage and used as cash for transactions; for example, a $25 cell phone card.

DISPOSAL: The final disposition of health or other electronic data, or the hardware on which electronic data is stored.

DISTANCE LEARNING: Obtaining online distance education from a remote teaching site; usually but not always live and asynchronous, but absent a united physical location (www.CertifiedMedicalPlanner.com and www.HealthDictionarySeries.com).

DISTRIBUTED COMPUTER ENVIRONMENT (DCE): Independent client server platform with separate operating system and network that is geographically dispersed but connected by a wide area network (WAN), or local area network (LAN).

DISTRIBUTED COMPUTING: A web of many computer users connected to a specialized medical system, programs, or applications, usually with broadband connectivity.

DISTRIBUTED DATABASE: Database protected and stored in more than one physical location ad server; databank implemented on a computer system server.

DISTRIBUTED DENIAL OF SERVICE ATTACK (DDOSA): Occurs when hundreds of computer systems attempt to simultaneously connect with a network, denying access to legitimate users.

DISTRIBUTED INTELLIGENCE: A database, medical, or other databank distributed among several computer system servers used to function as part of a larger enterprise-wide clinical decision support system; medical specialty specific; distributed network; distributed process or list; distributed health workplace or medical group.

DISTRIBUTED INTRANET: A health organization's intranet typically dispersed physically and interconnected by circuits that are frequently not controlled by the medical organization, or HIPAA covered entity, as illustrated in Figure 3.

DISTRIBUTED PROCESSING: Multiple-linked computer servers using a WAN or LAN architecture.

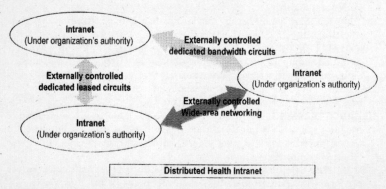

Figure 3: Distributed health intranet.

DISTRIBUTED SECURITY SERVICES: Health care organization schematic or cognitive understanding of how medical data services rest upon other services as they are logically and physically distributed across a computer network; such services depend on operating system assurance as a key element surrounding the entire enterprise; a coordinated management approach by IT team, CIO, database administrator, network administrator, and all hardware and software engineers and applications that integrate the area (Figure 4).

DISTRO: A ready-to-use version of a complicated software program or sophisticated computer application; slang term.

DITHER: The use of a color pallet outside of the standard 216 browser safe selection; slang term.

DO: The execution keyword in the C computer programming language.

DOARN, CHARLES R., MD: Associate Professor of Bioengineering and Executive Director for the Center of Surgical Innovation, University of Cincinnati, OH; co-Editor-in-Chief of *Telemedicine and e-Health* journal.

DOCK: To move subordinate computer programs to a new viewing window; MAC OS X® feature that keeps track of frequently used programs, applications, or files; to connect a mobile or laptop computer to a base station.

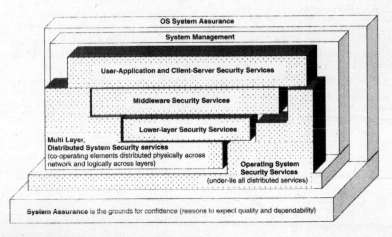

Figure 4: Distributed health security services.

DOCKING STATION: Laptop accessory used at a fixed location to charge a battery, connect to a larger monitor screen, or access a network or other peripheral devices, and so forth.

DOCTOR: A simulated computerized psychotherapy program version of ELIZA bundled into an eMacs® editor.

DOCUMENT: A created computer file that can be modified, stored, transmitted, and so forth.

DOCUMENTATION: Written security plans, rules, procedures, and instructions concerning all components of an entity's security.

DOCUMENT EXCHANGE SOFTWARE: Software program that allows a file to be viewed by those without the original creation application.

DOCUMENT IMAGING: The online storage, retrieval, and manipulation of electronic photographs such as those used in radiology.

DO-GOODER: A computer worm, trojan, or virus that is released on a network in order to find security flaws, exploits, or access points in order to fix, patch, or seal them; slang term.

DOMAIN: A collection of networked computers and servers that share a common communications address; the last two parts of an e-mail address or URL signifying an organizations name on the Internet; for example, 'aol. com' refers to America On Line.

DOMAIN ADDRESS: Internet address in readable form.

DOMAIN CONTROLLER: Authentication management device for Windows-NT© servers and workstations.

DOMAIN HIJACK: To register a domain name for resale; hoard or poach.

DOMAIN HOARD: To register multiple unused domain names for resale; hijack or poach.

DOMAIN NAME (ADDRESS): Exact TCP/IP network name for an electronic or computing device connected to the Internet; system of IP addresses developed in 1984.

DOMAIN NAME (COUNTRY): Any country Web address format within the Internet field:

- United States .us
- United Kingdom .uk
- France .fr
- Finland .fi
- Germany .de
- Canada .ca
- Australia .au
- New Zealand .nz
- Singapore .sg

DOMAIN NAME (DOMESTIC): Any type of haphazard domestic Web address format within the Internet field:

- commercial .com
- organization .org
- Internet related .net
- international .int

DOMAIN NAME (GLOBAL): Any type of global top-level Web address format within the Internet field:

- air transport .aero
- business .biz
- cooperatives .cop
- information .info
- museum .museum
- individuals .name
- professionals .pro

DOMAIN NAME SYSTEM (DNS): An Internet friendly name that converts IP numerical addresses into a URL name.

DOMAIN PARKING: Registered Internet domain names whose main purpose is to secure revenues through pay-per-click advertising.

DOMAIN POACH: To register an Internet domain name for resale; hoard or hijack.

DOMAIN REGISTRAR: A company that registers domain names for profit; usually parked site with pay-per-click advertising models; for example, Godady©.

DOMAIN SYNCHRONIZATION: Authentication device for Widows-NT© servers and workstations where a primary domain controller (PDC) updates all back-up domain controllers (BDCs); manual back-up also possible.

DONGLE: A mechanism for ensuring that only authorized users can copy or use specific software programs or applications; especially very expensive programs or those that contain PHI; common protective mechanisms include a hardware key that plugs into a parallel or serial port on a computer and that a software application accesses for verification before continuing to run; special key diskettes accessed in a similar manner; and registration numbers that are loaded into some form of read-only memory at the factory or during system setup.

DOORWAY: An Internet page that acts as an entry or access point for an Internet site; home page; front page; slang term.

DOS: A single user disk operating system first used for the PC as the underlying control program for Windows© 3.1, 95, 98© and ME©; Windows NT©, 2000©, XP©, Vista©, and other versions emulate DOS in order to support existing DOS applications; DOS prompt is the visual cursor indicator for user input for the MS-DOS® and WINDOWS® operating system.

DOT: The character (.) or period used in Internet address and files names.

DOT BOMB: A failed Internet business; bust.

DOT BUST: Period of bankruptcy for many Internet companies (1999–2001); failed Internet or technology companies; bomb.

DOT COM: A lawful and successful Internet commercial business enterprise.

DOT COMPOST: A failed Internet business; humorous.

DOT CON: Internet money-making scheme; fraudulent; humorous.

DOT GONE: A failed Internet business; humorous.

DOT MATRIX: Type of pin-head impact printer technology.

DOT NET: A business strategy from Microsoft© and its collection of programming support for what Web service, or the ability to use the Web rather than a computer for various services; its goal is to provide individual and business users with a seamlessly interoperable and Web-enabled interface for applications and computing devices and to make computing activities increasingly browser-oriented, the .NET platform includes servers, building-block services, such as Web-based data storage, and device software; it also includes Passport©, Microsoft's fill-in-the-form-only-once identity verification service.

DOT PITCH: Space between computer monitor pixels; smaller is a better indication of clarity.

DOUBLE BUFFER: The net graphic frame in an animation memory displayed while the first is still visible.

DOUBLE CLICK: Left mouse button push and release twice in rapid sequence for program or system input activation.

DOUBLE CLICK SPEED: Time lag allowed in a double-click mouse input process.

DOUBLE POST: To reply to one's own wiki, Web site post, blog, and so forth; to speak to ones' self; slang term.

DOWN: A computer system not available for use.

DOWN LINK: The path from a satellite to the Earth stations that receive its signals; to send electronic information from an earth-orbiting satellite to a land station; down remote load server-to-client.

DOWNLOAD: To copy and save files on a computer from the Internet or intranet; the process of transferring files or software from another computer to your computer.

DOWNLOADER: Computer program that automatically downloads and runs and/or installs other software without the user's knowledge or permission; it may download updated versions of itself or constantly check for updated files.

DOWN STREAM: Unidirectional health data or other information sent from server to client.

DOWN TIME: Nonfunctional computer or network system time.

DOWN TIME POLICY: Protocol used when a health or medical information system is inoperable.

DOWNWARD COMPATIBLE: The ability of a computer system to work with older hardware or software; backward compatible.

DRAFT STANDARDS FOR TRIAL USE (DSTU): Older terminology for standard X12 formats.

DRAG: To move an icon, file, program, or other object across a computer desktop to a new location by using a mouse input device.

DRAG-DROP: To use a computer mouse to move icons, files, or applications on the screen and select commands from a menu; to their destination.

DRAW: Software program to create plans, tables, graphs, diagrams, flow charts, and so forth: MSFT Visio©, Corel Draw©, Audodesk AutoCAD©, and Adobe Illustrator©.

DRG 468–470: Diagnostic Related Groups that are especially common in medical workload financial analysis:

- 468—extensive operating room procedures unrelated to primary diagnosis
- 469—primary diagnosis invalidated or not matched to discharge summary
- 470—medical records with ungroupable diagnosis
- 477—simple OR procedure not related to primary diagnosis

DRG CREEP: Slang term for Diagnostic Related Group coding creep, or upgrading / up-coding or exaggeration in order to increase reimbursement in a fee-for-service environment.

DRG RATE: Fixed monetary payment (diagnostic related group) amount based on patient averages in a based year for comparison and adjusted for factors such as inflation, bad debt, specialty, acuity, or other economic factors.

DRG RISK POOL: A hospital's diagnostic related group economic uncertainty.

DRG SPECIFIC PER-CASE PRICE: Fixed diagnostic related group payment rate used by Medicare, with risk-limits through the identification of long length of stay (LOS) cases; global fee or category DRG pricing.

DRG WEIGHT: Diagnostic Related Group assigned index used to reflect relative hospital costs.

DRIBBLEWARE: Software that is previewed and displayed before release; in need of multiple fixes, patches, and corrections; vaporware; slang term.

DRILL DOWN: To follow an algorithm, menu, or series of steps; checklist of increasingly finer points.

DRIVE: A mechanical-electrical device that spins tapes and computer disks at a specific speed.

DRIVER: A utility program that links an operating system to a computer peripheral device.

DROP: Releasing a mouse button in order to allow a dragged electronic icon or object to fall into its new place.

DROP DOWN LIST BOX: The list of available options from a drop down computer memory box, or icon; menu.

DRUM: A photosensitive cylinder for image receipt and paper transfer; laser printer.

DRUM STORAGE: Addressable computer data storage with magnetic rotating cylinder.

DUAL BOOT: To start-up a bidirectional computer operating system.

DUAL CORE PROCESSOR: Two CPUs that are built into one; Intel®; duo-core; coprocessor.

DUAL HOME: Primary and secondary mission critical enterprise computerized health system networked fault-tolerance level, for increased security beyond primary failure.

DUAL HOME FIREWALL: Security protocol with two different networks (public and private) and simultaneously acting as a gatekeeper for health data traffic access and/or secure medical information denial.

DUAL-IN-LINE PACKAGE: (DIP): Two lines used in computers and associated devices to configure hardware options.

DUE CARE: Health administrators and their organizations have a duty to provide for information security to ensure that the type of control, the cost of control, and the deployment of control are appropriate for the system being managed.

DUMB NETWORK: Term for a network or intranet without Graphical User Interface (GUI), memory, storage, or processing functionality and usually associated with older mainframes and centralized computing architectures; slang term.

DUMB TERMINAL: Term for a computer without Graphical User Interface (GUI), memory, storage, or processing functionality and usually associated with older mainframes and centralized computing architectures; slang term.

DUMP: To transfer large amounts of health or other data without regard for significance or security; to copy on a large scale.

DUMPSTER DIVING: Trashcan and garbage physical searches for security information such as bank account ID numbers, SSNs, passwords, e-mail addresses, and so forth.

DUPLEX: Electronic bidirectional communications; a transmission system permitting data to be transmitted in both directions simultaneously.

DUPLICATE DATABASE: A health information system using a central repository of clinical, nonclinical, or other health data.

DURABLE: Health data and storage that is permanent and must sustain attacks and power interruptions, and so forth.

DURON©: An Intel Pentium© compatible CPU made by AMD®.

DURRANT, CAMERON, MD, MBA: President of PediaMed Pharmaceuticals, Inc., of Greater Cincinnati, OH.

DUSTY DECK: Legacy older hardware, software, or peripheral electronic computer components that are still in use; slang term.

DVD: Digital Video Disk optical storage device.

DVD RECORDER: A Digital video disk (DVD) recording and storage device copies analog or digital audio/visual (A/V) signals in a digital format onto a DVD. DVD recorders differ from digital video recorders (DVRs) in that they record medical or other information onto a removable disk (the DVD) instead of a hard disk.

DVD ROM: A DVD containing health data or other information files, rather than video files.

DVD+RW: A DVD that can record and write for storage; compatible.

DVD WRITER: Speeds beyond 16X for DVDs and 48X for CDs.

DWEEB: An unsophisticated individual; dufus; nerd; geek; slang term.

DXPLAIN: A clinical decision support system from the Massachusetts General Hospital that uses signs, symptoms, and physical diagnosis to rank associated clinical diagnoses.

DYADIC: A computer mathematical operation on two numbers.

DYNAMIC: An operation performed while a computer program is functional.

DYNAMIC HOST CONFIGURATION PROTOCOL (DHCP): Operating system protocol for IP network information that retains the assigned address for a timed-period or lease.

DYNAMIC IP: A nonpermanent IP address automatically assigned to a host by a DHCP server.

DYNAMIC LINK: The runtime connection from one computer program to another.

DYNAMIC MEMORY ALLOCATION: Computer memory segmentation without prior specification.

DYNAMIC NETWORK: A computer health information system that delivers interactive mobile and fixed access points to freely and securely facilitate medical EDI, both on and off-site.

DYNAMIC PAGE: An HTML Web page or Web site with animated icons, JPEGs, JAVA applets, GIFS, audio, visuals, and so forth; medical specialty specific or user preferred and variable Web content and information.

DYNAMIC RAM: The most common type of computer transistor-capacitor memory, which loses content when power is terminated.

DYNAMIC RANDOM ACCESS MEMORY (DRAM): Volatile and unstable RAM that needs continuous refreshment.

DYNAMIC RANGE: The characteristic of a communications or imaging system to reproduce or transmit various brightness levels.

E

e: Electronic, or electrical.

EARTH STATION: The ground equipment essential for receiving and transmitting satellite telecommunications signals.

EASTER EGG: Undocumented code hidden in a software program without direct user knowledge; usually not malicious; slang term.

e-BAY®: A popular online auction house started in 1995 in San Jose, California, by Pierre Omidyar.

e-BOOK: A medical text or other tome distributed electronically.

e-BUSINESS: The use of electronic information systems (especially health Internet technologies) in business processes.

ECHO: Signal repetition in an electronic communication or computer systems line.

ECKERT, JOHN PRESPER (1919–1995): Professor from the University of Pennsylvania who collaborated with John Mauchly in the construction of the Electronic Integrator and Computer (ENIAC) and Binary Automatic Computer (BNAIC) using data storage on magnetic tape instead of punch cards.

ECKSTEIN, JULIE: Director, Missouri Health Information Technology Task Force.

ECLIPSE©: A JAVA language open source program development tool.

e-CODE: International Classification of Diseases, Ninth Edition, Clinical Modification© code that describes an external injury or adverse medicine reaction, rather than disease or illness for medical reimbursement purposes.

e-COMMERCE: The use of electronic information systems (especially health Internet technologies) to perform buy–sell transactions.

EDIT: To make changes, additions, or deletions to a computer file.

EDITOR: A computer or HIT systems utility program to create and modify text files.

e-DOCUMENT: Information intended to be displayed and read on a computer monitor.

EFFECTOR KEY: A keyboard button that changes the meaning of other buttons or keys.

EFFICIENCY: The promises of e-health to increase medical care delivery speed, thereby decreasing costs; for example, the formation of medical error database, electronic health claims submission, through enhanced communication possibilities between health care establishments, and through patient involvement; use of these systems decreases medical errors and morbidity especially as related to prescription interactions.

e-FORM: Any electronically automated application, medical invoice, super-bill, and so forth.

EGO SURF: An Internet search for one's own name; narcissi-surf; slang term.

e-GOVERNMENT: The delivery of government services using electronic information systems (especially medical care, politics, and health Internet technologies).

EGRESS FILTERING: The blockage of harmful traffic from leaving a secure network.

e-HEALTH: Emerging field in the intersection of medical informatics, public health, and business, referring to health services and information delivered or enhanced through the Internet and related technologies; characterizes not only a technical development, but also a state-of-mind, attitude, and a commitment for networked, global thinking, to improve health care worldwide by using information and communication technology.

e-HIM: Electronic health information management.

e-HIR: Electronic health information records; medical data and PHI.

EHR COLLABORATIVE: Trade association of health IT professionals supporting the HL7 initiatives for electronic health records.

EHR SECURITY SERVICE MODEL: Electronic Health Records (EHR) security framework that integrates HIPAA security requirements and takes into account transaction privacy, which is where many of the privacy regulations overlap with the security regulations; according to the following purposes:

- support: generic and underlie most IT security capabilities.
- prevent: focused on preventing a security breach from occurring.
- recover: focused on detection and recovery from a security breach. (Figure 5)

EJECT: To remove a diskette, CD, memory stick, peripheral devices, and so forth, from a computer or similar device.

e-JOURNAL: A personal or professional Web-based diary similar to a blog; or more traditional journal format delivered electronically to subscribers.

e-LEARNING: Education by means of the Internet and distant education electronic platforms (www.CertifiedMedicalPlanner.com).

ELECTRONIC ATTESTATION: Signature certified and computer systems linked verification of medical data or PHI transmission.

ELECTRONIC BILLING: Medical, Durable Medical Equipment (DME), and related health insurance bills or premiums submitted though Electronic Data Interchange (EDI) (nonpaper claims) systems.

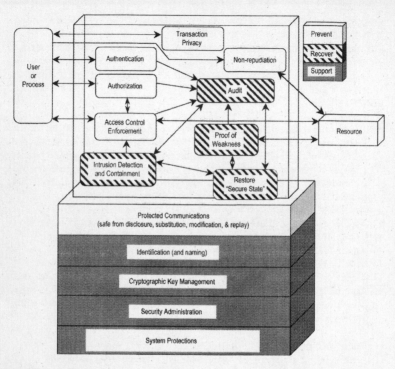

Figure 5: EHR security services model.

ELECTRONIC CLAIM: The digital or electrical representation of a medical bill or invoice; the HIPAA 837 transactions.

ELECTRONIC COMMERCE: The purchase of products or services with online payment.

ELECTRONIC DATA INTERCHANGE (EDI): Intercompany, computer-to-computer transmission of business or health information in a standard format; direct transmission from the originating application program to the receiving, or processing, application program; an EDI transmission consists only of business or health data, not any accompanying verbiage or free-form messages; a standard format is one that is approved by a national or international standards organization, as opposed to formats developed by health industry groups, medical practices, clinics, or companies; the electronic transmission of secure medical and financial data in the health care industrial complex; X12 and similar variable-length formats for the electronic exchange of structured health data. The Centers for Medicare and Medicaid Services (CMS) regulates security and Electronic Data Interchange (EDI, Table 4).

ELECTRONIC DATA INTERCHANGE STANDARDS (EDIS): The American National Standards Institute (ANSI) set of EDI standards known as the *X12 standards*. These standards have been developed by private sector standards development organizations (SDOs) and are maintained by the Accredited Standards Committee (ASC) X12. ANSI ASC X12N standards, Version 4010, were chosen for all of the transactions except retail pharmacy transactions, which continue to use the standard maintained by the National Council for Prescription Drug Programs (NCPDP) because it is already in widespread use. The NCPDP Telecommunications Standard Format Version 5.1 and equivalent NCPDP Batch Standard Version 1.0 have been adopted in this rule (health plans will be required to support one of these two NCPDP formats). The standards are designed to work across industry and company boundaries. Changes and updates to the standards are made by consensus, reflecting the needs of the entire base of standards users, rather than those of a single organization or business sector. Specifically, the following nine health care transactions were required to use X12N standard electronic claim formats by October 16, 2003. (Table 5)

1. Health care encounter claim and coordination of benefits (COB)
2. Claim payment and remittance advice
3. Health care claim status
4. Eligibility for a health plan
5. Referral certification and authorization
6. Enrollment and disenrollment in a health plan
7. Premium payments
8. First report of injury

ELECTRONIC DISCOVERY: Refers to any process in which electronic health or other data is sought, located, secured, and searched with the intent of using it as evidence in a civil (malpractice) or criminal (fraud) legal case; court-ordered or government sanctioned hacking for the purpose of obtaining critical evidence is also a type of e-discovery.

Table 4: EDI Transaction Explanations

Transaction	Title and Use
270	**Health Care Eligibility, Coverage, or Benefit Inquiry** Provider uses to request details of health care eligibility and benefit information or to determine if an information source organization has a particular subscriber or dependent on file.
271	**Health Care Eligibility, Coverage, or Benefit Response** Payer uses to respond to 270 requests.
276	**Health Care Claim Status Request** Provider uses to request the status of health care claims.
277	**Health Care Claim Status Notification** Payer uses to respond to 276 requests.
278	**Health Care Services Review Information—Request and Response** Health care providers use *request* transactions to request information on admission certifications, referrals, service certifications, extended certifications, certification appeals, and other related information. Review entities use *response* transactions to respond to inquiries regarding admission certifications, referrals, service certifications, extended certifications, certification appeals, and other related information.
820	**Payment Order/Remittance Advice** Insurance companies, third-party administrators, payroll service providers, and internal payroll departments use to transmit premium payment information.
834	**Benefit Enrollment and Maintenance** Benefit plan sponsors and administrators use to transmit enrollment and benefits information between each other.
835	**Health Care Claim Payment/Advice** Used by the payer and the provider to make payments on a claim, send an Explanation of Benefits (EOB) remittance advice, or to send both the payment and EOB in the same transaction.
837	**Health Care Claim** There are three separate Implementation Guides for 837 Health Care Claims: • Dental • Institutional • Professional Each is used by the provider—dentist/dental group, clinic/hospital, and physicians/surgeons—or between payers to submit and transfer claims and encounters to the payer.

Table 5: EDIS Transaction Claim Formats

Transaction	Electronic Claim Format
Provider—plan and payer transactions	
Health care encounter claim and coordination of benefits (COB)	837
Claim payment and remittance advice	835
Health care claim status	276/277
Eligibility for a health plan	270/271
Referral certification and authorization	278
Sponsor—plan and payer transactions	
Enrollment and disenrollment in a health plan	834
Premium payments	820
***Future transactions (identified in HIPAA)**	
First report of injury	148
Health care claim attachment	275

* Denotes the actual publication date. All other NPRM (Notice of Proposed Rulemaking) dates are expected publication dates.

ELECTRONIC ERASABLE PROGRAMMABLE READ ONLY MEMORY (EEPROM): An electronic storage and memory chip.

ELECTRONIC FORMS MANAGEMENT (EFM): Automatic and populateable data gathering systems for medical and PHI or other information.

ELECTRONIC FUNDS TRANSFER (EFT): The nonpaper-based transfer of funds by electronic means.

ELECTRONIC HEALTH *AND* ELECTRONIC MEDICAL RECORD: The 2003 Institute of Medicine (IOM) *Patient Safety Report* describes an EMR as encompassing:

1. a longitudinal collection of electronic health information for and about persons;
2. [immediate] electronic access to person- and population-level information by authorized users;

3. provision of knowledge and decision-support systems [that enhance the quality, safety, and efficiency of patient care]; and
4. support for efficient processes for health care delivery. [IOM, 2003]

A 1997 IOM REPORT, *THE COMPUTER-BASED PATIENT RECORD: An Essential Technology for Health Care* provides the following definition that is more extensive:

A patient record system is a type of clinical information system, which is dedicated to collecting, storing, manipulating, and making available clinical information important to the delivery of patient care. The central focus of such systems is clinical data and not financial or billing information. Such systems may be limited in their scope to a single area of clinical information (e.g., dedicated to laboratory data), or they may be comprehensive and cover virtually every facet of clinical information pertinent to patient care (e.g., computer-based patient record systems). [IOM, 1997]

The EHR definitional model document developed by the Health Information and Management Systems Society (HIMSS) [HIMSS, 2003] includes "a working definition of an EHR, attributes, key requirements to meet attributes, and measures or 'evidence' to assess the degree to which essential requirements have been met once EHR is implemented."

Another IOM report, *Key Capabilities of an Electronic Health Record System* [Tang, 2003], identified a set of eight core care delivery functions that EHR systems should be capable of performing in order to promote greater safety, quality, and efficiency in health care delivery:

The eight core capabilities that EHRs should possess are:

1. Health information and data. Having immediate access to key information—such as patients' diagnoses, allergies, lab test results, and medications—would improve caregivers' ability to make sound clinical decisions in a timely manner.
2. Result management. The ability for all providers participating in the care of a patient in multiple settings to quickly access new and past test results would increase patient safety and the effectiveness of care.
3. Order management. The ability to enter and store orders for prescriptions, tests, and other services in a computer-based system should enhance legibility, reduce duplication, and improve the speed with which orders are executed.
4. Decision support. Using reminders, prompts, and alerts, computerized decision-support systems would help improve compliance with

best clinical practices, ensure regular screenings and other preventive practices, identify possible drug interactions, and facilitate diagnoses and treatments.

5. Electronic communication and connectivity. Efficient, secure, and readily accessible communication among providers and patients would improve the continuity of care, increase the timeliness of diagnoses and treatments, and reduce the frequency of adverse events.

6. Patient support. Tools that give patients access to their health records, provide interactive patient education, and help them carry out home monitoring and self-testing can improve control of chronic conditions, such as diabetes.

7. Administrative processes. Computerized administrative tools, such as scheduling systems, would greatly improve hospitals' and clinics' efficiency and provide more timely service to patients.

8. Reporting. Electronic data storage that employs uniform data standards will enable health care organizations to respond more quickly to federal, state, and private reporting requirements, including those that support patient safety and disease surveillance.

ELECTRONIC HEALTH CARE NETWORK ACCREDITATION COMMISSION (EHC-NAC): An organization that tests transactions for consistency with HIPAA requirements and that accredits health care clearinghouses.

ELECTRONIC HEALTH RECORD (EHR): A real-time patient health record with access to evidence-based decision support tools that can be used to aid clinicians in decision-making; the EHR can automate and streamline a clinician's workflow, ensuring that all clinical information is communicated; prevents delays in response that result in gaps in care; can also support the collection of data for uses other than clinical care, such as billing, quality management, outcome reporting, and public health disease surveillance and reporting; electronic medical record.

ELECTRONIC MEDIA: Refers to the mode of electrical health data transmission for collaborating purposes, regardless of method or medium. Health data or medical information that includes:

- electronic memory devices in computers (hard drives) and any removable/transportable digital memory medium, such as magnetic tape or disk, optical disk, or digital memory card; or
- transmission media used to exchange information already in electronic storage media; includes the Internet (wide-open), extranet (using Internet technology to link a business with information accessible only to collaborating parties), leased lines, dial-up lines, private networks, and

the physical movement of removable/transportable electronic storage media.

Note: Certain health data transmission, including of paper via facsimile and of voice via telephone, are not considered to be transmissions via electronic media, because the information being exchanged did not exist in electronic form before the transmission.

ELECTRONIC MEDICAL (MEDIA) CLAIMS (EMC): Usually refers to a flat file format used to transmit or transport medical claims, such as the 192-byte UB-92 Institutional EMC format and the 320-byte Professional EMC-NSF.

ELECTRONIC MEDICAL RECORD (EMR): Hospital, clinic, or medical office information systems that involves accessibility at the patient site or bedside either through bedside terminals, portable workstations, laptops, wireless tablets, and handheld computers and personal digital assistants (e.g., PDAs, e.g., 3Com®, Palm Pilot®); inputs can either be uploaded into the main computer system after rounds or transmitted immediately to the system in the case of wireless technology; bedside technology obviates the need to re-enter data from notes after rounds are complete, improves recall, and avoids redundancy in the work process, saving time that can instead be devoted to patient care; EMRs are not without drawbacks as listed below:

- Operator dependence: The term "garbage in, garbage out" (GIGO) applies to EMRs.
- Variable flexibility for unique needs: A "one size fits all" misses the target; even within a hospital whose needs may change rapidly over time given the continued onslaught of external initiatives and measurement demands; systems vary in flexibility and customizability; more flexible systems are expensive.
- Data entry errors: Most notably, patient data can more easily be entered into the wrong chart due to errors in chart selection; in general, simple double-checking and "sanity checks" in the system usually catch such errors, but if unchecked the impact can be significant.
- Lack of system integration: Interconnectivity of systems becomes more important with EMRs than with any other system. Personnel use the data in many different areas. If there are isolated departmental systems without connectivity, redundant data entry occur leading to confusion in the different departments. (Figure 6)

ELECTRONIC MEDICATION ADMINISTRATION RECORD (EMAR): An electrical file keeping computerized system for tracking clinical medication

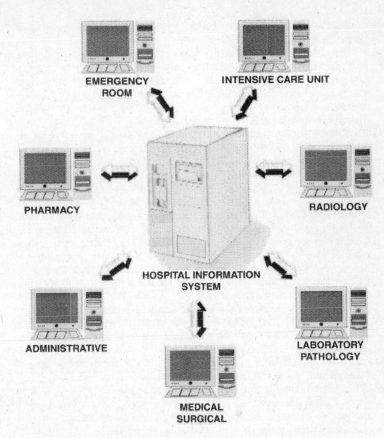

Figure 6: Electronic medical records schematic for a large health system.

dispensation and use; integrated with TPAs, PBMs, robotic dispensing devices, CPOEs, and so forth.

ELECTRONIC PRESCRIBING (ERX): A type of computer technology whereby physicians use handheld or personal computer devices to review drug and formulary coverage and to transmit prescriptions to a printer or to a local pharmacy; e-prescribing software can be integrated into existing clinical information systems to allow physician access to patient-specific information to screen for drug interactions and allergies.

ELECTRONIC PREVENTIVE SERVICES SELECTOR (EPSS): A digital tool for primary care clinicians to use when recommending preventive services for their patients unveiled by the Department of Health and Human Services' Agency for Healthcare Research and Quality (AHRQ), in November 2006; designed for use on a personal digital assistant (PDA) or desktop computer to allow clinicians to access the latest recommendations from the AHRQ-sponsored U.S. Preventive Services Task Force; designed to serve as an aid to clinical decision-making at the point of care and contains 110 recommendations for specific populations covering 59 separate preventive services topics; a real time search function allows a clinician to input a patient's age, gender, and selected behavioral risk factors, such as whether or not they smoke, in the appropriate fields, while the software cross-references the patient characteristics entered with the applicable Task Force recommendations and generates a report specifically tailored for that patient.

ELECTRONIC PROTECTED HEALTH INFORMATION (EPHI): All individually identifiable health information that is transmitted or maintained in electronic media.

ELECTRONIC REMITTANCE ADVICE (ERA): Any of several electronic formats for explaining the payments of health care claims.

ELECTRONIC SIGNATURE: Various date and time stamped electronic security verification systems, such as passwords, encryption, ID numbers, biometrics identifiers, and so forth; electrical transmission and authentication of real signatories; signatory attribute that is affixed to an electronic health document to bind it to a particular entity; an electronic signature process secures the user authentication (proof of claimed health identity, such as by biometrics [fingerprints, retinal scans, hand written signature verification, etc.], tokens, or passwords) at the time the signature is generated; creates the logical manifestation of signature (including the possibility for multiple parties to sign a medical document and have the order of application recognized and proven) and supplies additional information such as time stamp and signature purpose specific to that user; and ensures the integrity of the signed document to enable transportability, interoperability, independent verifiability, and continuity of signature capability; verifying a signature on a document verifies the integrity of the document and associated attributes and verifies the identity of the signer; there are several technologies available for user authentication, including passwords, cryptography, and biometrics (ASTM 1762–95).

ELECTRONIC SOFTWARE DISTRIBUTION (ESD): Providing new software and upgrades by the Internet or over a network instead of individual packaged (shrink-wrapped) installations on each machine.

ELEVATOR: A vertical roll page and square box scroll bar used to change computer text or screen pages; scroll box; scroll bar.

ELITE HACKER: Highly trained and experienced professional engineer who possesses great computer system security intrusion skills; intermediate and novice hackers.

ELLIPSES: The use of three dots (...) to indicate a trailing thought.

ELLISON, IKE: Chairman of MS-HUG® and VP Business Dev NextGen Healthcare Information Systems®.

ELLISON, LAWRENCE J.: The cofounder and CEO of Oracle Corporation® since June 1977; MSFT SQL Server is a major product competitor; Linux OS distributor.

e-MAIL: Electronic message transmission from one user to another; not private; uses Internet or intranet technologies to send messages and documents to and from computers around the world in a matter of seconds; sending or receiving e-mail requires Internet access and an e-mail address; electronic mail usually using an Internet Service Provider (ISP); created by Ray Tomlinson in the 1970s; health data can be transmitted to anywhere in the world for the price of a local telephone call; an e-mail address is typically made up of a part of your name (your account name), the 'at' sign (@), and your domain name.

e-MAIL ADDRESS: Either a personal or Web site format in the model of username @ domain name or the Web site address of an URL; e-mail address filter.

e-MAIL ATTACHMENT: A file, occasionally malicious, sent with an e-mail message.

e-MAIL BROADCAST: To send the same message to many recipients; blast.

e-MAIL CODE (AGENCY): Traditionally: .gov; .edu; .com; and .net.

e-MAIL CODE (COUNTRY): .au, .fr, .it, .uk, .jp, and so forth.

e-MAIL FORWARDING: Sending an e-mail message to another destination.

e-MAIL PROGRAM: Software to enable e-mail functionality; Mozilla's Thunderbird©; MSFT's Outlook and Outlook Express©, and Eudora by Qualcomm©.

e-MAIL TENNIS: Pinging or sending e-mail messages back and forth.

e-MAIL WORM: Blast e-mail delivered malicious code that may be disguised as an anti-virus program, for example, the Sober worm delivered in both English and German, in 2003.

EMBEDDED FONT: Print style or format included in a transmitted file to ensure correct production.

EMBEDDED HYPERLINK: A clickable link as part of a menu or e-mail message.

EMBEDDED LINK: A hyperlink within a text page or Web page.

EMC CORPORATION®: Maker of enterprise-wide intelligent storage and retrieval technology designed for all major server environments; Hopkinton, MA.

EMERGENCY MODE OPERATION: Access controls in place that enable an enterprise to continue to operate in the event of fire, vandalism, natural disaster, or system failure.

EMERGENCY MODE OPERATION PLAN (EMOP): A pro-active action plan that defines how a health care business entity will operate under less than optimal conditions. The intent is to train and prepare employees in what is required to maintain operational integrity throughout the enterprise.

EMOTAG: An e-text, e-mail message emoticon, or attitude, usually within angled brackets, for example, <humorous>.

EMOTICON: Sideways viewed e-mail or text message characters that convey an attitude, or emotion; emotional message typed in an e-mail using standard keyboard characters; a form of electronic smiley or small face made out of keyboard characters; for example, 9 or sad ;-).

EMPLOYEE: One who works for another entity, or employer.

EMPLOYEE TERMINATION PROCEDURE: Establishes a procedure for changing physical or electronic locking mechanisms, both on a recurring basis and when personnel knowledgeable of combinations no longer have need to know or require access to a protected health facility or medical system; includes the removal from access lists to establish a procedure to ensure physical eradication of an entity's access privileges; remove user accounts and ensure terminating employees turn in keys, tokens, or cards that allow access (preferably before termination).

EMPLOYER: The covered health entity for whom an individual performs or performed any service, of whatever nature, as the employee of that entity except that:

- if the entity for whom the individual performs or performed the services does not have control of the payment of wages for those services, the term "employer" means the entity having control of the payment of the wages;
- in the case of an entity paying wages on behalf of a nonresident alien individual, foreign partnership, or foreign corporation, not engaged in trade or business within the United States, the term "employer" means that entity; and

- any entity acting directly as an employer, or indirectly in the interest of an employer, in relation to an employee benefit plan and includes a group or association of employers acting for an employer in that capacity.

EMPOWERMENT: Patient- and evidence-based access to health care knowledge; an AMA review of Internet-based health information suggested that not all medical information is reliable, and that one needs multiple sites for a correct view of a particular medical condition.

EMULATION: Software program that allows one operating system to mimic another and uses both systems; PC to Macintosh® bridge program.

ENABLE: Health care information exchange and communication in a standardized way between health care establishments; HIPAA implementation standardizes health information communication formats and e-health coding conventions.

ENABLING TECHNOLOGY: Any new electronic software or hardware device that facilitates health or other data interchange.

ENCAPSULATED POSTSCRIPT: A file format that supports both vector graphics and bitmap images and is usually used for combination artwork or charts and graphs; encapsulated security payload.

ENCAPSULATION: The technique of embedding or imprinting one network protocol inside of another; to set up a virtual tunnel by using header and trailer transmission packets.

ENCODE: To designate a health data code or to encrypt a message containing PHI or other medical information, and so forth.

ENCODER: A device that assigns a data code for protected health information.

ENCOUNTER: Face to face interaction between a medical provider and patient; now may be facilitated electronically and in real-time with audio, visual, Web cameras, and so forth.

ENCOUNTER DATA: Detailed data about individual services provided by a capitated managed care entity; the level of detail about each service reported is similar to that of a standard claim form; sometimes referred to as medical "shadow claims."

ENCRYPTED VIRUS: Malicious software that is coded to prevent removal or detection; Cascade variant.

ENCRYPTION: The ability to securely change, transmit, and receive medical health or other data and to reconstitute it into useable information, regardless of methodology; the most common form of wireless encryption is Wired Equivalent Privacy (WEP) and Wi-Fi Protected Access (WPA); to encode, mix, or garble an electronic message for health care or other security and authentication purposes; transforming confidential plaintext into cipher medical text to protect it; encipherment; an algorithm combines plaintext with other values called keys, or ciphers, so the data becomes unintelligible; once encrypted, data can be stored or transmitted over unsecured lines; decrypting data reverses the encryption algorithm process and makes the plaintext available for further processing.

ENDPOINT SECURITY: Security strategy where software is distributed to end-user devices but centrally managed and works on a client-server that verifies logins and sends updates and patches when needed; doctors, nurses, medical technicians, and so forth.

ENGINE: A computer systems program that determines how another program manages or manipulates health or medical data or other electronic and archived information.

ENIAC (ELECTRONIC NUMERICAL INTEGRATOR AND COMPUTER): The first computer, built in 1946, with 18,000 vacuum tubes, 8 by 100 feet wide, and 80 tons; it could perform 5,000 summation problems in 360 multiplications per second.

ENTERPRISE: An entire health care or other organization (including subsidiaries) that implies a large corporation or government agency, but may also refer to an entity of any size with many systems and health information technology users to manage.

ENTERPRISE ARCHITECTURE (EA): A strategic resource that aligns health business and technology, leverages shared assets, builds internal and external partnerships, and optimizes the value of information technology services; Clinger-Cohen Act of 1996.

ENTERPRISE MASTER PATIENT INDEX (EMPI): Electronic communications system used to integrate patient medical, administrative, and PHI across multiple business platforms associated with ID management and access.

ENTERPRISE NETWORK: Multiple computers and servers connected over small or large geographic areas; LAN, MAN, and WAN.

ENTERPRISE RESOURCE PLANNING (ERP): The use of medical information technology to facilitate all health care entity-wide operations and tasks.

ENTERPRISE SEARCH: Internet/intranet enabled premium and meaning-based, information and access solution search engine; such as Vivisimo©, Oracle Search©, Endeca©, Fast©, and Autonomy©.

ENTERPRISE USER AUTHENTICATION (EUA): An access control computer management system using secure sign-in verification and identification; based on the Kerberos (RFC 1510) Needham-Schroeder protocol and Health Level 7 CCOW standard.

ENTITY: Either a subject (an active element that operates on information or the system state) or an object (a passive element that contains or receives information); a legal business structure type (PC, Inc, LLC, S or C corp., etc.).

ENTITY AUTHENTICATION: The corroboration that a medical or health care entity is the one claimed (ISO 7498–2); a communications/

network mechanism to irrefutably identify authorized users, programs, and processes, and to deny access to unauthorized users, programs, and processes.

ENUMERATOR: HIPAA issued identification numbers; to identify hardware and peripheral devices of a computer system.

ENVELOPE: The almost invisible outline enclosing an object, icon, or symbol.

ENVIRONMENT: A specific hardware or software configuration with operating system.

ENVIRONMENTAL VIRUS: A relatively harmless newsgroup computer code that locates directories where targets reside; first appeared in 1994 as the KAOS4 variant.

E-OFFICE: Electronic and paperless medical practice.

EPHI RISK ANALYSIS: Protected Health Information in Electronic Form (PHIEF) protocol that suggests basic steps be considered when conducting a health IT risk analysis, such as an inventory to determine assets needing protection; by using the following as a starting point to identify where EPHI is received, stored, and transmitted, and who has access to it:

- Hardware: computers, radiology storage devices, medical equipment, front-end processors, workstations, modems
- Information networks: servers, communication lines, internal and external connectivity, remote access
- Applications: database and application software, operating systems, utilities, compilers, encryption tools, procedure libraries
- Physical facilities: heating, ventilation and cooling systems; furniture; supplies; machinery; fire control systems; storage
- Other assets: records and data, policies and procedures, customer confidence

e-PRESCRIBING: The use of electric computer systems to enter, modify, review, output, and store patient and DEA controlled-medication information.

e-PUBLISH: The creation, production, and distribution of electronic medical, health care, and other documents.

EQUAL ACCESS: The ability to choose between various long distance telephone carriers; in more remote areas, some local exchange carriers are still serviced by only one long distance carrier.

EQUIPMENT CONTROL (INGRESS-EGRESS): Documented security procedures for bringing hardware and software into and out of a health facility and for maintaining a record of that equipment; includes, but is not limited to, the marking, handling, and disposal of hardware and storage media.

EQUITY: Suggestion that e-health may deepen the gap between those with technology access and those without; possibility that underdeveloped nations or domestic economic sectors that would benefit the most from e-health technology will not be able to access the systems.

ERASE: To delete a medical, health care, or other data file on an operating system; or to make it available for new data.

ERGONOMICS: Functional Product design and use based on human physical work requirements.

ERISA: Employment Retirement Income Security Act (U.S.C. Title 29, U.S. Code sections 1001). Enacted in 1974, it governs how private employers and pension or insurance companies must administer employee benefit plans, including employee health care plans.

ERROR MESSAGE: Text that indicates computer system malfunction.

ESCAPE CODE: Computer code for a character or symbol that cannot be typed or inputted with a normal keyboard.

ETHERNET: LAN transmission standards, such as 10BASE-T, developed jointly by DEC, Intel, and Xerox with wired network IEEE 802.3 specifications; developed by Robert Metcalfe in the 1970s.

ETHICAL HACK: Attempting to break into a computer system in order to find errors, holes, or other security hazards to improve security; protection technique; white hat hacker; slang term.

ETHICS: Form of e-health that involves patient–physician interaction and poses new challenges and threats, such as online professional practice, informed consent, privacy, and equity issues; for example, some suggest that physicians limit e-mail because of liability and security reasons; legal debates for patients and physicians to conduct online health systems.

EUDORA®: An early free e-mail program developed by Steven Dorner in 1988.

EUREKSTER: An online amateur search-engine or mashup; slang term.

EUROPEAN TECHNICAL COMMITTEE FOR NORMALIZATION (CEN): An international agency responsible for setting standards in health care informatics and medical data manipulation.

EVALUATION AND MANAGEMENT: Medical provider patient contact code for diagnosis, assessment, and counseling reported with CPT-4 Codes for payment.

EVEN PARITY: Data parity method set at an even number of "1" bits or words; checksum.

EVEN SMALLS: An all-lower-case-typed message.

EVENT: Computer end-user generated response; action or occurrence.

EVENT DRIVEN PROGRAM: A computer system that responds to incidents rather than following a program or application; machine controlled computers.

EVENT LOG: Journal of electronic data, information, and error messages; event log.

EVENT REPORT: Any computer or network message indicating operational irregularities in physical elements of a network or a response to the occurrence of a significant task, typically the completion of a request for information.

EVIDENCED-BASED MEDICINE (EBM): Scientific evidence of intervention effectiveness that replaces traditional health care assumptions; a public-academic collaboration to provide empirical medicine models; only 20% of medical protocols follow EBM, integrating individual clinical experience with the best available external clinical evidence from systematic research and health informatics when making decisions about patient care.

EVIL TWIN: A malicious wireless computer hotspot that appears credible.

EVIL TWIN INTERCEPT: Unauthorized wireless access point used to connect and disclose sensitive medical data or PHI.

EVOLUTION DATA OPTIMIZED (EVDO): A wireless radio broadband standard that takes the form of a PC card slipped into a laptop computer to obtain Internet connectivity anywhere cell phone service is available.

EXABYTE: 1024 terabytes capacity.

EXCEL®: An electronic spreadsheet program from MSFT, first released in 1985.

EXCEPTION: An unauthorized electrical data transmission, void of secure protocol.

EXCHANGE SERVER©: A MSFT collaborative program for e-mail.

EXCITE®: An Internet search engine using Intelligent Concept Extraction (ICE) technology.

EXECUTE: To initiate computer systems instructions for work product; a computer program that can be run or used.

EXE FILE: An executable machine language file program for DOS and Windows©.

EXECUTIVE DASHBOARD: Electronic synopsis of real-time managerial data and information; physician, nurse, or medical provider specific dashboard.

EXIT: To close a computer file, program, application, and so forth.

EXL®: Commercial grade Internet access, often bundled with VPNs, anti-spam, virus and pop-up blockers, firewalls, and so forth.

EXPANDED MEMORY: Additional memory beyond the typical DOS or Windows/Intel©-based computer; beyond standard Wintel systems, greater than 1–10 MB.

EXPERT SYSTEMS: Software application program with a distinct and deep subject matter knowledge base; as in medicine and health care; computer program developed to simulate human decisions in a specific field, or fields; branch of artificial intelligence; medical or clinical decision-making algorithm; cookbook medicine; slang term.

EXPLOIT: To crack, hack, or breach into a secure computer system; sploit; slang term.

EXPORT: To convert or move medical data from one application to another.

EXTENDED ASCII: ASCII 8-bit standard processing code with 256 characters.

EXTENDED MEMORY: Additional memory storage capacity beyond 1-MB DOS computers.

EXTENSIBILITY: The ability to add additional computer system hardware, software, peripherals, or communication functionality, and so forth; extension.

EXTENSIBLE MARKUP LANGUAGE (XML): Data interchange as structured text as a W3C-recommended general-purpose language for creating special-purpose markup languages, capable of describing many different kinds of medical, health, and other data. Its primary purpose is to facilitate the sharing of data across different systems, particularly systems connected via the Internet. With the help of data analysts, database developers, and database administrators versed in structured query language, the identification, method of entry, and formatting of protected health information is accomplished. There are multiple vendors well versed in practice management and electronic medical record software, but the successful use of their services depends heavily on the interoperability of your current data scheme and the ability to successfully import it. This new security standard will require covered entities to implement security measures that could be technology-neutral and scalable, and yet integrate all the components of security (administrative safeguards, physical safeguards, and technical safeguards) that must be in place to preserve health information confidentiality, integrity, and availability (three basic elements of security).

EXTENSION: To expand the scope of health care beyond conventional boundaries; for example, clinical trial in Europe, or world information access applied to a certain situation; also, the three character terminus to a DOS file name.

EXTENT: The contiguous area on a computer disk containing a file or a portion of a file consisting of one or more clusters.

EXTERNAL STORAGE: Storage media that is physically separated from a computer or network.

EXTERNAL TRANSACTIONS: Distinction made between health data transactions that are outside an organization, and those that are inside; use of end-to-end encrypted paths, as illustrated in Figure 7.

EXTORTIONWARE: A malicious computer pop-up program that demands online monetary payment to allow closure.

EXTRACT: To remove medical data, health files, or other information from a larger database, to a smaller one.

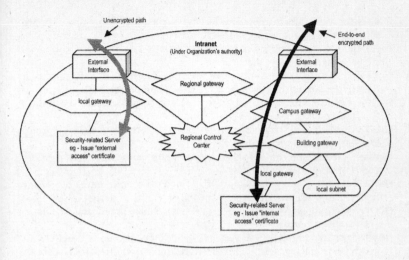

Figure 7: External health care entity transactions.

EXTRANET: A Web site that links a health organization with other specific organizations or people; extranets are only accessible to those specified organizations or people and are protected via passwords; intranet.

EYEBALLS: Web page or Web site end users; doctors, nurses, administrators, teachers, laymen and patients, and so forth; Web page or Web site viewers.

e-ZINE: An electronic newsletter, journal, or magazine; slang term.

F

F2F: Face to Face.

FACE TIME: Personal patient–physician or medical provider health care interaction; patient, clinic, hospice, or hospital visit, and so forth.

FACILITY SECURITY: The safeguarding of both the exterior and interior of a health care building and equipment from those unauthorized to access health information.

FACILITY SECURITY PLAN: A scheme to safeguard health premises, clinics, hospitals, and building(s) (exterior and interior) from unauthorized physical access, and to safeguard the equipment therein from unauthorized physical access, tampering, and theft.

FACSIMILE: The transmission of printed pages between remote locations; tele-copying; fax.

FAILSAFE: The avoidance of enterprise-wide health computer system compro-mise in the face of shutdown failure; fail-safe computer health system.

FAISON, FOREST, MD, CAPT., MC, USN: Director, Navy Medicine Technology Integration Office.

FALSE NEGATIVE / POSITIVE: Inappropriately or incorrectly denying or grant-ing computer network security access.

FAMILY SET: A single run of backed-up computer tapes, disks, CD, memory sticks, or other storage devices.

FARBER, DAVID: Carnegie-Mellon University Professor, "grandfather of the Internet" and opponent of federal meddling with the Internet.

FAST: Asynchronous communication over high-quality broadband-like Inter-net lines; slang term.

FAT: The original file allocation system used in DOS, Windows©, and OS/2©, which keeps track of where data are stored on a disk; directory list, which contains file name, extension, date, and so forth, points to the FAT entry where the file starts, and if a file is larger than one cluster, the first FAT entry points to the next FAT entry where the second cluster of the file is stored, to the end of the file. If a cluster becomes damaged, its FAT entry is marked as such and that cluster is not used again.

FAT 16: A 16-bit file cluster used by MS-DOS©, WINDOWS©, and WINDOWS-NT©.

FAT 32: The 32-bit version of the FAT file system, used on most PCs, which supports larger disk partitions and file sizes and has more safeguards than the earlier version of FAT (FAT16).

FAT 64: A 64-bit file cluster used by WINDOWS VISTA© edition and WINDOWS-NT© series.

FATAL ERROR: An electronic process halting or termination condition.

FAT CLIENT: A client/server machine with little or no server input.

FATHER FILE: A medical file that contains the last validated and secure set of health information; preceded by a grandfather health file and succeeded by its son.

FAT SERVER: A server that performs most all functions with little input from the client.

FAULT: Usually a physical computer system defect.

FAULT TOLERANCE: The ability of a health information technology system to respond gracefully to an unexpected hardware or software failure; there are many levels of fault tolerance, the lowest being the ability to continue operation in the event of a power failure; many fault-tolerant systems mirror all operations as every operation is performed on two or more duplicate systems, so if one fails the other can take over.

FAVORITE PLACE: An ISP feature that allows quick identification of frequently visited Web sites.

FAX: Electronic reproduction and transmission of a document or image on a telecommunications network; facsimile machine.

FAX BROADCAST: A blast fax; sending the same message to different recipients.

FAX MODEM: A computer with an internal fax modem.

FAX SERVER: LAN, MAN, or WAN workstation access to outgoing or incoming electronic fax transmissions.

FDISK COMMAND: A "format disk" input that does not erase health data, but eliminates the operating system's ability to locate it, while the original data still exists on a hard drive; retrieved using available tools.

FEDERAL HEALTH ARCHITECTURE (FHA): A collaborative body composed of several federal departments and agencies, including the Department of Health and Human Services (HHS), the Department of Homeland Security (DHS), the Department of Veterans Affairs (VA), the Environmental Protection Agency (EPA), the U.S. Department of Agriculture (USDA), the Department of Defense (DOD), and the Department of Energy (DOE). FHA provides a framework for linking health business processes to technology solutions and standards and for demonstrating how these solutions achieve improved health performance outcomes.

FEDERAL HIPAA FEATURES: The Federal government required compliance with HIPAA security regulations by April 2005 with the following HIS features:

- Secure password protection performed at multiple levels to ensure that access to PHI is restricted to those who need the information at that time needed.
- Encrypted health data for transmission between systems in order to prevent data intercept and corruption.

FEDERAL PRIVACY ACT 1974 (FPA): HIPAA USC Sec 522a frame for the PHI Statutes.

FEDERATED IDENTITY MANAGEMENT (FIM): An arrangement that can be made among multiple health enterprises that lets subscribers use the same identification data to obtain access to the networks of all enterprises in the group; such a system is sometimes called identity federation.

FIBER DISTRIBUTED DATA INTERFACE: A high-speed fiber optic network containing state-of-the art bandwidth.

FIBER OPTIC CABLE: Glass line that is more efficient than copper and used for the electronic transmission of digital signals over long distances; wide area networks; produces LEDs or ILDs; cable that is insulated, flexible, and consists of a glass core that relies on light sources rather than electricity to transmit audio, medical images, video, and health data signals; permits high-capacity transmission at extreme speeds, sometimes billions of bits per second, with very low error rates.

FICHE: Plastic analog data and information image film and data repository method; a microfilm preserving printed text in reduced form; microfiche; ultra-fiche.

FIELD: Unit of medical, health information, or other data within a recorded area.

FIELD LEVEL SECURITY: Authorization for use within a specific electronic sector rather than enterprise wide access.

FIFTH GENERATION: A computer system with integrated large scale circuits to use vector processing or pipelining.

FIFTY TERABYTE DVD: Harvard Medical School (HMS) initiative to make a high-capacity storage device a reality by using genetically altered proteins from salt marsh microbes that temporarily react to light by converting it to molecules with unique shapes in order to make a binary system for data storage.

FILE: A cohort of computer electronic information; written, graphics, video, audio, and so forth; electronic data collected in related records usually described by its suffix (.doc, .ppt, .pdf, or .exe, etc.).

FILE ALLOCATION TABLE (FAT): A 16-, 32-, or 64-bit file cluster used by MS-DOS©, WINDOWS©, and WINDOWS-NT©.

FILE CORRUPTION: Alteration of health care, medical information, or other data on a computer network or program due to hardware or software failure, viruses, or power failure.

FILE EXTENSION: Characters that appear at the end of a computer file name; usually a dot (full stop) with one to three letters.

FILE FORMAT: Rules or methods of storing computer health, medical, or other information.

FILE INFECTOR: A computer virus that is launched upon program file installation; the Frodo virus variant.

FILE PROTECTION: Any physical or electrical method, such as a diskette notch or copyright protect mechanism, to prevent unauthorized file duplication, transfer, modification, or mirroring.

FILE RECORD SEGMENT. AN MFT (MASTER FILE TABLE): File record, or metadata file, indexes all files on a volume and contains the attributes of each file and the root of any index.

FILE SERVER: File handling and storage functionality for networked computers and controlled by server file software and not the embedded operating system.

FILE SHARE: A resource such as a folder or printer that has been made sharable with other computer system users; Gnutella®.

FILE SHARING WORM: Fast spreading file sharing malicious code, as with the MyDoom variant of 2004.

FILE SYSTEM: (1) The way in which files are named and where they are placed logically for storage and retrieval; the DOS, Windows©, OS/2©, Macintosh, and UNIX-based operating systems all have file systems in which files are placed somewhere in a hierarchical (tree) structure; a file is placed in a directory folder in Windows® or subdirectory at the desired place in the tree structure; file systems specify conventions for naming files and include the maximum number of characters in a name, which characters can be used, and, in some systems, how long the file name suffix can be; a file system also includes a format for specifying the path to a file through the structure of directories. (2) May refer to the part of an OS or added-on program that supports a file system, such as the Network File System (NFS) and the Andrew file system (AFS). (3) The hardware used for nonvolatile storage, the software application that controls the hardware, and the architecture of both the hardware and software.

FILE TRANSFER PROTOCOL (FTP): Method used to upload or download files from one networked computer or server to another; anonymous FTP is a file transfer between locations that does not require users to identify themselves with a password or log-in; an anonymous FTP is not secure, because it can be accessed by any other user of the Web.

FILM ALTERNATOR: A radiology imaging device powered by a motor that displays multiple films for interpretation and moves them under the control of an operator; may be thought of as multiple banks moving medical view boxes.

FILM DIGITIZER: An instrument that permits scanning of existing static medical images so that the images may be stored, manipulated, or transmitted in digital form.

FILMLESS RADIOLOGY: Use of devices that replace film by acquiring digital images and related patient information and transmit, store, retrieve, and display them electronically.

FILO, DAVID: Cofounder of YAHOO!, with Jerry Yang.

FILTER: To change electronic data or mask selected data; to securely change input-output health or medical data, or other information.

FINDBUGS®: Free software program that uses statistical analysis to identify problems in JAVA® programs and applications, such as difficult language features, misunderstood variants or API methods, typos, or incorrect Boolean operator.

FINE GRAIN SECURITY: Computer system that allows user access control and tiered levels of security clearance.

FINGER: UNIX utility identification program.

FIREFOX©: Popular Internet browser by Mozilla introduced in 2004; version 2.0 released in 2007.

FIREWALL: The software and hardware systems used to protect computers, servers, and networks from malicious mischief and unauthorized access and intrusion; security protection; program that hides a computer's ports from outside viewing, slang term; Zone Alarm©, Norton©, MSFT, AVG, Avast©, Panda©, McAfee®, and so forth. Generally, sits between a remote user's workstation or client and the host network or server. As the user's client establishes the communication with the firewall, the client may pass authentication data to an authentication service inside the perimeter. A known trusted person, sometimes only when using trusted devices, can be provided with appropriate security privileges to access resources not available to general users. An example of this application layer firewall would be TCP Wrapper.

FIREWALL SANDWICH: A firewall for both inbound and outbound medical information.

FIREWIRE: A high-speed bus interface that connects hardware for very fast electronic transmissions, video, and other real time applications; IEEE 1394.

FIRMWARE: Read-only ROM, PROM, EPROM chip, and so forth.

FIRST GENERATION: Computers built in the 1950s with vacuum tubes.

FISHBOWEL: To actively monitor a computer system end-user in real time; to electronically or physically watch; security system methodology; slang term.

FIXED DISK: A nonremovable computer disk.

F-KEY: A computer keyboard input function button.

FLAG SHIP: The best or most important product, idea, program, or computer application that a health care or other organization owns or produces.

FLAME: Excessive and harassing e-mail or text messages; flamer; flame war; flame-bait; flame-fest; slang term.

FLASH: Animated, multimedia, and interactive Vector Graphics® file format for the Internet and related URLS and Web pages.

FLASH DRIVE: Portable memory device; jump drive, memory key, memory stick, thumb drive, removable drive, and so forth; developed by Macromedia© for Web content and interactive, rather than HTML, presentations.

FLASH MEMORY: Nonvolatile, solid-state rewritable memory with read-only functionality that is durable and low-voltage; used for Linux, MAC-OS, Windows©, and handheld computer boot-up; Macromedia©, Adobe©, and so forth; type of EEPROM storage device.

FLAT FILES: Noncompressed computer files with similar lengths, regardless of actual data quantity; space not conserved.

FLAT PANEL: Computer or laptop monitor with plasma or LCD technology; flat screen; slang term.

FLAT RATE: An unmetered subscription ISP connection.

FLAW: Security or software error or computer system malfunction; a bug.

FLEURON: An electronic typographic error used as a decorative ornament; slang term.

FLEXIBLE DISPLAY: Portable computer radiology monitor with roll-up ability.

FLICKR: Picture and image sharing collaborative Web site first launched in 2004.

FLIP FLOP: One-bit memory that can store data or remain in a clear state.

FLOOD: Overwhelming a computer or network system with input data or information in order to crash it; overload.

FLOPPY DISK: Magnetic circular portable electronic storage medium in a variety of older sizes and capacities: 3.5 inch 720 KB; 5.25 inch 360 KB; 8 inch 270 KB storage (CP/M OS); floppy disk drive.

FLOW CHART: A symbolic graphical representation of expressions or data.

FLUSH: Computer or print screen dialog placed against a margin; flush left or flush right.

FLY OUT: A secondary or tertiary computer menu that appears on the side of a primary menu when activated for viewing.

FOCUS: An active operating computer system screen window.

FOLDER: Subset or collection of stored computer files, such as health data or medical records.

FONALITY: Open source telephone software.

FONT: Characteristic type face, size, or style.

FONT MANAGEMENT SYSTEM: A software code for the scaleability and change of computer fonts.

FOOTPRINT: The amount of electronic device-occupying desk space; or the geographic range on the earth beneath a satellite that is in the scope to receive that satellite's information.

FOREFRONT (FF): The brand for all technical security products from the Microsoft Corporation (antigen e-mail security: FF Security for Exchange Servers©, FF Client Security©, FF Security for SharePoint©, FF Edge and FF IM©, and Forefront Client Security© (FCS).

FOREGROUND: Multimedia functionality or simultaneous use computer application; for example, Internet surfing while using a spreadsheet.

FOREIGN KEY: Primary instrument of one data table that is placed within another data table to support relationship navigation.

FORENSIC HEALTH ACCOUNTANT (FHA): Forensic health care accounting has increased in prominence in recent years as the electronic and financial activities of corporations are more intensely scrutinized by shareholders and government agencies; FHAs are trained to prevent and detect corporate financial fraud such as embezzlement, securities fraud, tax scams, and money laundering, HIPAA, STARK, and U.S. Patriot Act violations; accounting firms, security companies, multinational corporations, and even the FBI rely on these professionals, who may be called on to examine a health firm's accounting statements or tapped as expert witnesses at divorce proceedings or intellectual property trials; FHAs usually begin as a certified public accountant (CPA) and learn the health trade through hands-on work while others have a background in law enforcement or investigation; the most marketable professionals have earned the certified health fraud examiner (CHFE) designation.

FORMAT: To prepare a disk to accept written computer files; to wipe a disk clean or erase prior information; data elements that provide or control the enveloping or hierarchical structure, or assist in identifying data content of a transaction; health care information data element structure.

FORMAT STANDARD: HIPAA specificity for electronic health data element security transmissions; does not apply to paper.

FORMATTING: The process used to format a computer disk with tracks and sectors to locate data accurately.

FORM HTLM: A Web site that allows data entry, which is returned to its server for later retrieval.

FORMULA TRANSLATOR: A language compiler computer program system that allows software to be written in any type of mathematical language.

FORTEZZA CARD: A plastic data encryption or security authorization pass; low cost cryptographic token used in the military, NSA, and federal government.

FORTH: A threaded interpretative computer language developed by Charles Moore in the early 1970s that is known for simple statements that require few machine resources.

FORTRAN: IBM developed formula transmission computer language of the late 1950s with mathematical calculations.

FORWARD: To send along an e-mail message to another recipient with notification of same.

FOURTH GENERATION: Computers built with integrated circuits instead of vacuum tubes.

FRACTAL: A lossy color image compression method; infinite amount of fine detail.

FRACTIONAL T-1 LINE: A small portion of a first level broadband T-Carrier information transmission trunk or telephone line.

FRAGMENT: A piece of data file often written in multiple fragments because there is no contiguous space available large enough to store the file.

FRAGMENTATION: A condition where health or other data is stored in noncontiguous areas on a computer disk; as files are updated, new data are stored in available free space, which may or may not be contiguous; fragmented files cause extra head movement, which slows disk accesses.

FRAME: A 64–1518 byte packet with header/data/trailer information to mark the initiation and cessation of transmitted or relayed information; synchronous serial communication; 'framed'; a Web site that divides a Web browser's screen into smaller sections; each area displays different data, usually to help the user navigate the site, or to display advertisements.

FRAME RELAY: Created to improve the rate of health data transfer compared to previous transmission protocols, frame relay is a streamlined process of sending and acknowledging transmitted packets of medical data; a packet orientated method of communication used in public and private LAN, MAN, and WAN networks; switch; router type device.

FRAMES PAGE: Web site or browser screen that divides a Web page into independent scrolling areas.

FRAPPER: A mash-up or combination of Web site groups for Google® maps.

FRAUD AND ABUSE: Federal and state Medicare and Medicaid violations of the Internal Revenue Code, Stark I and II laws, or other codes that proscribe patient referrals to entities in which a family member has a financial interest; abuse is unneeded, harmful, or poor-quality health care delivery or services; including e-health and e-medicine.

FRAUD AND ABUSE LEGISLATION: The original Social Security Act, Congressional legislation of 1977, 1981, 1987, OBRA, Stark I, Stark II, HIPAA, and so forth; including e-health and e-medicine.

FREE: Software void of error checking and debugging codes.

FREE SOFTWARE: Web-based software received without monetary charge in return for information, revealed or not; commercial programs, trials, demonstration programs, upgrades, and add-on programs; shareware; drivers and freeware; freeware; slang term.

FREE SOFTWARE MOVEMENT: Philosophy that began in 1983 when Richard Stallman announced the GNU project, and the Free Software Foundation in 1985 to support the movement; its philosophy is to give freedom to computer users by replacing proprietary software under restrictive licensing terms with free software, with the ultimate goal of liberating everyone in cyberspace.

FREESPIRE®: An open, community driven, and free computer operating system by Linspire, Inc.

FREE TEXT DATA: Health or medical information in narrative form; unstructured and uncoded.

FREEWARE: Downloadable software free of charge; slang term.

FREEZE: To seize, stop working, or stall; slang term.

FREEZE DATE: Date of the last computer software modification after which no additional changes can be made.

FREEZE FRAME: A way to transmit still images over regular telephone lines; a single image is transmitted every 8 to 30 seconds; slow scan.

FREQUENCY: The rates at which an electromagnetic signal alternates, denoted in Hertz.

FRESNEL EFFECT: Occurs when direct visual line sight obstructs radio frequency line of transmissions.

FRINGEWARE: Questionable or potentially unreliable software; slang term.

FRITTERWARE: Time wasting and unproductive software, game, or application; slang term.

FRONTPAGE®: A MSFT Windows®-based Web authoring program.

FULFILLMENT: To deliver e-commerce products, equipment goods, or medical services; DME delivery; telemedicine.

FULFILLMENT SERVICE PROVIDER: Firm that provides or outsources e-commerce goods or services; patient access management; admissions department, and so forth.

FULL DUPLEX: Electronic transmission channel that allows simultaneous two-way data communication; a standard telephone line is one example of this because both parties can simultaneously speak while listening to the voice on the opposing end.

FULL MOTION VIDEO: A standard video signal, conventionally requiring 6 MHz in analog format and 90 Mbps when digitally encoded, that is able to be transmitted by a variety of ways including television broadcast, microwave, fiber optics, and satellite.

FULLY SPECIFIC NAME: Complete concept text in SNOMED-CT.

FUNCTION KEY: Computer keyboard buttons F1–F12 that perform software program or special application functions.

FURL: To send an Internet e-mail or Web site address without explanation; forward URL; slang term.

FUSION®: Software bridge for Oracle acquired programs and applications from companies such as Siebel Systems© and PeopleSoft©.

FUZZY DATA: Health, medical, or other information that is vague, ambiguous, or incomplete.

FUZZY LOGIC: Loose artificial intelligence decision-making methodology based on heuristic data and incomplete information that falls between absolute values; imprecise feelings; gut feeling.

FUZZY SET LOGIC: Artificial intelligence theory of logic, disease, or treatment tracking that sets heuristic upper and lower data set boundaries; thought process employed before hard data, true statistics and stochastic dampening methods are available; educated guess.

G

<g>: e-mail emoticon for a grin.

GAMMA: A root-kit kernel OS anti-virus detection tool from Komoku, College Park, Maryland; nonlinear response to a computer video screen or game.

GAMMA TEST: A software functionality test done after beta testing, but before commercial product release.

GANTT CHART: Bar chart with horizontal time line depiction used for project management.

GARCIA, GREGORY: U.S. Department of Homeland Cyber Security Czar.

GARETS, DAVID E.: President and CEO of HIMSS Analytics, in Chicago, Illinois.

GAS LINE BROADBAND: High computer system bandwidth frequency ability of natural gas lines to provide Internet access through wireless ultra-wideband technology that maintains signal strength.

GATES, WILLIAM H.: Chairman, Cofounder, and Chief Software Architect for the Microsoft Corporation, and Microsoft Health User's Group (MS-HUG), whose mission is to provide value through education, communication, and access to health care information and medical technology experts.

GATEWAY: Method of interconnecting two dissimilar computers, servers, operating systems, or complex networks; router or bridge; a computer used to provide translations between different types of standards or complex protocol suites; for example, different e-mail messaging systems; may describe a 'door' from a private data network to the Internet.

GB (GIGABYTE): A measure of the storage capacity and memory of a computer. One gigabyte is equivalent to 1.074 billion bytes or 1,000 MB; used to express a data transfer rate (1 gigabit/second = 1 Gbps); the bandwidth of optical fiber is often in the gigabit or billion-bits-per-second range.

GBPS (GIGABITS PER SECOND): A measure of bandwidth and rate of data flow in digital transmission.

GEEK: An electronic stereotype for nerd; slang term.

GELLO: An object-orientated expression language for a medical, health, or other clinical decision support system.

GENERATIONS OF PROGRAMMING COMPUTER LANGUAGES:

1st: machine language
2nd: assembly language
3rd: procedural language
4th: problem orientated language
5th: artificial intelligence
6th: self-adapting applications

GENIE®: An ISP of the General Electric and IDT Company.

GENOME@HOME: A large scale multicomputer distributed system that analyzes DNA, chromosomal, and genome information; Stanford University.

GENUINE ADVANTAGE®: Anti-piracy program from MSFT alleged to be a type of computer spy ware software.

GEOSTATIONARY ORBIT: Refers to the orbit of a satellite whose location relative to the earth's surface is constant so it seems to hover over one spot on the earth's equator.

GESTURE RECOGNITION TECHNOLOGY: The recognition of intelligent characters by electrical methods.

GHOST: To mirror, duplicate, or burn; secondary monitor or computer screen image.

GHZ (GIGAHERTZ): One billion cycles per second; measures analog signal transmission.

GIGABIT: One billion bits of electronic storage capacity.

GIGABYTE: One billion bytes; GB, Gbyte, gig and G-byte.

GIGAHERTZ: One billion cycles per second; computer speed measurement unit; GHz.

GINSBURG, PAUL, PHD: President, Center for Studying Health Systems Change.

GLASER, JOHN, PHD: CIO, Partners Healthcare System.

GLITCH: A software error, communications, peripheral device, or computer system malfunction.

GLOBAL DOMAIN NAME: Top three include: education (edu.), military (mil.), and government (gov.).

GLOBAL INFORMATION GRID (GIG): A globally connected computer information system for managing information and health data, on-demand.

GLOBAL INTERNET COMMUNICATION: Architecture systems and protocols that include e-mail, voicemail, video-mail, and videoconferencing, as well as Internet and holographic telephony, i-pod broadcasts, and so forth.

GLOBAL MEDICAL DEVICE NOMENCLATURE (GMDN): International standard for medical device descriptors.

GLOSSARY: List of terms, definitions, abbreviations, acronyms, and explanations; data dictionary; www.HealthDictionarySeries.com.

GLUE LOGIC: Computer interconnecting logic circuits.

GLYPH: Any electronic or printed character or symbol.

GNOME: Linux open source computer code licensing initiative.

GNU: Copy-left free software of the GNU foundation that must be distributed intact and with its source code included.

GNU'S NOT UNIX (GNU): A project sponsored by the Free Software Foundation that develops and maintains a complete software environment including operating system kernel and utilities, editor, compiler, and debugger; many consultants and organizations provide support for GNU software; Richard Stallman.

GNUTELLA: P2P file sharing standard protocol.

GODWIN'S (MICHAEL) LAW: Online discussion or thread that is circuitous, rambling, or meaningless.

GOLD: A CD or DVD ready to be commercially sold to the public; slang term.

GOLDBEG, MARK, MD: CMIO of Perceptive Informatics, Inc., of Waltham, MA.

GOODMAN, JOHN C.: President and CEO, National Center for Policy Analysis, father of Health Savings Accounts.

GOOGLE: Mathematical name for a very large number followed by 10 zeros.

GOOGLE©: A popular Internet search engine/director started by Larry Page and Sergey Brin of Stanford University in 1996; ranking system driven.

GOOGLE® HACKING: The use of the search engine to locate security vulnerability on the Internet, such as software vulnerabilities and misconfigurations. Although there are some sophisticated intruders who target a specific system and try to discover vulnerabilities that will allow them access, the majority of intruders start out with a specific software vulnerability or common user misconfiguration that they already know how to exploit, and simply try to find or scan for systems that have this vulnerability; Google© is of limited use to the first attacker, but invaluable to the second; cracking.

GOOGLE® WACK: A word so obscure that it is found on only one indexed Web page after engine search.

GOOGLE WRITELY©: An Internet-based word processing tool.

GOPHER: Virtually obsolete menu-driven text and document retrieval system that predates Graphical User Interface (GUI) architecture; old HTML protocol; gopher server, gopher site; a predecessor to the World Wide Web using a method of storing and retrieving text and software files on the Internet; more user friendly than FTP, but less so than the Web.

GOSLING, JAMES, PHD: Father of the Java programming language whose achievements include engineering the news window system and the original Unix Emacs; researcher at Sun labs whose primary interest is software development.

GOTCHA: A computer system "feature" that leads to mistakes; slang term.

GOULDE, MICHAEL: Author of the downloadable seminal white paper "Open-Source Software: A Primer for Healthcare Providers" (Forrester Research).

GOYAL, PAWAN, MD, MHA: Electronic Data Systems (EDS) Functional Analyst for Healthcare Information Technology.

GRANDFATHER TAPE: A computer system back-up that is two generations older than the current health or other input data; slang term.

GRANGER, RICHARD: CIO, National Health Service, United Kingdom.

GRANULARITY: Level of specific information and discrete data detail; drill down; course-to-more fine medical data or information.

GRAPHIC: Computer screen arrangement of lines, bars, details, and so forth, to symbolize a picture or image; software programs to create, use, and edit pictures, for example, Adobe Photoshop® and Paint Shop Pro®.

GRAPHICAL INTERCHANGE (INTERFACE) FORMAT (GIF): An image style generated specifically for computer use as its resolution is usually very low, making it undesirable for printing purposes; a common medical graphics or radiology image file commonly used on the Web that is most effective when the graphic or image is not a photograph or X-ray.

GRAPHICAL USER INTERFACE (GUI): The use of window screens and graphic icons and a mouse, pointer, or other input device to issue commands to a computer operating system; post-dates DOS command line demand entry.

GRAY, WILLIAM: Deputy Commissioner of Systems for the U.S. Social Security Administration.

GRAY SCALE: A file created by electronically scanning a continuous tone original and saving the information as shades of gray; also, an image containing a series of tones stepped from white to black; refers to the quantity of various tones or levels of gray that can be stored and displayed by a computer system; the number of gray levels, or gray scale, is directly related to the number of bits used in each pixel, with the number of gray levels doubling for each added bit; for example, there are 64 gray levels in a 6 bits system, 128 gray levels for 7 bits, 256 gray levels for 8 bits, and so forth.

GRAY SCALE MONITOR: A visual display with varying shades of gray, extending up to thousands, making it capable of displaying an image; a monochrome monitor.

GREENBERG, ROSS: Creator of one of the first commercial anti-virus programs; Flu_Shot©, in 1987.

GREENES, ROBERT A., MD, PHD: Medical Informaticist at Harvard Medical School.

GREEN PC: An energy limiting electronic device or computer; slang term.

GRID COMPUTING: The use of many separate but connected computers to solve large scale enterprise-wide problems; networked computers.

GRIEFER: One who goes online to participate in chat rooms, newsgroups, or other collaborative activities for the purposes of causing misery; slang term.

GROK: To understand and appreciate; coined by Robert A. Heinlein; slang term.

GROKSTER: An online file sharing service found liable for copyright violations in 2005.

GROUP: Collection of program items within the Windows® OS Program Manager.

GROUPER: The automatic assignment of medical reimbursement based on clinical codes.

GROUPWARE: Computer software applications that are linked together by networks, allowing health care workers to share electronic communications and documents.

GRUNGE: Dead, incorrect, or obsolete computer code, medical, health, or other database information; slang term.

GUEST: The common name for a newsgroup; wiki, BBS, and so forth; generic account; generic name.

GUILTYWARE: A software program or online application that repeatedly asks for information, donations, and so forth; nagware; slang term.

GUNK: Anything that degrades a computer systems performance or security; adware, spy ware, cookies, and so forth; slang term.

GURU SITE: A powerful or otherwise popular Web site created by a single expert authority; slang term.

GUTTER: The white space between Web site, book, or newspaper columns; slang term.

GZIP: Software utility used for GNU file compression.

H

H4X: A malicious computer hacker, exploiter, or cracker; slang term.

HACK: To gain unwanted, unauthorized, unethical, and often illegal access for malicious purposes into a computer, server, or online network; hacker; hacktivist; hack attack; cracker; slang term.

HACKER: One who hacks; cracker; hack-attacker; honker; slang term; for example Legion of Doom; hacktivist; slang term.

HACK SPEAK: A type of colloquial communications where one replaces letters with numbers or other characters or symbols; hak-speak; leetspeak; slang term.

HALAMKA, JOHN, MD: The CIO of Harvard Medical School.

HALF DUPLEX: Bidirectional electronic communications that is not simultaneous; a channel of communication that is capable of both transmitting and receiving information, but only in one direction at a time.

HALF TONE: A method of generating on press or on a laser printer an image that requires varying densities or shades to accurately render the image and achieved by representing the image as a pattern of dots of varying size; larger dots represent darker areas, and smaller dots represent lighter areas of an image.

HALTING PROBLEM: The difficulty in determining if a computer system bug will terminate or continue repetition in an endless loop.

HAMMOND, EDWARD: Professor Emeritus of Biomedical Engineering, Pratt School of Engineering at Duke University.

HAMR©: Seagate Systems© technology to heat assist magnetic recordings by adding a reserve to disk casings that contains nano-tube based lubricant molecules in order to boost disk capacity by a factor of 10 while data writing to disks; about a terabyte of information.

HANDHELD PC: A pocket PC or Personal Digital Assistant (PDA) that is portable using the Windows Mobile©, Windows CE, or other condensed operating systems.

HANDLE: Identification nickname for e-mail addresses, URLs, links, files, or other types of communication; slang term.

HAND OFF COMMUNICATIONS: JCAHO recommendation for patient movement to another unit or turned over to a new nurse or doctor during a shift change, with a communication model known as SBAR—Situation, Background, Assessment, and Recommendation—adapted from a program used to quickly brief nuclear submariners.

HANDSHAKE: High squealing communication signals that establish network connectivity; slang term.

HANG: To lock, freeze, disconnect, or stop responding; slang term.

HAPTICS: Human interaction, or the sense of touch, between computer system and end user.

HARD: A permanent, fixed, real, or physically defined asset.

HARD CODE: Software code applied throughout an entire health care ERP network.

HARD CODED: Unchangeable features built into hardware or software in such a way that they cannot be modified.

HARD COPY: A traditional paper file, medical chart, or printed document.

HARD DISK: Circular sealed magnetic digital data storage device platter; speeds may exceed 15,000 RPM with higher SCSI speeds; and/or ATA (IDE, Ultra ATA, or SATA) interface.

HARD DRIVE: Electronic storage platter and area for PC contents; in Windows® contains documents and settings folder (My Documents, My Pictures©, systems and applications settings, favorites, Outlook Express©, and e-mail), program and applications file folder, and Windows folder for XP and Vista© OS.

HARD PAGE BREAK: A word processing forced page break or separation.

HARDWARE: Physical tangible components of a computer, server, or networked system; not software, programming code, or application related.

HARDWARE ADDRESS: Low level identification address burned into a PC, servers, or networked hardware device.

HARDWARE KEY: A security device to prove that a computer system is licensed; may be an alphanumeric code or string.

HARDWARE/SOFTWARE INSTALLATION MAINTENANCE AUDIT: Formal, documented procedures for (1) connecting and loading new equipment and programs; (2) periodic review of the maintenance occurring on that equipment and programs; and (3) periodic security testing of the security attributes of that hardware/software.

HARDWIRED: Physical connection to a computer or network.

HARMON, BART, MD: Deputy Director and Colonel, CMIO Medical Corps, U.S. Army.

HARMONIZATION: The prevention or elimination of technical differences in trade, traditional commerce, health care technology, e-commerce, and so forth; standardization.

HARRIS, MARTIN C., MD: CIO and Chairman of the Information Technology Division for the Cleveland Clinic Foundation.

HASH: To convert a string of computer characters into a number; encryption; hash search, hash code, hash value; slang term.

HASHEM, AHMAD, MD, PHD: Medical informatics consultant, speaker, futurist, author, and former Global Manager for Microsoft's Healthcare and Life Sciences Group; former MS-HUG© advisor; advisor with Informatics Unlimited in Maple Valley, WA.

HASHING: Encrypted security code iterative value for data intrusion alerting; slang term.

HAYMAKER, MICHAEL: Sun Microsystems, Inc.® global health care industry manager.

HCFA 1450: Health Care Financing Administration (Center for Medicare and Medicaid Service) name for the institutional uniform claim form, or UB-92.

HCFA 1500: Health Care Finance Administration's (CMS) standard form for submitting physician service claims to third party (insurance) companies.

HCFA COMMON PROCEDURAL CODING SYSTEM (HCPCS): A medical code set that identifies health care procedures, equipment, and supplies for claim submission purposes; selected for use in the HIPAA transactions; HCPCS Level I contain numeric CPT codes that are maintained by the AMA; HCPCS Level II contains alphanumeric codes used to identify various items and services that are not included in the CPT medical code set; maintained by HCFA, the BCBSA, and the HIAA; HCPCS Level III contains alphanumeric codes that are assigned by Medicaid state agencies to identify additional items and services not included in levels I or II; usually known as "local codes, and must have "W," "X," "Y," or "Z" in the first position. HCPCS Procedure Modifier Codes can be used with all three levels, with the WA–ZY range used for locally assigned procedure modifiers.

HEAD: A hardware device that reads (senses) and writes (records) health or other data on a magnetic disk (hard disk, floppy disk, tape, etc.); the writing surface of the disk or tape is moved past the read/write head and by discharging electrical impulses at the appropriate times, bits are recorded as tiny, magnetized spots of positive or negative polarity; when reading, the surface is moved past the read/write head, and the bits that are present induce an electrical current across the gap.

HEADER: Early, introductory, or preceding health, medical data, or other information; usually on a Web page or file.

HEALTH AND HUMAN SERVICES (HHS): The federal government department that has overall responsibility for implementing HIPAA.

HEALTH CARE: Medical services or supplies related to the health of an individual; Health care includes, but is not limited to preventive, diagnostic, therapeutic, rehabilitative, maintenance, mental health, or palliative care and sale or dispensing of a drug, device, equipment, or other item in accordance with a prescription.

HEALTH CARE CLEARINGHOUSE: A public or private entity that performs functions including, but not limited to, billing services, re-pricing companies, community health management information systems, or community health information systems; and "value-added" networks and switches are health care clearinghouses if they perform these functions: (1) Processes or facilitates the processing of information received from another entity in a nonstandard format or containing nonstandard data content into standard data elements or a standard transaction; (2) Receives a standard transaction from another entity and processes or facilitates the processing of information into nonstandard format or nonstandard data content for a receiving entity; HIPAA protocol.

HEALTH CARE CODE MAINTENANCE COMMITTEE: An organization administered by Blue Cross Blue Shield of America that is responsible for maintaining certain coding schemes used in the X12 transactions; includes the Claim Adjustment Reason Codes, the Claim Status Category Codes, and the Claim Status Codes.

HEALTH CARE COMMON PROCEDURAL CODING SYSTEM (HCCPCS): Medicare and other payer codes to describe medical procedures and supplies for payment:

- Level I CPT: Payment for a wide spectrum of medical services and procedures
- Level II CPT: Alphanumeric and initiated by a single letter with four numbers
- Level III CPT: Local and regional codes phased out in 2003
- CDT: Current Dental Terminology codes
- Health standards for CPT codes; noncovered equipment, supplies, services, and modifiers developed by CMS; and the local codes of Medicare B carriers

HEALTH CARE COMMON PROCEDURAL CODING SYSTEM MODIFIERS: Codes that identify or augment circumstances that change HCPCS supply or medical service descriptions for payment.

HEALTH CARE FINANCIAL MANAGEMENT ASSOCIATION (HFMA): An organization for the improvement of the financial management of health care–related organizations; CMS.

HEALTH CARE FINANCING ADMINISTRATION (HCFA): The former name for the agency within the Department of Health and Human Services that administers federal health financing and related regulatory programs, principally the Medicare, Medicaid, and Peer Review Organization; maintains the UB-92 institutional EMC format specifications, the professional EMC NSF specifications, and specifications for various certifications and authorizations used by the Medicare and Medicaid programs; maintains the HCPCS medical code set and the Medicare Remittance Advice Remark Codes administrative code set; now CMS.

HEALTH CARE INFORMATICS (HI): The scientific management of health data and information using secure electrical means.

HEALTH CARE INFORMATION: Personal, medical, and financial information obtained from patients, health care providers, payers, and third party intermediaries, as a result of a clinical encounter; protected health care information (PHI).

HEALTH CARE INFORMATION FRAMEWORK (HIF): A high level and logical electrical model of health care for a modern delivery system.

HEALTH CARE INFORMATION INFRASTRUCTURE (HCII): A subset of the National Information Infrastructure (NII).

HEALTH CARE INFORMATION MANAGEMENT SYSTEMS SOCIETY (HIMSS): A professional organization for health care information, CIOs, CTOs, and management systems professionals; based in Chicago, Illinois.

HEALTH CARE INFORMATION STANDARDS PLANNING PANEL (HCISPP): Established by ANSI to coordinate the evolution of standards using standard-setting organizations in health care.

HEALTH CARE LEADERSHIP COUNCIL: Consortium of chief executives of the country's largest health care organizations who are pressing for new rules to allow medical groups to share their expertise and investments in electronic records with doctors' offices and CEs.

HEALTH CARE OPERATIONS: Includes any of the following activities:

- conducting quality assessment and quality improvement activities.
- reviewing the competence or qualifications of health care professionals.
- evaluating practitioner and provider performance, health care plan performance, and conducting training programs of nonhealth care professionals, accreditation, and certification, licensing, or credentialing activities.
- underwriting, premium rating, and other activities relating to the creation, renewal, or replacement of a contract of health insurance or health benefits and ceding, securing, or placing a contract for reinsurance of risk relating to claims for health care.

- conducting or arranging for medical review, legal services, and auditing functions including fraud and abuse detection and compliance programs.
- business planning and development, such as conducting cost-management and planning-related analyses related to managing and operating the entity, including formulary development and administration, development, or improvement of methods of payment or coverage policies.
- business management and general administrative activities of the entity.

HEALTH CARE ORGANIZATIONS: Financial Management Strategies: Two volume, quarterly health economics, IT, and institutional management periodical that

promotes and integrates academic and applied research, and serves as a multi-disciplined forum for the dissemination of economic, financial management, and health administration information to all healthcare organizations; both emerging and mature. Its goal is to be the pre-eminent interpretive guide for financial management strategies, and the enduring business analytics guide for all healthcare organizations; and to promote related enterprise-wide health economics initiatives. (www.HealthCareFinancials.com)

HEALTH CARE OVERSIGHT: An agency or authority of the United States, or a political subdivision of a state, or a person or entity acting under a grant of authority from such public agency that is authorized by law to oversee the health care system or government programs in which health information is necessary to determine eligibility or compliance, or to enforce civil rights laws for which health information is relevant; health care auditor.

HEALTH CARE PLAN: An individual or group plan that provides, or pays the cost of, medical care; includes:

- a group health care plan (created pursuant to the Employee Retirement Income Security Act of 1974 [ERISA]);
- a health insurance issuer;
- an HMO;
- Part A or Part B of the Medicare program;
- the Medical Assistance program;
- an issuer of a Medicare supplemental policy;
- an issuer of a long-term-care policy, excluding a nursing home fixed-indemnity policy;
- an employee welfare benefit plan;
- the health care program for active military personnel;
- Veterans Administration health care program;

- Civilian Health and Medical Program of the Uniformed Services (CHAMPUS);
- Indian Health Service program under the Indian Health Care Improvement Act;
- Federal Employees Health Benefits Program;
- an approved State child health care plan; and
- the Medicare+Choice program. A high-risk pool that is a mechanism established under State law to provide health insurance coverage or comparable coverage to eligible individuals.

HEALTH CARE PROVIDER: A provider of medical services and any other person or organization who furnishes, bills, or is paid for health care in the normal course of business and who transmits any health information in electronic form in connection with a covered function; physician, dentist, podiatrist, osteopath, optometrist, psychologist, nurse, or other allied health care provider, and so forth.

HEALTH CARE PROVIDER TAXONOMY COMMITTEE: An organization administered by the NUCC that is responsible for maintaining the Provider Taxonomy coding scheme used in the X12 transactions; also done in coordination with X12N/TG2/WG15.

HEALTH CARE STANDARDS LANDSCAPE: A repository (prototype) that provides information on health care standards, medical standards development organizations, and health organizations that use or implement health care and related IT and similar standards.

HEALTH CARE TECHNICAL SERVICE (HCTS): A national organization and structure that supports the technology used in the delivery of health care.

HEALTH CARE TECHNOLOGY ASSESSMENT (HCTA): The systematic evaluation of properties, effects, and impacts of health care technology; may address the direct, intended consequences of technologies as well as their indirect, unintended consequences; its purpose is to inform technology-related policymaking in health care; conducted by interdisciplinary groups using explicit analytical frameworks drawing from a variety of methods.

HEALTH CARE TECHNOLOGY PACKAGE (HCTP): The range of input needs to be addressed if technology is to be successfully transferred into the health care environment, including: management and planning, allocation of financial resources, selection of technology, procurement, preparation for technology use, continued operation, maintenance and repair, personnel, training, technology assessment and research and development, and local production.

HEALTH CLAIM ATTACHMENT: Additional medical or clinical information submitted with a primary claim or invoice for reimbursement.

HEALTH DICTIONARY SERIES© (HDS©): First conceived as an ambitious and much needed project by the Institute of Medical Business Advisors Inc. (iMBA) in 2006, the illustrated Health Dictionary Series™ contains more than 50,000 entries in four volumes; electronically coupled as an interactive Wiki with iMBA's *Collaborative Lexicon Query Service®*; a social network to maintain continuous subject-matter health expertise and peer-reviewed user input (www.HealthDictionarySeries.com).

HEALTH INDUSTRY BUSINESS COMMUNICATIONS COUNCIL (HIBCC): A council of health care industry associations that develops technical standards used within the health care IT industry; subgroup of ASC X12.

HEALTH INFORMATICS STANDARDS BOARD (HISB): An ANSI-accredited standards group that has developed standards for possible HIPAA inclusion.

HEALTH INFORMATION (HI): Any medical or related administrative information, whether oral or recorded in any form or medium, that is created or received by a health care provider, health care plan, public health authority, employer, life insurer, school or university, or health care clearinghouse; or relates to the physical or mental health or condition of an individual, the provision of health care to an individual, or payment for the provision of health care to an individual.

HEALTH INFORMATION EXCHANGE (HIE): Commonly used to describe a RHIO as its precursor and used interchangeably with RHIOs.

HEALTH INFORMATION MANAGEMENT SYSTEMS SOCIETY (HIMSS): A health care industry membership organization exclusively focused on providing leadership for the optimal use of health care information technology and management systems for the betterment of human health; founded in 1961 with offices in Chicago, Washington, D.C., and other locations across the country, HIMSS represents more than 14,000 individual members and some 220 member corporations that employ more than 1 million people. HIMSS frames and leads health care public policy and industry practices through its advocacy, educational, and professional development initiatives.

HEALTH INFORMATION STANDARDS BOARD (HISB): ANSI subcommittee for all those interested in developing HIT and medical data transmission standards.

HEALTH (HOSPITAL) INFORMATION SYSTEMS (HIS): The enterprise-wide computer networking system for the gathering, manipulation, verification, dissemination, retrieval, and storage of medical and PHI.

HEALTH (HOSPITAL) INFORMATION TECHNOLOGY (HIT): The application of information processing involving both computer hardware and software that deals with the storage, retrieval, sharing, and use of health care information, medical data, and knowledge for communication and decision making.

HEALTH INFORMATION TECHNOLOGY AUDITOR (HITA): An expert who evaluates a health organization's computer systems to ensure the proper safeguards are in place to protect and maintain the integrity of the firm's data. While the position has existed since the mid-1960s, companies that previously employed just a handful of HIT auditors are now significantly adding to their ranks, sometimes doubling, tripling, or quadrupling current staff levels; much current demand is due to the Sarbanes-Oxley Act and other legislation aimed at improving corporate governance in the wake of major accounting scandals earlier in the decade; publicly traded hospital systems require the expertise of HIT auditors to meet ongoing compliance requirements; the Gramm-Leach-Bliley Act and the Health Insurance Portability and Accountability Act (HIPAA), among other regulations, also are fueling the need for HIT auditors. Health IT auditors must have a general understanding of accounting principles and the strategic vision to ensure a health organization's HIT systems allow it to achieve its short- and long-term objectives. Many hospitals promote from within for this role. Health facilities which look outside the organization for these professionals usually seek candidates with experience, knowledge of health care of emerging technologies and issues, and increasingly, certifications such as the certified information systems auditor (CISA) designation.

HEALTH INFORMATION TECHNOLOGY PROMOTION ACT (HITPA): Legislation to accelerate the adoption of interoperable electronic health records by ensuring uniform standards, championed by Rep. Nancy Johnson, R-Conn (H.R. 4157), which would: codify the Office of the National Coordinator for Health Information Technology in statute and delineate its ongoing responsibilities; create exceptions to the fraud and abuse statutes to allow certain providers to fund health information technology equipment and services for other providers; and provide for a study of federal and state health privacy policies.

HEALTH INSURANCE ASSOCIATION OF AMERICA (HIAA): An industry association that represents the interests of commercial health care insurers; participates in the maintenance of some HIPAA code sets, including the HCPCS Level II codes.

HEALTH INSURANCE ISSUER: 2791(b)(2) of the PHS Act, 42 U.S.C. 300gg-91(b)(2) Any insurance company, insurance service, or insurance organization (including an HMO) that is licensed to engage in the business of insurance in a State and is subject to State law that regulates insurance; does not include a group health plan.

HEALTH INSURANCE PORTABILITY AND ACCOUNTABILITY ACT (HIPAA): Also known as the Kennedy-Kassebaum Act of 1996, HIPAA is federal legislation that mandates the electronic: (1) connectivity, (2) transmission, (3) storage/retrieval, and (4) confidentiality of health care information for all covered entities (CE). The shift to Electronic Data Interchange (EDI) was planned by the federal government and the Health Care Financing Administration for more than a decade; its goal is to reduce the 17% administrative cost of health care through the standardization of electronic transactions into a single format, replacing the 400-plus disparate platforms previously used. For purposes of HIPAA, the definition of a covered entity includes three classes:

- Individual health care providers, pharmacies, hospitals, skilled nursing facilities (SNFs), and home health care agencies.
- Medicare, Medicaid, insurance companies, HMOs, MCOs, and other health plans.

Health care vendors, clearinghouses, billing firms, Internet service providers (ISPs), Web servers, and hosting companies, as well as computer software and hardware companies and other third-party vendors facilitating EDI. Full implementation of the EDI components of HIPAA occurred in August 2005 with the following updates for 2006–2008:

- April 2006: Security compliance for small health plans who must meet HHS standards for the administrative, technical, and physical security of electronic health records (EHRs).
- May 2007: National Provider Identifier (NPI) for all covered entities except small health plans.
- May 2008: National Provider Identifier (NPI) for small health plans presenting a unique identifying number to be used by all insurers and health care organizations.

Although nonpunitive in nature, civil penalties may be as high as $100 per violation, with a cap of $25,000 per year. Criminal penalties include fines of up to $250,000 and/or imprisonment for up to 10 years (Table 6).

HEALTH IT RISKS: The net medical mission/ health care business impact (probability of occurrence combined with impact) from a particular threat source exploiting, or triggering, a particular information technology vulnerability. Information technology related uncertainties risks arise from legal liability or mission/business loss due to:

- unauthorized (malicious, nonmalicious, or accidental) disclosure, modification, or destruction of information;

Table 6: HIPAA Standards Compliance Calendar

Standard	Publication of NPRM	Publication of Final Rule	Effective Date	Compliance Date
Privacy Rule	11/03/1999*	12/28/2000*	02/26/2001	04/14/2003
Privacy Modifications	03/27/2002*	08/14/2002*	10/15/2002	04/14/2003
Transaction and Code Sets (TCS) Rule	05/07/1998*	08/17/2000*	10/16/2000	10/16/2003**
TCS Implementation Guide Addenda	05/31/2002*	02/20/2003*	03/20/2003	10/16/2003
TCS Modifications	05/31/2002*	02/20/2003*	03/20/2003	10/16/2003
TCS Modifications	January 2007			
HIPAA Code Sets Revisions	February 2007			
Security Rule	08/12/1998*	02/20/2003*	04/21/2003	04/21/2005
National Employer Identifier Rule	06/16/1998*	05/31/2002*	07/30/2002	07/30/2004
National Provider Identifier Rule	05/07/1998*	01/23/2004*	05/23/2005	05/23/2007
Interim Enforcement Rule; expired 03/16/2006	N/A	04/17/2003*	05/19/2003	05/19/2003
Enforcement Rule—Final	04/18/2005*	02/16/2006*	03/16/2006	03/16/2006
Electronic Signature Rule	08/12/1998*			
National Health Plan Identifier Rule	On hold			
Claims Attachment Rule	09/23/2005*	09/2008	TBD	TBD

(Continued)

Table 6: HIPAA Standards Compliance Calendar (*Continued*)

First Report of Injury Rule	TBD
National Individual Identifier Rule	On hold

* Denotes the actual publication date. All other NPRM (Notice of Proposed Rule-making) dates are expected publication dates.
** Compliance was required by October 16, 2002 for the TCS rule. CDHS filed for an extension under the Administrative.

- nonmalicious errors and omissions;
- IT disruptions due to natural or man-made disasters; and
- failure to exercise due care and diligence in the implementation and operation of the health care informatics.

HEALTH LEVEL SEVEN (HL7): An international community of health care subject matter experts and information technology physicians and scientists collaborating to create standards for the exchange, management, and integration of protected electronic health care information; the Ann Arbor, Mich.–based Health Level Seven (HL7) standards developing organization has evolved Version 3 of its standard, which includes the Reference Information Model (RIM) and Data Type Specification (both ANSI standards); HL7 Version 3 is the only standard that specifically deals with creation of semantically interoperable health care information, essential to building the national infrastructure; HL7 promotes the use of standards within and among health care organizations to increase the effectiveness and efficiency of health care delivery for the benefit of all patients, payers, and third parties; uses an Open System Interconnection (OSI) and high level seven health care electronic communication protocol that is unique in the medical information management technology space and modeled after the International Standards Organization (ISO) and American National Standards Institute (ANSI); each has a particular health care domain such as pharmacy, medical devices, imaging, or insurance (claims processing) transactions. Health Level Seven's domain is clinical and administrative data. Goals include:

- develop coherent, extendible standards that permit structured, encoded health care information of the type required to support patient care, to be exchanged between computer applications while preserving meaning;

- develop a formal methodology to support the creation of HL7 standards from the HL7 Reference Information Model (RIM);
- educate the health care industry, policymakers, and the general public concerning the benefits of health care information standardization generally and HL7 standards specifically;
- promote the use of HL7 standards worldwide through the creation of HL7 International Affiliate organizations, which participate in developing HL7 standards and which localize HL7 standards as required;
- stimulate, encourage, and facilitate domain experts from health care industry stakeholder organizations to participate in HL7 to develop health care information standards in their area of expertise;
- collaborate with other standards development organizations and national and international sanctioning bodies (e.g., ANSI and ISO) in both the health care and information infrastructure domains to promote the use of supportive and compatible standards; and
- collaborate with health care information technology users to ensure that HL7 standards meet real-world requirements and that appropriate standards development efforts are initiated by HL7 to meet emergent requirements.

HL7 focuses on addressing immediate needs but the group dedicates its efforts to ensuring concurrence with other U.S. and International standards development activities. Argentina, Australia, Canada, China, Czech Republic, Finland, Germany, India, Japan, Korea, Lithuania, The Netherlands, New Zealand, Southern Africa, Switzerland, Taiwan, Turkey, and the United Kingdom are part of HL7 initiatives.

HEALTH MAINTENANCE ORGANIZATION (HMO): A legal corporation that offers health insurance and medical care. HMOs typically offer a range of health care services at a fixed price (see capitation); types of HMOs include:

- Staff Model—Organization owns its clinics and employs its doctors.
- Group Model—Contract with medical groups for services.
- IPA Model—Contract with an IPA that contracts individual physicians.
- Direct Contract Model—Contracts directly with individual physicians.
- Mixed Model—Members get options ranging from staff to IPA models.

2791(b)(3) of the PHS Act, 42 U.S.C. 300gg-91(b)(3) means a federally qualified HMO, an organization recognized as an HMO under State law, or a similar organization regulated for solvency under State law in the same manner and to the same extent as such an HMO.

HEALTH (HOSPITAL) MANAGEMENT INFORMATION SYSTEM (HMIS): Computerized data-gathering, collating, and reporting system for management indicators throughout the health care industrial complex.

HEALTH OVERSIGHT AGENCY: Any person or entity acting under the authority of the federal government, state, region, or political subdivision to oversee the health care system of enforcement, relevancy, or health information rights, and so forth; HHS, OCR, CMS, and so forth.

HEALTH PLAN: An individual or group that provides or pays the cost of medical care (2791(a)(2) of the PHS Act, 42 U.S.C. 300gg-91(a)(2)), and includes the following, individually or collectively:

- a group health plan,
- a health insurance issuer,
- an HMO,
- Part A or Part B of the Medicare program under title XVIII of the Act,
- Medicaid program under title XIX of the Act, 42 U.S.C. 1396,
- an issuer of a Medicare supplemental policy (as defined in section 1882(g)(1) of the Act, 42 U.S.C. 1395ss(g)(1)),
- an issuer of a long-term care policy, excluding a nursing home fixed-indemnity policy,
- an employee welfare benefit plan or any other arrangement that is established or maintained for the purpose of offering or providing health benefits to the employees of two or more employers,
- the health care program for active military personnel under title 10 of the United States Code,
- Veterans Administration health care program under 38 U.S.C. Chapter 17,
- Civilian Health and Medical Program of the Uniformed Services (CHAMPUS) (10 U.S.C. 1072(4)),
- Indian Health Service program under the Indian Health Care Improvement Act, 25 U.S.C. 1601, et seq,
- Federal Employees Health Benefits Program under 5 U.S.C. 8902,
- an approved State child health plan under title XXI of the Act, providing benefits for child health assistance that meet the requirements of section 2103 of the Act, 42 U.S.C. 1397,
- Medicare + Choice program under Part C of title XVIII of the Act, 42 USC 1395 w-21 through 1395w-28,
- a high-risk pool that is a mechanism established under State law to provide health insurance coverage or comparable coverage to eligible individuals, and

- any other individual or group plan, or combination of individual or group plans, that provides or pays for the cost of medical care (as defined in section 2791(a)(2) of the PHS Act, 42 U.S.C. 300gg-91(a)(2).

HEALTH RECORD NUMBER: Unique alphanumeric identifier assigned to a patient chart or other medical record.

HEALTH RECORD OWNERSHIP: Legal theory suggesting that the health entity owns a medical record, but the patient has certain rights of control and confidentiality.

HEALTH SCIENCE LIBRARIAN: One who administers or manages a medical library.

HEAP: A block of computer program or reserved application memory not yet given a formal use.

HEAVY BROADBAND: Commercial users of massive amounts of broadband communications networks such as EarthLink©, Amazon, eBay©, Google©, and Microsoft©; slang term.

HEDIC: Healthcare Electronic Data Interchange Coalition and nonprofit association for the collaborative improvement of electronic business (EBusiness) efficiencies in the health care industry; promotes the use of compatible electronic data processes, standards, and rules to automate information sharing and transactions between trading partners with minimum human intervention.

HEEKIN, MICHAEL, JD: Chair, Health Information Infrastructure Advisory Board, FL.

HEISENBURG: An application or computer program bug that alters its affectations upon discovery or investigation; humorous term.

HELLMAN, MARTIN E., PHD: Professor Emeritus of Electrical Engineering, Stanford University, and best known for his invention, with Diffie and Merkle, of public key cryptography as the basis for secure transactions on the Internet and related computer privacy issues.

HELLO-WORLD: A computer program or application that merely greets the user with a singular salutation to demonstrate functionality; humorous term.

HELMS, DAVID W., PHD: President and CEO of Academy Health, Inc.

HELP: A computer system assistance button, key, or function; onscreen; online or live.

HELP DESK: Administrative, financial, technical, or customer/patient support for a PC, server, network, or other online encounter; hardware, software, or peripheral electronic components.

HENDRICKS, CARL: CIO for the Military Health Systems, DoD.

HERTZ (HZ): Channel speed meter for a Central Processing Unit (microchip); one cycle per second unit of frequency; bits per second.

HEURISTIC: Intelligent trial and error; gut feelings.

HEWLETT-PACKARD©: A leading manufacturer of computers and printers, based in Palo Alto, CA.

HEXADECIMAL: Base 16 number system that represents 4 bits per digit; A–F letters and 0–9 digits to represent 10–15 digits.

HIBERNATE: To power-down and temporarily suspend computer system operations; sleep mode; slang term.

HICOM®: Algorithm-based survey that provides answers to more than 400 questions dealing with mandatory HIPAA compliance privacy, transaction code sets, and security areas; HIPAA Compliance; Duane Morris, LLP.

HIDDEN FILE: User-concealed data usually present only on the operating system.

HIDDEN LAYER: Neurons clocked and located between input and output neurons in a neural computer network.

HIDE: To briefly remove an onscreen computer system display.

HIEB, BARRY, MD: Research Director for Gartner Healthcare and member of ASTM-E.31.

HIERARCHY: The arrangement of computer routing levels; hierarchical file system; hierarchical menu, and so forth.

HIESTER, GEORGE, MD: Medical director and COO of Midcoast Care, an independent physician practice association in Santa Maria, CA.

HIGH-DEFINITION TELEVISION (HDTV): A television system with 1125 lines of horizontal resolution, with the ability of creating high-quality video images.

HIGH-DEFINITION VIDEO OVER NET (HDVON): High-bandwidth connections and compression formats, such as H.264, which make radiology images and video over the Internet possible.

HIGH DENSITY MEDIA INTERFACE: A method used to link high-definition video components and graphics cards to a PC, radiology, or HDTV monitor; teleradiology and imaging enhancement.

HIGH DYNAMIC-RANGE DISPLAY (HDRD): Brightside Technology DR37-P providing a full range of digital colors and shades, for telemedicine, imaging, and radiology.

HIGH LEVEL LANGUAGE: Computer language that combines several PC languages into a single abstracted instruction set; BASIC©, Pascal©, C, JAVA©, and so forth.

HIGH LIGHT: A color coded and/or selected computer item, file, or application activated for further use.

HIGH-PERFORMANCE COMPUTING AND COMMUNICATIONS (HPCC): A program of research coordinated by the Federal Government focused on research and development, created to expedite the introduction and use of the next generation of high-performance computer systems; especially for health care and HI.7 initiatives.

HIGH RESOLUTION DISPLAYS UNLIMITED COLORS (HRDUC): Medical imaging technology developed by the Institute of Technology in Zurich that can reproduce the entire visible spectrum of light.

HIJACK: The ability to use one's IT talents, or malicious software that takes over a computer or network browser; usually in order to redirect the user to pay-per-click search engines; hijackware.

HIJACKER: One who hijack's computer systems; cracker; exploit; sploit; hijackware.

HINT: Digitally encoded information for computer printing output; slang term.

HIPAA ACCOUNTABLE ORGANIZATIONS: Office of Civil Rights within the Department of Health and Human Services (DHHS) regulates privacy rules; while security and EDI rules are regulated by the Centers for Medicare and Medicaid Services (CMS).

HIPAA COMPLIANT: Following the HIPAA standards of 1996 for health data and information electronic interchange.

HIPAA COSTS: All the direct and indirect expenses associated with the Health Insurance Portability and Accountability Act, such as:

- HIPAA Privacy Official Costs: The final rules required covered entities to designate a privacy official who will be responsible for the development and implementation of privacy policies and procedures; the primary cost affiliated with this function was the personnel-hours to train and to develop detailed policies and procedures, as well as the oversight management such as coordinating between departments, evaluating procedures, and assuring compliance; depending on the size of the hospital or covered entity, and the diversity of activities involving privacy issues, staff involved with privacy related issues will need to devote several hours per week to ensure compliance with this effort.
- HIPAA Internal Complaints Costs: The Privacy Rule required that each hospital and covered entity have an internal process to allow an individual to file a complaint concerning the covered entity's compliance with its privacy policies and procedures; requires covered entities and hospitals to designate a contact person who is responsible for receiving and documenting the complaint as well as the disposition.
- HIPAA Disclosure Tracking and History Costs: The Privacy Rule that required hospitals, covered entities, and providers to produce a record of all disclosures of protected health information, except for such items as treatment, payment, health care operations, or disclosures to individuals; required the documentation of a note in the electronic or manual record of when, to whom, and what information was disclosed, as well as the purpose of the disclosure; hospitals must provide an accounting of disclosures to the patient, if requested; a rare occurrence.

- HIPAA De-identification of Certain Information Costs: Hospitals and covered entities are required to assess what information needs to be de-identified, such as information related to driver's license numbers, specific age, and research data; required hospitals to review and modify existing agreements or reprogram automated systems to remove key information that needed to be excluded.
- HIPAA Policy and Procedures Development Costs: Required covered entities and hospitals to develop policies and procedures to establish and maintain compliance with the regulation, such as copying medical records or amending records.
- HIPAA Training Costs: The privacy regulation provided each hospital or covered entity with a great deal of flexibility in developing training programs for its staff; each hospital's training program varied based on the size of the facility, number of staff, types of operations, worker turnover, and in general the experience of the workforce.
- HIPAA Notice Costs: The Privacy Regulation required each covered entity and hospital to provide a notice at each admission, regardless of how many visits an individual had to the hospital in a given year; initial cost was training the staff and the only ongoing cost was the cost related to printing the notices.
- HIPAA Consent Costs: Required that all hospitals and covered entities obtain an individual's consent for use or disclosure of protected health information for treatment, payment, or health care operations; most hospitals had already been obtaining consents from patients therefore; the only additional cost to the hospital was in changing the language in the document to conform to the rule; there is no new cost for records maintenance in that the consent form had already been filed in the paper or electronic medical record.
- HIPAA Business Associates Costs: Requires a written contract or arrangement that documents satisfactory assurance that business associates will appropriately safeguard protected health information in order to disclose it to a business associate based on such an arrangement.
- HIPAA Inspection and Copying Costs: Estimated and will continue to be a significant cost to all hospitals and covered entities; the degree of inspection and copying of medical records is not expected to change in the future; most states have given patients' rights (in varying degrees) to access medical information; the primary cost to hospitals was initially developing the procedures of what information was accessible and who had the right to request that information and the affiliated copying costs.
- HIPAA Law Enforcement/Judicial and Administrative Proceedings Costs: This provision allows disclosure of protected health information without patient authorization under four circumstances: (1) legal process or required by law; (2) to locate or identify a suspect, fugitive, material witness, or missing

person; (3) conditions related to a victim of crime; and (4) protected health information may be related to a crime committed on its premises.

HIPAA DATA DICTIONARY (HIPAA DD): A data dictionary that defines and cross-references the contents of all X12 transactions included in the HIPAA mandate; maintained by X12N/TG3.

HIPAA GROUPS: Health plans, health maintenance organizations, physicians, hospitals, pharmacies, and any organization that offers health, dental, and/ or insurances. In August of 2002, the U.S. Department of Health and Human Services (HHS) published amended regulations to HIPAA governing Standards of Privacy of individual identifiable health information. In April of 2003, the privacy rules went into effect. The Privacy Standards control the use and disclosures of protected health information (PHI) and establishes safeguards that must be achieved to protect the privacy of PHI. This includes past, present, or future physical or mental conditions of an individual or payment for health care for that individual, either in an electronic, written, or oral format. Presently, information related to treatment, payment, and health care operations, such an insurance billing, can be used and disclosed without employee authorization. Since April 2005, hospitals and covered entities must also achieve compliance in five areas:

- Administrative safeguards
- Physical safeguards
- Technical safeguards
- Organizational safeguards
- Security policies and procedures

HIPAA IMPLEMENTATION GUIDELINES: Requirements for HIPAA compliance for standard transactions set forth by the Washington Publication Company (WPC) or the National Council for Prescription Drug Programs (NCPDP).

HIPAA INTENT: Signed into law by President Clinton in 1996 was part of a broad attempt at health care reform. Its intent was:

- curtail health care fraud and abuse;
- enforce standards for health information;
- guarantee the security and privacy of health information; and
- assure health insurance portability for employed persons.

HIPAA PRIVACY RULES: Regulations mandated for the delivery of high-quality health care, because the entire health care system is built upon the willingness of individuals to share the most intimate details of their lives with their health care providers, insurers, lawyers, and so forth; the major impacts on the privacy regulation that had an effect on time and cost to the hospital are:

- defining protected health information that relates to maintaining or transmitting information;
- determining exactly when an authorization is needed by patients;
- establishing a policy and guideline for determining what parts of the health record are owned by the patient;
- ensuring that privacy procedures and agreements are adhered to and updated on a regular basis;
- mandating and assuring that all outside entities meet the same standards as the hospital; and
- determining what can and cannot be released for research.

HISTORY: A list of visited Web hypertext links as a Web browser feature.

HISTORY FOLDER: A computer file of Web sites and pages visited.

HIT: An item found using a Web site search engine or a Web site/page visit; recorded each time a Web browser display a page, a hit refers to a single access of a Web page; it is common for a user's homepage to display the number of hits it has received, and this number is used by Webmasters to determine the popularity of any given Web site and thus how much attention it should receive.

HIT ANALYSIS: Web site visitor data collection numerics for benchmarks such as hits, downloads, page views, time, clicks, and so forth.

HIVE: Computer information registry stored in a file on the computer's hard disk; located on a specified volume or in the user profiles: slang term.

H KEY CLASS-ROOT: One of the five Windows-NT© registry keys that contains object linked and embedding information (OLE).

H KEY CURRENT-CONFIG: One of the five Windows-NT© registry keys that contains current computer configuration information.

HOAX: An electronically delivered piece of misinformation; meme virus; deliberate prank, worm, trojan, urban legend; hoax virus; hoax worm.

HOLE: Any online, software, communications, or Internet security breach; bug; slang term.

HOLLOWELL, TODD A.: Director of Information Technology for the University of Chicago Hospitals.

HOLOGRAM: The reconstruction of any individual electrical component into the whole; laser image or light imprint; three dimensional visual image of health, medical, or other data or information.

/HOME: The home directory for the UNIX operating system.

HOME BREW: Computer system network, hardware, software, or peripheral devices developed by a hobbyist.

HOMELAND SECURITY PRESIDENTIAL DIRECTIVES-12 (HSPD-12): October 2006 mandate that required standard forms of identity verification for all federal employees and contractors.

HOME PAGE: A Web page or Web site point of welcome or point of entry to a series of embedded sounds, documents, images, or links.

HONEY POT: A preset security trap for malicious computer system hackers, crackers, and so forth.

HONKER: Hacker, cracker, or hijacker; Lion worm; slang term.

HOOK: Programming instructions that provide breakpoints for future expansion; may be changed to call some outside routine or function, or may be placed where additional processing is added.

HOP: Distance between one router to another router, or network system node to node; slang term.

HOP COUNT: Number of hops from one router node to another; slang term.

HOPPER, GRACE BREWSTER, PHD (1906–1992): Rear Admiral and computer scientist from Vassar College and Yale University who coined the term computer "bug" and developed the language COBOL, as a simple linguistically based computer language program.

HOSPITAL IDENTIFICATION: Unique health care entity identifier.

HOSPITAL INFORMATION SYSTEM: A secure computer system used to store and retrieve patient information and medical data; integrated computer-based system may include or be linked to laboratory and radiology information systems (LIS and RIS).

HOST: A central PC connected to terminals or a network for processing and control that acts as a source of information or signals; can refer to nearly any type of computer, such as a centralized mainframe that is a host to its terminals, a server that is acting as a host to its clients, or a desktop or networked PC that is acting as a host to its peripherals; in network architecture it is a client station (the health care user's machine) and is considered to be a host, because it is a source of health data and related information to the network (in contrast to a device such as a router or switch, which directs traffic).

HOST COMPILER: CPU system that provides services such as database management, word processing, medical, or other special programs.

HOST FILE: Text file that maps host names to IP addresses.

HOST NAME: The identifier of a specific computer network server.

HOT BACK-UP SITE: Real-time duplication of health care entities' critical IT systems stored in a remote location.

HOT BOT: Inktomi® and HotWired Inc® search engine with Slurp® Web-robot database tool.

HOT DESK: Medical office or other operational strategy that allows fewer employee desks than employees often leaving them adrift among phone and Web connections linked to specific desks.

HOTELING: Medical office or other operational strategy that allows fewer employee desks than employees through the use of VOIP and WiFi LAN access.

HOT FIX: A rapidly delivered software update or fast security patch; slang term.

HOT LINK: A continuously updated shared program connection; slang term.

HOT LIST: A compilation of electronic bookmarks or favorite URLs; slang term.

HOT MAIL®: MSFT Internet-based e-mail server launched in 1996.

HOT PLUG: To add or remove peripheral devices while a computer is still running; USB and FireWire standards support hot-plugging; slang term.

HOT SITE: An alternative backup site that contains the same equipment as found in the health care organization's actual IT center.

HOT SPOT: Specific nonsecure (surf and sip) geographic location in which an access point provides public wireless broadband network services; wireless hot spot for Wi-Fi functionality (e.g., iPas® and Boingo®).

HOT SWAP: A computer system item or device that is replaceable while running; slang term.

HOT SYNC: Palm synchronization and communication application for computer and Palm Pilot®; cable or wireless connection.

HOT ZONE: End of line word processing feature that triggers a hyphen.

HOURGLASS: Microsoft© "busy-waiting" icon.

HOVER(ING): To move the mechanical, optical, or infrared mouse pointer to a specific location of a computer screen; pointing; hover button.

HOWARD, ROBERT: The VA System's first centralized CIO.

HSIAO, WILLIAM: Researcher form Harvard University who established the relative value appropriateness of CPT codes, along with Peter Braun.

HTML: Abbreviation for HyperText Markup Language; the major language of the Internet's World Wide Web; Web sites and Web pages are written in HTML, which basically comprises a set of instructions for creating Web pages.

HTML VALIDATOR: A quality assurance program used to check Hypertext Markup Language elements for errors.

HUB: Electronic computer network communications device that divides one data channel into two or more channels; a concentrator or receptor; slang term.

HUFFMAN CODE: Statistical compression conversion method for character data into bit strings.

HUMAN COMPUTER INTERFACE: A human being-to-computer network input access device.

HUMAN FIREWALL: An employee who practices good security techniques to prevent any security attacks from passing through them.

HUMMEL, JOHN: CIO and Senior Vice-President of Information Services for Sutter Health.

HUNT AND PECK: Untrained typing or keyboard operating style; slang term.

HURD: A collection of servers that run on top of a microkernel (such as Mach) to implement different features.

HYBRID FIREWALL: Computer network security protection technology with firewall features such as circuit level proxy, packet filtering, application level proxies, and so forth, in order to protect against multidimensional attacks.

HYBRID NETWORK: A LAN, MAN, or WAN ring, star, and topology nodule computer network; computer systems network architecture.

HYBRID RECORD: A combined paper, computer system, and electronic health care chart or medical record; medical information multiple formats.

HYBRID SMART CARD: A plastic card with both optical and smart card magnetic tape storage technologies for data transference.

HYBRIS VIRUS: Self-updating e-mail attachment and Internet worm released in 2000.

HYPE CYCLE: Gartner Group flow-sheet for emerging technology stages: trigger, inflated expectations, trough of disillusionment, slope of enlightenment, and productivity plateau.

HYPERCARD: Visual tool for building hyperlinked applications.

HYPERLINK: A predefined data element link between electronic objects; basic Web site navigator; hyper media; Weblink.

HYPERTEXT: Nonlinear access language that allows entry to and through many different software applications; hyper media; coined by Ted Nelson in the 1960s for document linkage.

HYPERTEXT LINK: A link or visual aid, usually signified by highlighting, underlining, or graphics, instructs the computer to display a specific Web document; permits users to move easily within a Web site or across Web sites residing on different computers; a 'bad' link refers to one that does not work properly and will display an error message rather than the Web page the user was attempting to visit; bad links are caused because a Web site has changed location without leaving a forwarding address or because the page was simply removed from the Web.

HYPERTEXT MARKUP LANGUAGE (HTML:): Descriptive ASCII-based computer language that creates Internet hyper text documents for online display; HTML documents comprise the core of a Web site and can be identified by a .shtml or .shtm suffix.

HYPERTEXT TRANSPORT PROTOCOL (HTTP): Technology enabling hypertext link usage; the standard by which the World Wide Web operates.

HYPERTHREAD: The ability of a CPU to follow two instruction streams.

HYPERVISION: Open source language and OS from Xen© and VMware© that can run a microkernel attached to the metal of a CPU and can host virtual computers with different operating systems running next to each other.

HYPERWAVE: An Internet server that specializes in multimedia events, health, medical, or other data manipulation.

HYSTERESIS: The tendency of a computer system to operate differently depending merely on input change and/or direction.

I

I2: The Internet.

IA-16: Intel© 16-bit architecture for the 80286 CPU series.

IA-32: Intel© 32-bit architecture for the 80386, 80486, and Pentium CPU series.

IA-64: Intel© 64-bit architecture for the Itanium© microprocessor series with explicit parallel instruction computing and backward hardware capacity.

I-BAR: Mouse pointer icon shape.

IBM PC®: The first open architecture personal computer that invited third party innovation and transformed the IT and health care industry.

iBOOK: Apple® notebook computer of 1999; a portable iMAC®.

ICF LOG FILE: Internet Connection Firewall (ICF) that contains information about lost transmission packets or successful connections in time sequence, and usually in six field records: date, time, action, protocol, source IP address, and destination IP address.

ICON: A small visual image or representation used in a graphical user interface (GUI) environment to interface with a computer operating system, application, or program.

ICON: A high-level, general-purpose programming language with a large repertoire of features for processing data structures and character strings; imperative, procedural language with a syntax reminiscent of C and Pascal, but with semantics at a much higher level.

ICONIC INTERFACE: The manipulation of icons to achieve designated application, online, or computer program navigation results.

ICON NURSING: Nursing clinical and management tool.

IDENTIFICATION NAMING: In order to implement many health care IT services, it is essential that both subjects and objects be identifiable; provides the capability to uniquely identify users, processes, and information resources.

IDENTITY: Information that is unique within a security domain and that is recognized as denoting a particular entity within that domain.

IDENTITY-BASED SECURITY POLICY: A security policy based on the identities or attributes of the object (system resource) being accessed and of the subject (user, group of users, process, or device) requesting access.

IDENTITY MANAGEMENT: Policies and procedures for personal or master patient index verification.

IDEOGRAM: A symbol or character that represents an idea.

IDLE: A computer system that is in operation, but not currently in use.

IEEE 802.2–802.5: Institute of Electrical and Electronic Engineers standard for Internet IT data transmissions.

IGLEHART, JOHN: Founding Editor, *Health Affairs*.

IGNORE LIST: A table of blocked e-mail, IM, or IRC instant chat addresses.

ILLEGAL OPERATION: A computer system operation that a current user is not authorized to access or use.

iMAC®: Apple Corporation® Macintosh computer line with distinctive style and flat screened computer monitor for Internet browsing, first introduced in 1998.

IMAGE: Visual computer representation; electronic picture or icon in three file-formats: .gif, .jpeg, and .png.

IMAGE COMPRESSION: To reduce the amount of memory needed for electronic pictures by using methods such as JPEG, iVEX, MPEG, or Wavelet technology®.

IMAGE EDITOR: Software program designed for capturing, creating, editing, and manipulating radiology or other images.

IMAGE MAP: Several electronic pictures with more than one link.

IMAGE PROCESSING: Process of modifying medical data representing an image, typically to ameliorate diagnostic interpretation, using algorithms.

IMAGE SETTER: A device that uses laser light to expose film at high dpi resolution, usually 1200 dpi or higher; maximum dpi of 4000.

IMAGE TECHNOLOGY: The components of computer applications that transform documents, medical illustrations, photographs, and other health care images into data that computers and special-purpose workstations are capable of storing, distributing, accessing, and processing.

IMAGING: The process of scanning, capturing, archiving, and transmitting digital medical or other images, x-rays, CT or PET scans, and so forth.

i-MEDICAL BUSINESS ADVISORS, INC.© (iMBA, INC): Health education institution with online virtual university located in Norcross, GA; one of North America's leading professional health care consulting firms and provider of textbooks, CDs, tools, templates, and onsite and distance education for the health economics, administration, and financial management policy space; as litigation support activities increase and the cognitive demands of the global marketplace change, the firm is well positioned, with offices in five states and Europe, to meet the needs of medical colleagues, related advisory clients, and corporate customers.

IMPLANTABLE COMPUTER: A surgically placed computing device, similar to a pacemaker.

IMPLEMENTATION GUIDE (IG): A document explaining the proper use of a standard for a specific health business purpose; X12N HIPAA IGs are the primary reference documents used by those implementing the associated transactions and are incorporated into the HIPAA regulations by reference.

IMPLEMENTATION SPECIFICATION: Refers to the HIPAA guidelines published by WPS or the NCPDP.

IMPORT: To load a file from one native format to another format.

INCIDENT RESPONSE TEAM: An employee team charged with gathering and handling the digital evidence of an attack.

INCREMENTAL BACKUP: Partial file copying (back-up) since the last modification.

INDEO: Intel® technology for digital video file compression; code name.

INDEPENDENT HEALTH RECORD BANK ACT (IHRBA): Proposal that allows individual patients to view and edit their own health and medical records.

INDEPENDENT SOFTWARE VENDOR (ISV): Those smaller medical technology vendors who develop solutions using larger computer system development tools from SUN®, Oracle®, Microsoft® technology, and so forth, for the health care industry, or to showcase how organizations are using technology to enhance and transform the quality of patient care, reduce costs, streamline clinical and business processes, drive interoperability, improve productivity and workflow, enable informed decisions, and so forth:

- Clinical Records—inpatient
- Clinical Records—ambulatory
- Delivery Transformation
- Disease Surveillance
- Interoperability
- Outcomes Reporting

INDEPENDENT TELEPHONE COMPANY: A local exchange carrier that is independent of the Bell system of operating companies (BOCs); in rural locations, many of the independent telephone companies are cooperative.

INDEPENDENT VERIFIABILITY: The capability to verify the signature without the cooperation of the signer; accomplished using the public key of the signatory, and it is a property of all digital signatures performed with asymmetric key encryption.

INDEX: An organized list of health, medical, or other data; usually alphanumeric.

INDEXED COLOR: A format that contains a palette of 256 colors or less to define an image and can reduce file size while maintaining visual quality; reduction in file size makes it an ideal format for radiology multimedia or Web graphics.

INDIGO: Microsoft Corp© design tool for creating Windows Communications Foundation® (WCF) applications; code term.

INDIRECT TREATMENT RELATIONSHIP: Third party medical diagnosis, intervention, or treatment, as seen in a provider-2-provider environment; rather than a provider-2-patient environment.

INDIVIDUAL: A person or patient who is the subject of protected health information according to HIPAA statutes.

INDIVIDUALLY IDENTIFIABLE DATA (IID): Person or patient specific medical or health information.

INDIVIDUALLY IDENTIFIABLE HEALTH INFORMATION (IDHI): Information that is created or received by a covered entity; relates to the physical or mental health condition of an individual, provision of health care, or the payment for the provision of health care; identifies the individual, or there is reasonable belief that the information can be used to identify the individual.

INDUCTIVE REASONING: The process of observations leading to conclusions.

INFECTION: The presence of malicious computer code, such as virus, trojan worm, or other electronic miscreant.

INFERENCE ENGINE: The electronic matching of data to preselected information.

INFERENTIAL STATISTICS: The ability to make cohort generalizations based on sample characteristics; mathematical statistics.

INFILTRATION: Unauthorized entry into a computer, server, or network online application without detection, usually with malicious intent.

INFOBAHN: The German information superhighway; Internet.

INFOBUTTON: An on-demand computer information alerting system.

INFORMATICS: The study of the impact that technology has on people, or the science of information and information technology; refers to the creation, recognition, representation, collection, organization, transformation, communication, evaluation, and control of information in various health contexts; health informatics.

INFORMATION: Meaningful fractal data for decision support purposes; data to which meaning is assigned, according to context and assumed conventions (National Security Council, 1991).

INFORMATION ACCESS CONTROL: Established formal, documented policies and procedures for granting different levels of access to health care information; includes information on who gives authorization for access, to what types of information, and to what groups of individuals; policy should state any access limitations and ensure that users have access to information needed to perform their jobs.

INFORMATION ARCHITECTURE: A useful combination of computers, programs and applications, servers, networks, peripherals, Internet, and mainframes legacy systems.

INFORMATION ASSET: Data with organizational or enterprise benefit.

INFORMATION COMPROMISE: The degradation or disclosure of information.

INFORMATION EXTRACTION: Computer-assisted human language retrieval and ultimate interpretation.

INFORMATION HIGHWAY (SUPER): The Internet; the National Information Infrastructure; Infobahn; slang term.

INFORMATION INFRASTRUCTURE TASK FORCE (IITF): An organization, established by the Clinton Administration, and comprised of Federal agencies specializing in information and telecommunications technology development and application, with the goal of outlining and implementing a plan for the National Information Infrastructure (NII).

INFORMATION MODEL: Business concept to support a commercial health function or other system.

INFORMATION SECURITY: The effective safeguard of protected health care information; digital, analog, or paper platforms; a computer or network that is free from threats against it.

INFORMATION SYSTEMS: All the components of a network, server, or computerized knowledge management and data platform; mainframe, PC, legacy, Mac, UNIX, open source, or other; an interconnected set of health information resources under the same direct management control that shares common functionality.

INFORMATION TECHNOLOGY (IT): Processing information by use of a computer, network, or Internet; information processing industry term used after other titles such as electronic data processing (EDP), management information systems (MIS), and health information systems (HIS).

INFORMATION WARFARE: A deliberate attack in order to compromise protected health care or medical information.

INFOSEEK®: An Internet full-text search engine.

INFRARED: Invisible light with computer ports for laptop and wireless machines and printers.

INFRARED FILE TRANSFER: Wireless medical, health data, or other information file transfer.

INHERITANCE: One similar computer object defined in a slightly dissimilar fashion compared to another.

INITIALIZE: To store a health data variable, medical information segment, or other information for the first time; to prepare for use.

IN-LOOP: To have some control in a medical, health IT, or other decision-making process; slang term.

INOCULATE: To protect a computer system against worms, viruses, intruders, sploits, malicious conduct, and so forth; HIPAA security measure.

INPRISE CORPORATION®: The Borland International Company.

INPUT: Medical data or other information to be processed or manipulated.

INPUT DEVICE: An instrument that makes information available for computer or network data processing; keyboard, mouse, finger-pad, joystick, game-pad, wheel, voice recognition, and so forth.

INPUT LAYER: Input form examples and cases in a neural computer network; not networked neurons.

INPUT/OUTPUT: Transferring data between computer CPU and a peripheral device.

INPUT/OUTPUT EXPRESS: Executive Software's Automatic Data Caching utility for Open VMS.

INPUT/OUTPUT WAIT MONITOR UTILITY: A utility available from Executive Software® used to determine I/O bottlenecks on an open VMS system.

INSERTION ATTACK: The ability to connect a wireless computer client to an access point without authorization because of password authentication absence.

INSERTION POINT: Blinking vertical cursor identification and location bar within a program or application.

INSTANTIATE: To create or initialize computer systems operations.

INSTANT MESSAGE(ING) (IM): Real time instantaneous e-mail communications and conversation; text messaging from a computer, cell phone, pager, and so forth; files, voice, or video; ICQ, AOL, or Windows Messenger®; IMing; slang term.

INSTITUTE OF ELECTRICAL AND ELECTRONICS ENGINEERS (IEEE): Group that sets Ethernet or wired computer network standards.

INSTITUTE OF MEDICAL BUSINESS ADVISORS©: A leading professional health economics consulting and valuation firm and focused provider of text-books, CDs, tools, templates, and onsite and distance education for the health economics, administration, and financial management policy space (www.MedicalBusinessAdvisors.com).

INSTRUCTION: Set of characters with addresses that define a computer or network operation.

INTEGRATE: The combination of programs, applications, or archives into a functional computer system unit.

INTEGRATED CALL MANAGEMENT: Electrical system to improve the speed and efficiency of medical and health care information and support services.

INTEGRATED CIRCUIT (IC): A single silicone, germanium, or similar wafer chip that contains many millions of transistors and circuit elements; a solid state microcircuit comprised of interconnected semiconductor components diffused into a single instrument.

INTEGRATED CLIENT: Seamlessly meshed technology applications to support health care organization electronic record functionality using HL7 v3 messaging and standards and protocols.

INTEGRATED PROGRAM: A combination or suite of software applications, such as MSFT Office® 2007.

INTEGRATED SERVICES DIGITAL NETWORK (ISDN): Digital landline telephone network with channels for high-speed video and voice and data transmission over public phone lines; a completely digital telephone system, enjoying more popularity throughout the United States, that permits the integrated transmission of voice, video, and data to users at a higher speed than would be possible over typical telephone lines; provides connections to a universal network; currently requires special installation and equipment.

- ISDN: Basic Rate: 128 kbps, 64K-B channels with one 16-K channel that replaced conventional phone lines.
- ISDN: Primary Rate: 65K-B channels with one 16-K D-channel for control signaling.

INTEGRATION TESTING: To benchmark computer systems and components for use-ability, functionality, performance, and efficiency.

INTEGRITY: The security objective that generates the requirement for protection against either intentional or accidental attempts to violate data integrity (the property that data has not been altered in an unauthorized manner) or system integrity (the quality that a system has when it performs its intended function in an unimpaired manner, free from unauthorized manipulation); to determine if medical information or PHI has been accessed, altered, or tampered.

INTEGRITY CONTROLS: Security mechanism employed to ensure the validity of health information being electronically transmitted or stored.

INTEL®: A first and leading manufacturer of 8080, Z80, 4004, and 8008 CPUs, and then of PC compatible CPUs from the 8088, 8026, 8036, 846, Pentium®, Celeron®, and Centrino® series, to the Duo® and Quad-Core processor series, and so forth; Santa Clara, CA.

INTEL® 4004: Manufacturer that produced the first microprocessor chip in 1972; programmable, handled 4-bit word processor that contained 2,250 transistors; designed by engineer Marcian "Ted" Hoff; computer on a chip.

INTEL® 8086: A 16-bit microprocessor introduced in June 1978 and followed a year later with the 8088, a lower-cost and slower version; IBM® used the 8088 for its first PC.

INTEL® I386 PROCESSOR: Defined the 32-bit standard and paved the way for desktop computer virtualization in multitasking formats.

INTEL® CELERON® CPU: A 90-nanometer microprocessor built in a 478-pin package and an FC-LGA775 land package that expanded Intel's series of

CPUs into the value-priced PC market with an integrated L2 cache, fast system bus, and multimedia power.

INTEL® CENTRINO® CPU: Mobile technology laptop CPU that features fully integrated wireless LAN+ capabilities while enabling significant battery life.

INTEL® CHIP ARCHITECTURE (PROPOSED CPU CIRCUITRY DESIGNS):

- 2006: 65-nanometer; core microarchitecture
- 2007: 45-nanometer; penryn
- 2008: 45-nanometer; nehalem
- 2009: 32-nanometer; nehalem-c
- 2010: 32-nanometer; gesher

INTELLECTUAL PROPERTY: Works created by others such as books, music, plays, paintings, photographs, and so forth.

INTELLECTUAL PROPERTY LITIGATOR (IPL): An attorney diligent about protecting health or other patents, copyrights, and trademarks; previously the exclusive realm of small boutique firms, IP litigation is increasingly being handled by large national and global firms.

INTELLIGENT AGENT: A software program or utility that offers intuitive suggestions and judgments based on prior use; spiders, bots, and so forth.

INTELLIGENT HUB: A central computer network connecting device.

INTELLIGENT TERMINAL: Network or computer peripheral that allows input and output functionality.

INTEL® PROCESSORS: Central Processing Unit (CPU) list that includes:

Desktop
- Intel® Core™ Duo Processor
- Intel® Pentium® Processor Extreme Edition
- Intel® Pentium® D Processor
- Intel® Pentium® 4 Processor Extreme Edition Hyper-Threading Technology
- Intel® Pentium® 4 Processor supporting Hyper-Threading Technology
- Intel® Pentium® 4 Processor
- Intel® Celeron® D Processor
- Intel® Celeron® Processor

Laptop
- Intel® Core™ Duo processor
- Intel® Core™ Solo processor
- Intel® Pentium® M Processor
- Mobile Intel® Pentium® 4 Processor
- Intel® Celeron® M Processor

Server
- Intel® Itanium® 2 Processor
- Intel® Xeon® Processor
- Intel® Xeon® Processor MP
- Intel® Pentium® D Processor
- Intel® Pentium® 4 Processor Hyper-Threading Technology
- Intel® Pentium® 4 Processor

Work Station
- Intel® Xeon® Processor
- Intel® Pentium® D Processor
- Intel® Pentium® 4 Processor Hyper-Threading Technology
- Intel® Pentium® 4 Processor

Network
- Intel® IXP465 Network Processor
- Intel® IXP460 Network Processor
- Intel® IXP425 Network Processor
- Intel® IXP422 Network Processor
- Intel® IXP421 Network Processor
- Intel® IXP420 Network Processor
- Intel® IXP2855 Network Processor
- Intel® IXP2805 Network Processor
- Intel® IXP2400 Network Processor
- Intel® IXP2325 Network Processor
- Intel® IXP2350 Network Processor
- Intel® IXP1200 Network Processor

Wireless
- Intel® Application Processors
- Intel® Cellular Processors

Embedded
- Intel® Architecture Processors
- Intel® Xeon® Processors
- Intel® Pentium® M Processors
- Intel® Pentium® 4 Processors
- Intel® Pentium® III Processors
- Intel® Pentium® II Processors
- Intel® Celeron® M Processors
- Intel® Celeron® Processors
- Intel® Pentium® Processors MMX™ Technology

- Intel® Pentium® Processors
- Intel 486™ Processors
- Intel 386™ Processors
- Intel® 186 Processors
- Intel® Application Processors
- Intel® PXA270 Processor
- Intel® PXA255 Processor

Network Processors
- Intel® IXP465 Network Processor
- Intel® IXP460 Network Processor
- Intel® IXP425 Network Processor
- Intel® IXP422 Network Processor
- Intel® IXP421 Network Processor
- Intel® IXP420 Network Processor

I/O Processors
- Intel® IOP333 I/O Processor with XScale® Microarchitecture
- Intel® IOP332 I/O Processor with XScale® Microarchitecture
- Intel® IOP331 I/O Processor
- Intel® IOP321 I/O Processor
- Intel® IOP315 I/O Processor Chipset
- Intel® IOP310 I/O Processor Chipset
- Intel® IOP303 I/O Processor
- Intel® 80219 General Purpose PCI Processor
- Classic Intel® i960® Processors

INTERACTIVE: Immediate communication between computer/network or user and its output/input.

INTERCAP: Upper case letters in the middle of a single word.

INTEREXCHANGE CARRIER (IXC): A long-distance telephone carrier; a telephone company that carries long-distance calls.

INTERFACE: The boundary that two computer systems cross and function; hardware, software, peripheral, programs and applications, LANs, WANs, MANs, Internet, and so forth; connection between two devices; applies to both hardware and software.

INTERIX: MSFT utility application joining the Windows® and UNIX operating systems for improved functionality.

INTERLACED: An illuminated CRT screen that displays odd then even lines with noticeable motion.

INTERLACED GIF: A downloaded and optimized BITMAP file.

INTERNAL AUDIT: The in-house review of the records of system activity (for example, logins, file accesses, security incidents) maintained by a health or other organization; part of administrative procedures to guard data integrity, confidentiality, and availability on the matrix.

INTERNAL STORAGE: Electronic storage capability or device that is physically integrated with a computer or network.

INTERNATIONAL BUSINESS MACHINES© (IBM): The former industry leading mainframe computer maker of the 1950s and leading PC industry icon based in Armonk, NY, until PC division sale to Lenovo® in 2006; introduced the IBM PC in 1981.

INTERNATIONAL CLASSIFICATION OF DISEASES (ICD): A medical code set maintained by the World Health Organization (WHO), whose primary purpose is to classify causes of death; the U.S. extension, maintained by the NCHS within the CDC, identifies morbidity factors, or diagnoses; ICD-9-CM codes were selected for use in HIPAA transactions.

INTERNATIONAL CLASSIFICATION OF DISEASES, NINTH EDITION: Numeric (usually) codes used for statistical and payment reporting in the United States.

INTERNATIONAL CLASSIFICATION OF DISEASES, TENTH EDITION: Alphanumeric codes used for statistical reporting by the World Health Organization (WHO), but not the United States.

INTERNATIONAL CLASSIFICATION OF DISEASES, TENTH EDITION—CLINICAL MODIFICATION: Clinical modifications of ICD-10 codes developed for the United States.

INTERNATIONAL ORGANIZATION FOR STANDARDIZATION (ISO): An organization that coordinates the development and adoption of numerous international standards.

INTERNATIONAL ORGANIZATION FOR STANDARDIZATION / OPEN SYSTEMS INTERCONNECTIONS (ISO/OSI): A typical reference archetype for a local area network (LAN) architecture model made up of several hierarchical levels (physical, data link, network, transport, session, presentation, and application) that address LAN design, from the specification of the physical transmission medium to the abilities of user interaction with LAN services.

INTERNATIONAL TELECOMMUNICATIONS UNION (ITU): Governed by a treaty and comprised of government telecommunications agencies responsible for setting standards for radio, telegraph, telephone, and television.

INTERNATIONAL TELECOMMUNICATIONS UNION CONSULTATIVE COMMITTEE FOR TELECOMMUNICATIONS (ITUCCT): Formerly the Consultative Committee on International Telephone and Telegraph (CCITT); an international agency responsible for developing standards for telecommunications, including FAX and video coder–decoder devices.

INTERNET: Global network of interconnecting computers and systems interfaced with hypertext markup code, JAVA, or similar languages; a vast system of computers that are networked (linked together) to exchange health information and resources; the Internet makes it easy for people all over the world to communicate with each other through telephone lines or wirelessly; a shared global resource that is not owned or regulated by anyone; Internetwork.

INTERNET 2: A group of businesses, governments, and universities collaboratively working to create a high-performance next generation successor to the Internet, since 1996; based in Ann Arbor, MI.

INTERNET ADDRESS: A unique 32-bit, four-octet moniker assigned to each computer accessing the Internet.

INTERNET APPLIANCE: A single purpose non-PC device built solely for Web access and related tasks.

INTERNET BACKBONE: A group of commercial networked communication companies that provide national high-speed electronic links; National Science Foundation high-speed network; Cisco Systems®, Juniper Networks®, Lucent Technologies®, Sycamore Networks®, and so forth.

INTERNET BROWSER: Software client interface that supports messages, visuals, hyperlinks, searches, and audio information transmissions on the World Wide Web (WWW); for example, AOL, Firefox©, Mozilla©, Netscape Navigator©, and so forth.

INTERNET CAFÉ: Usually a coffee house or local pub selling Internet access or service, WiFi hotspots, and so forth.

INTERNET CONTROL MESSAGE PROTOCOL (ICMP): A computing network IP standard for control, error, and informational messaging; usually features PING command host detection functionality.

INTERNET DATAGRAM: The basic unit of digital information that passes across the Internet, with data, source, and destination information and security material.

INTERNET EXPLORER® (IE): Windows® GUI Web browser from Microsoft released in 1995; version 7.0 released in 2007; bundled with the Vista® OS, or as a free Internet download providing search functionality with sound, graphics, texts, movies, and JAVA® applets; available for UNIX and Macintosh environments.

INTERNET FAX: Facsimile server routing a digital fax server as a destination fax machine.

INTERNET KEY EXCHANGE (IKE): Network management protocol standard used with an IPS for security and authentication purposes.

INTERNET PROTOCOL (IP): Connectionless best-efforts digital packet delivery methodology for Internet access; based on the Web site's technical address, it is another way for accessing Web sites; the formal for this protocol is a four-part number, such as 206.17.253.48.

INTERNET PROTOCOL ADDRESS (IPA): The basic sequence of computer networking to locate a specific Web site (version IPv4 for 32-bit binary numbers grouped in four 8-bit octets); some are private and used only for internal networks and not into the Internet from a router.

INTERNET PROTOCOL SECURITY (IPSec): An encryption standard for Virtual Private Networks (VPNs).

INTERNET RADIO: The transmission of radio signals and waves to PCs over the Internet.

INTERNET RELAY CHAT (IRC): Real-time Internet computer conferencing by typing back and forth; "talking"; developed by Jarkko Oikarinen in 1988, IMing; a form of instant Internet communication designed for group (many-to-many) communication in discussion forums called channels, but also allows one-to-one communication; created to replace a program called MultiUser® talk on a Finnish BBS called OuluBox®; IRC chat room.

INTERNET SECURITY AND ACCELERATOR SERVICE: Security utility and SAAS from MSFT for enhanced Internet reliability and management.

INTERNET SECURITY ASSOCIATION AND KEY MANAGEMENT PROTOCOL (ISAKMP): An early precursor to IKE.

INTERNET SERVICE PROVIDER (ISP): Firm that provides Internet connectivity services to end users through an Internet dial-up connection, DSL, or cable modem, along with other services such as Web hosting, security features, domain names, and so forth; AOL, Comcast®, Microsoft®, InsideInternet©, BellSouth, Verizon®, Earthlink,® Qwest®, Net Zero©, Sympatico©, and so forth.

INTERNET SMALL COMPUTER SYSTEM INTERFACE (iSCSI). Ethernet network standard to boost data transfer speed among interconnected storage devices and computers running on traditional networks; avoiding more expensive fiber channel health data communications pipelines.

INTERNET SOCIETY: An Internet Architecture Board of members based in Reston, VA.

INTERNET TELEPHONY (IP): Digitized point-to-point telephone calls or video images (Internet TV and radio) transmitted over the Internet; VOIP; Vonage®, Skype®, and so forth.

INTEROPERABILITY: The ability of a computer to operate under different operating systems and platforms while maintaining the same functionality and interface experience; the applications used on either side of a communication, between health care partners or between internal components of a medical entity, being able to read and correctly interpret the information communicated from one to the other.

INTERPRETED LANGUAGE: Noncompiled, line-by-line, slowly functioning computer code.

INTERPRETER: High-level computer programming language that runs and translates simultaneously.

INTERPRETER RELIABILITY: Health or other data consistency between or among various abstractors.

INTERRUPT: A signal that gets the attention of the CPU and is usually generated when I/O is required; software interrupts are generated by a program requiring disk input or output; hardware interrupts are generated when a key is pressed or when the mouse is moved; control is transferred to the OS, which determines the prioritized action to be taken.

INTERSTITIAL: Pop-up Internet add between Web pages.

INTRANET: Digital communications network used solely within an organization as an enterprise-wide private application; LAN, MAN, and WAN functionality without the Internet and often used in hospital systems, HMOs, and so forth; any private health care network that uses some or all of the protocols of the Internet; intranet nodes interact in a hub–client relationship, nodes are identified by using (IP) addresses, and files are identified by universal resource locators (URLs); the health data being exchanged are typically formatted using HTML and are controlled and displayed using a browser; an intranet system may be connected to the Internet via firewalls, or it may be a totally separate schematic system, as illustrated in Figure 8.

INTRAWARE: Private health or other group middleware or software; value added program.

INTRUDER: An unauthorized or nonsecurity cleared, and usually malicious, computer system user; attacker; hacker, cracker, or honker.

INTRUSION CONTAINMENT: Detecting insecure computer or network situations in order to respond in a timely manner; effective response, isolation, and eradication.

INTRUSION DETECTION: Applications, tools, and code used to detect unauthorized and unwanted computer, server, or network break-ins or entries.

INTRUSION DETECTION SYSTEM (IDS): A type of security management system for computers and networks that gathers and analyzes information from various areas within a computer or a network to identify possible security breaches, which include both intrusions (attacks from outside the organization) and misuse (attacks from within the organization); ID uses

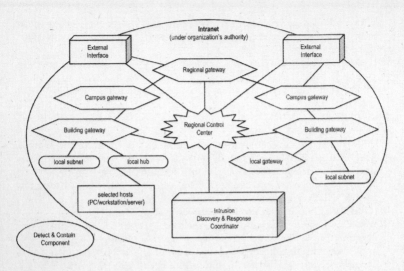

Figure 8: Health care enterprise intranet system.

vulnerability assessment (scanning), which is a technology developed to assess the security of a computer system or network.

INTRUSION PREVENTION: A preemptive approach to network security used to identify potential threats and respond to them swiftly; like ID, an intrusion prevention system (IPS) monitors network traffic, however, because an exploit may be carried out after the attacker gains access, intrusion prevention systems also have the ability to take immediate action, based on a set of rules established by the network administrator.

IOMEGA CORP®: Mass storage company and maker of portable electronic computer devices such as Zip© and Jazz© drives.

IOS: Programmable platform from Cisco Systems® that augmented computer networking and intelligence.

IOTUM: Presence management software.

IP ADDRESS: Physical binary number address of a computer TCP/IP network.

iPHONE®: Product from Apple, Inc®., that combines three products - a mobile phone, a widescreen iPod with touch controls and an Internet communications device with e-mail, Web browsing, maps- and Search — into a single device with unique multi-touch display.

I-PIX: Panoramic view image file with .ipx extension.

IP-NG: A unique 128-bit, 16-byte moniker assigned to each computer accessing the Internet; Internet protocol, next generation IP address.

IP NUMBER: Internet protocol address consisting of four numbers, separated by periods (dots).

iPOD®: A proprietary portable video and audio player from Apple Computer®; MP3 and other music file formats; Shuffle®; Jon Lech Johansen of Double Twist cracked Apple's FairPlay copy-protection technology in 2006, allowing other companies to offer content for iPods®.

IP-SEC: Minor Internet protocol (IP) encryption and authentication packet.

iPv6: Internet Protocol (IP) version 6 with improvement over version 4 (iPv4), such as better routing functionality and more addresses.

IRC CHAT WORM: Malicious IRC code infecting channels through Plug-n-Play modules in 2005.

ISM: License exempt Industrial, Scientific, and Medical radio band that is divided into 11 transmission channels in the United States and 13 in the United Kingdom.

ISO/IEC 17799: The Code of Practice for information security management is a generic set of best practices for the security of information systems and considered the foremost security specification document in the world; the code of practice includes guidelines for all organizations, no matter what their size or purpose; originally published in the United Kingdom as DT Code of Practice, and then later as BS 7799.

ISOLATION: A blind transaction that remains invisible until another transaction is executed.

ISS: Internet Security Systems®, Inc.; public company located in Atlanta that produced the Proventia© network protection software product and Real-Secure© server security system; recently acquired by IBM® to focus on end-to-end security for health care organizations and large enterprise-wide systems; Thomas Noonan CEO.

ITANIUM®: A 64-bit Intel® CPU implementing the IA-64 architecture first developed in 2001.

IT SECURITY ARCHITECTURE: A description of security principles and an overall approach for complying with the HIPAA and protection principles that drive a health care technology system design; for examples, guidelines on the placement and implementation of specific security services within various distributed computing environments.

iTUNES®: Electronic music download channel of distribution model launched by Apple Computer, Inc.® in 2001.

i-WAY: The Internet or information superhighway; i-away; slang term.

J

J#: A computer language similar to JAVA and C+.

JABBER: A random or continuous stream of medical or other transmitted computer network data transmissions; slang term.

JAGGIES: Effect caused by images or lines being rendered at too low a resolution and easily defined as a stair-stepped effect giving the line or images a rough appearance; increasing the resolution reduces the effect; slang term.

JAMMING: A wireless computer network 2.4 GHz-band shutdown attack with radio frequency interface; slang term.

JARGON FILE: The Stanford University collection of computer terms and definitions first begun in 1975, enlarged by MIT, and published as the *New Hacker's Dictionary* (MIT Press, 3rd edition, 1996), edited by Eric Raymond.

JAVA®: A powerful computer language from Sun Microsystems, Inc.©, that allows Web page and Internet interactivity across a whole host of different topologies, operating systems, languages, and software applications; Web page java virtual machine and applet production language; JavaScript is an interpreted programming language and Internet development tool; designed to have the "look and feel" of the C++ computer language, but it is simpler and enforces OOP applications that may run on a single computer, or be distributed among servers and clients in a network, or to build a small application module or applet for use as part of a Web page. Java Virtual Machine© (JVM) was introduced in 1995 and instantly created a new sense of the interactive possibilities of the Web. Both of the major Web browsers include a Java virtual machine, and almost all major operating system developers (IBM®, Lenovo®, Microsoft®, and others) have added Java compilers as part of their product offerings; JAVA applet, card, virtual machine, chip, browser, hotspot, mail page, and so forth; developed by James Gosling and code named "Oak."

JAVA BEAN: Any software component, application, or program written in the JAVA computer language; Sun Microsystems, Inc®.

JAVA CRYPTOGRAPHY EXTENSION (JCE): An application program interface that provides a uniform framework for the implementation of security features in JAVA, often using techniques such as:

- Symmetric ciphers
- Asymmetric ciphers
- Stream ciphers
- Block ciphers
- Key generation
- Key storage
- Key retrieval

- Secure streams
- Sealed objects
- Digital signatures
- Message Authentication Code (MAC) algorithms

JAVASCRIPT®: The executable commands of a Web page written in a slightly different JAVA code language combined with HTML; permits augmented functionality of, and enhancements to, a Web site; if one's browser is unable to use these languages, the enhancements or features found in the Web site will usually not be displayed; Netscape® and Microsoft® support this language.

J-CODES: A subset of the HCPCS Level II code set with a high-order value of "J" that has been used to identify certain drugs and other items; dropped from HCPCS; NDC codes are used to identify pharmaceuticals and supplies.

JIGSAW: An online electronic business contact database.

JINDAL, PAWAN, MD: Health Care Managing Consultant for Quiology® Inc.

JOILET FILE: ISO 9660 variant for CD-ROM recording made by Microsoft® to support longer file name extensions.

JOINS: A SQL database management operation performed on relationship tables combining elements into a common table.

JOINT COMMISSION ON ACCREDITATION OF HEALTHCARE ORGANIZATIONS (JCAHO): A subset of the HCPCS Level II code set with a high-order value of "J" that has been used to identify certain drugs and other items; the final codes were dropped from the HCPCS, and the NDC codes used to identify the associated pharmaceuticals and supplies.

JOINT CONSENT: An organized health care arrangement for health care Covered Entities to use and disclose PHI and IIHI for the treatment and payment of health care operations.

JOINT HEALTHCARE INFORMATION TECHNOLOGY ALLIANCE (JHITA): A health care industry association that represents AHIMA, AMIA, CHIM, CHIME, and HIMSS on legislative and regulatory issues affecting the use of health information technology.

JOINT PHOTOGRAPHIC EXPERTS GROUP (JPEG): A coding standard for transmitting and storing full color and echo grey-scale electronic images.

JONES, THOMAS M., MD: Member of HL7 and vice president and chief medical officer, Oracle Corp., Redwood Shores, CA.

JOO: The interrogative query, "you?"; slang term.

JOTSPOT: Online service provider of Wiki's, Web site services, and spreadsheets.

JOURNAL(ING): A list of the recording of all computer, server, network, and/or Internet browsing activities, such as video and e-mail, chat, Webcam functions, instant messaging, i-pod casts, and search functions.

JOY STICK: A computer game input device.

JOY, WILLIAM: Creator of the interactive UNIX format known as C-Shell, from the University of California; cofounder of Sun Microsystems, Inc®.

JPEG COMPRESSION: A generic computer algorithm that condenses and stores electronic images.

JUKEBOX: A mass storage device library of digitized music formats; slang term.

JUMPDRIVE®: A flash drive from Lexar®.

JUMP LINK: An Internet Web page that consists mainly of hyperlinks to other URLs.

JUNK FAX: Unsolicited facsimile transmissions.

JUNK MAIL: Unsolicited e-mail messages; slang term.

JYTHON®: The predecessor to Python®, a high-level, dynamic, object-oriented computer language based on JAVA®.

K

K: Kilobytes; Kb; Kbps; kilobytes per second.

K-6 CHIP: A CPU made by the AMD® Corporation in 1996, to compete with the Intel Pentium® CPU.

K-56 FLEX: Modem transmission standard of 56,600 bps, now replaced by the v90 standard.

KASPER, KARL: Touted ringleader of the formerly infamous, now often praised, security hacker organization known as the L0pht.

KB: Kilobyte; a measure of computer storage and memory capacity; equivalent to 1,024 bytes; often applied to 1,000 bytes as well.

KbPS: Kilobits per second; a measure of bandwidth and rate of data flow in digital transmission; one Kbps is 1,024 kilobits per second.

KEATON, BRIAN, MD: Director, Emergency Medicine Informatics, and Project Chair Northeastern Ohio, RHIO.

KENNEDY-KASSEBAUM BILL: The HIPAA Act of 1996.

KENTSFIED: Intel® quad-core extreme microprocessor chip series capable of executing four simultaneous threads; code name.

KERBEROS: Computer network security protection and authentication system for distributed environments and high-level applications; from MIT.

KERMIT: A health data or other information transmission protocol without using the Internet; developed by Columbia University; flexible X, Y, and Z modem.

KERNEL: The core key software component of a computer operating system (OS) that provides communication to manage files, memory resources, peripheral, and hardware devices.

KERNEL MODE TRAP: The (in)famous "blue screen of death" is a display image containing white text on a blue background generated by the Windows operating systems when suddenly terminated with an error; the system is locked up and has to be restarted; the blue screen may include hexadecimal values from a core dump (a display or printout of the contents of memory) that may help determine what caused the crash.

KETCHERSIDE, JOSEPH W., MD: Chief Medical Officer and VP of Corporate Strategies for Theradoc, Inc.

KEY: Data transmissions and input encryption controller; an input that controls the transformation of health data by an encryption algorithm (NRC, 1991); keyboard or computer button; key pair; key master.

KEYBOARD: Alphanumeric input buttons, such as a QWERTY typewriter, with function buttons, programmable keys, mice, and touch-pads; usual additions beyond the traditional typewriter include enter, control, enhance, escape, page up/down/insert/delete/home/end, arrow, and print screen buttons; keyboarding; keying.

KEY DISK: Noncopyable diskette needed to run a computer program or application; loaded disk.

KEY ESCROW: To place a cryptographic key with a trusted third party.

KEY FIELD: Each specific row in a database.

KEY-IN-KNOB LOCK: A basic lock that has the lock mechanism embedded in the knob or handle.

KEY LOG: Software that records computer keystrokes or other input information.

KEY LOGGER: One who logs computer input keystrokes.

KEY MANAGEMENT: The creation, storage, transmission, and maintenance of a secret electronic cryptographic key.

KEYSTROKE: A computer keyboard input execution; typing; keyboarding, keying.

KEYSTROKE LOGGER: A systems monitor device or small program that monitors each keystroke a user types on a specific computer's keyboard.

KEYSTROKE VERIFICATION: Data entry verification from a computer keyboard.

KEYWORD: A word assigned to a document, or in a text search, or reserved in a programming language; search engine tag; key pair; keyword master.

KILBOURNE, BRETT: Director of the United Power Line Council.

KILDALL, GARY: The first scientist to interface a disk system to a microcomputer and create an operating system for what had previously been a circuit; Intergalactic Research, Inc.

KILL: The UNIX language command to stop a microprocess.

KILLER APPLICATION: A massively popular computer program or Internet application that drives related products and life cycles; slang term.

KILL FILL: To automatically delete e-fax, e-mail, instant messages, and so forth.

KILOBYTE: Capacity; 1,024 bites.

KIN: To mark, title, and attach a significant image, note, file consult, and so forth; key image note.

KINGSHAW, RUBEN, JR.: Deputy Administrator and Chief Operating Officer at the Centers for Medicare and Medicaid Services (CMS), Baltimore, MD.

KLEINBERG, KEN: Former e-health analyst at Gartner, Stamford, CT, and now lead research for the health care group at Symbol Technologies, Holtsville, NY.

KLOSS, LINDA L.: CEO of the American Health Information Management Association.

KLUGE: An inelegant computer system, cobbled program, application, or patch; slang term.

K-NEAREST NEIGHBOR: Common associations between numeric data.

KNOWLEDGE: The objective, subjective, tangible, and intangible heuristic facts and assumptions used to formulate formal data interpretation and analysis; decision-making methodologies and inputs.

KNOWLEDGE-BASED SYSTEM: Expert computer system or network; medical decision-making algorithm.

KNOWLEDGE WORK(ER): One who relies on deep specific knowledge and subject matter expertise, rather than skills to perform a job; term coined by Peter Drucker.

KOLODNER, ROBERT M., MD: Chief Health Information Officer, U.S. Veterans Health Administration until September 2006; when he replaced David Brailer, MD as national coordinator for Health Care Information Technology (HCIT) for the Department of Health and Human Services in Washington, D.C.

KORN, DAVID: UNIX expert, computer scientist, and professional electronic engineer.

KORN SHELL: A higher-level Stephen Bourne Shell, developed by David Korn; UNIX $ prompt.

KRAKAUER, HENRY: Director, Office of Program Assessment and Health Information, Health Standards and Quality Bureau, Health Care Financing Administration, Baltimore, MD.

KRUEGERAPP: A downloaded computer application that diminishes performance; slang term.

KVEDAR, JOSEPH C., MD: CIO of Partners Telemedicine, Inc., of Boston, MA.

KYLIX®: A Delphi® C ++ programming environment under the Linux OS; Borland International®.

L

L@@K: To LOOK; humorous term.

L0PHT: Internet security organization that merged with @stake in 2000 and represented a group of sophisticated hackers that first assaulted the security of Microsoft's Windows NT® operating system by retrieving NT network-domain user names and passwords and displaying them in plain text.

L0PHT-CRACK: A graphical user interface-executable program that adds a spreadsheet-like interface that decrypts passwords; hacking tool from the L0pht group; slang term.

L1 CACHE: Memory that is closed to a computer's CPU.

L2 CACHE: Memory that is open to a computer's CPU.

L33T: Leetspeak, hackspeak, or hakspeak; from the word elite; slang term.

LABEL: An identified, name, number, character, or symbol in a computer program.

LABELER CODE: Initial portion of the National Drug Code assigned to a health care firm by the FDA.

LAG: A delayed computer network transmission; any time delay.

LANDHOLT, THOMAS, MD: Patient Care Director of Family Care for the Kryptiq Corporation®.

LANDSCAPE: The vertical or horizontal orientation of a Web page; background, color, designs, and so forth.

LANGUAGE: A standardized set of characters used to form meaningful symbols.

LANGUAGE TRANSLATOR: Program or application language conversion to computer language.

LANROVER: Shiva exemplar of the virtual private network technology that made public networks suitable for private transactions.

LAPTOP: A portable PC about the size of a sheet of paper with integrated keyboard, LCD screen, DVD/CD drive, PCI card, expansion slots, and input device; usually wireless enabled; a larger notebook computer that also may have a desktop docking station; Osborne I, 1981; handheld computer; pocket PC; pen-top computer.

LARENG, LOUIS, MD: Health care Informaticist at the Institute of European de Telemedicine.

LASER DISK: Optical recording medium with laser light interpreted pits burned into a plastic disk; CD-ROM or VD-ROM.

LASER-JET®: A popular ink jet printer, with built-in fonts, from the HP Corporation.

LASER PRINTER: A device that uses a xerographic printing process with dry toner to produce a hardcopy paper image.

LASER SMART CARD: An optical smart card.

LASSO: Highlighting a collection of icons or objects with a mouse for activation movement or further use; slang term.

LAST KNOWN GOOD (LKG): The most recent time period when a computer system was functioning optimally; a checksum slang term.

LAST MILE: The copper connection from computer to coaxial networks of telephone and cable companies; copper wire between POTS and end user; DSL, WiFi, WiMAX, and so forth.

LAST STAGE OF DELIRIUM: A hacking group that discovered the flaw that caused the Internet Blaster worm.

LAT: Nonroutable protocol by DEC® to support terminal bridged services; local area transport.

LATENCY: Time delay between initiation and actual data transfer.

LAVENTURE, MARTIN, PhD: Director, Center for Health Informatics, MN.

LAYER: IP suite or the class of health or other information exchange events of specific computer system functions: physical, data-link, network, transport, session, presentation, and application (low-to-high).

LAYER TWO TUNNELING PROTOCOL (L2TP): Network standard used to route non-IP traffic over an authenticated IP network; combined with IPSec for enhanced security features for protected health data or medical information.

LAYOUT PROGRAM: Software designed primarily for the creation of pages although they have the ability to create, draw, or manipulate images.

LEAK: Memory loss in a computer application or program, especially upon termination and reboot; slang term.

LEAPFROG ATTACK: To use a stolen ID or password to avoid hacker, or computer system intrusion detection.

LEASED LINE: Dedicated and permanent telephone line for computer transmissions; rented from a telephone company by a customer to have exclusive rights to it.

LEAVITT, MARK, MD, PhD: Certification Commission for Health Information Technology Chairman.

LEAVITT, MICHAEL O.: Secretary of the U.S. Department of Health and Human Services (HHSS).

LEETSPEAK: A type of colloquial communications where one replaces letters with numbers or other characters or symbols; hackspeak or hakspeak; slang term for elite speech.

LEFT CLICK: To press the left mouse button in the standard fashion.

LEGACY: Medical information or health data that was in existence prior to a certain point in time.

LEGACY FREE: Unburdened PC or software design requirement for backward compatibility needs.

LEGACY SYSTEM: Traditional mainframe computers, software, hardware, peripheral, storage, retrieval, and transmission integrated components; often non-PC based computers; older HIS configuration or software applications that may perform adequately.

LENOVO®: A Chinese manufacturer of computers; former IBM PC division.

LEOPARD: Mac OS X OS; slang code term.

LETTERBOMB: An e-mail message security breach; e-mail exploit, malicious intrusion, virus, or worm; slang term.

LEVEL 2 TUNNELING PROTOCOL (L2TP): PPTP variation used to secure a VPN.

LEXICON QUERY SERVICE® (LQS®): Read-only interface to access secure and standardized medical terminology database; electronic health collaborative dictionary; social health wiki (www.HealthDictionarySeries.com).

LICENSE: The formal authorization to use a software product or online subscription service.

LICENSE COMPLIANCE TRACKING: The act of using software or hardware according to the license as granted by the copyright owner of the product; violations include counterfeiting, corporate copying, and hard disk loading; license compliance tracking software, such as Executive Software's Sitekeeper® or MSFT-XP Activation® enables compliance simplicity.

LIEBER, STEPHEN H.: Healthcare Information and Management Systems Society (HIMSS) President and CEO.

LIGHT PEN: Mouse-like input and computer communication device.

LIGHTWEIGHT DIRECTORY ACCESS PROTOCOL (LDAP): A software protocol enabling anyone to locate organizations, individuals, and other resources such as files and devices in a network, whether on the public Internet or a corporate intranet.

LIMITED DATA SET: Protected Health Information (PHI) that excludes the following identifiers of the individual, or of relatives, employers, or household members of the individual: names; postal address information other than town or city; state and zip code; telephone numbers; fax numbers; electronic mail addresses; social security number; health plan beneficiary number; account number; certificate/license number; vehicle identifiers and serial numbers, including license plate numbers, device identifiers, and serial numbers; Web universal resource locators (URLs); Internet Protocol (IP) address numbers; biometric identifiers, including finger and voice prints and full face photographic images; and any comparable images.

LINDBERG, HENRY DONALD B.: Director, National Library of Medicine, National Institutes of Health, Bethesda, MD.

LINDOWS: A full featured computer operating system by Linspire Inc®; commercial LINUX; Freespire®.

LINE ART: Electronic computer artwork made of solid blacks and whites, with no tonal (gray) values.

LINE SIGHT: Electronic data propagation along a direct unobstructed straight line path; ISM band; Fresnel Effect.

LINES PER INCH (LPI): The number of lines per inch on a halftone computer screen/monitor—the higher the LPI, the higher the printed hard copy resolution.

LINK: Connection between two or more networked computer devices, LAN, MAN, WAN, Internet, and so forth; anchor; hotlink; hyperlink.

LINKROT: Tendency of hypertext links to become useless or broken as other sites cease to exist, or remove or reorganize their Web pages; slang term.

LINUX®: A free version of the UNIX operating system with Red Hat© open source systems offerings, designed by Finnish engineer Linus Torvalds and supported by thousands of programmers worldwide who continually update and improve it; a PC running the LINUX® operating system; slang term.

LINUX® KERNEL: Core software component that catalyzed a technology revolution in open GNU/Linux sourcing.

LION WORM: UNIX shellscript and password retrieving virus released in 2001 by Li()n.

LISP: A computer language developed in the 1950s used for complex structures and artificial intelligence needs.

LIST BOX: Window items list for computer programs, applications, files, and so forth.

LIST SERVE: An electronic mailing list management software program with "subscribe" and "unsubscribe" features for online discussions.

LIVE JOURNAL®: A free commercial online service for public journal and personal diaries; blog; blog site; blogger.

LIVE MEETING®: A MSFT Web conferencing service.

LOAD: To put medical or other data into internal storage.

LOADER: An offline to online computer program initiator.

LOCAL ACCESS TRANSPORT AREA (LOTA): The local telephone districts that were created by the divesture of the Regional Bell Operating Companies (RBOCs) formerly associated with AT&T.

LOCAL AREA NETWORK (LAN): A geographical small computer users group connected to a short-distance server, host, or network hub; wired 10BaseT Ethernet or wireless 802.11b or Wi-Fi connection; WAN; MAN.

LOCAL CODE: A nebulous term for code values that are defined for a state or other political subdivision, or for a specific payer; most commonly for HCPCS Level III Codes, but it also applies to state-assigned Institutional Revenue Codes, Condition Codes, Occurrence Codes, Value Codes, and so forth; eliminated in 2003 to comply with HIPAA.

LOCAL EXCHANGE CARRIER (LEC): A telephone company that carries local calls.

LOCAL HEALTH INFORMATION INFRASTRUCTURE (LHII): Used synonymously with RHIO by the Office of the National Coordinator of Health Information as the technology to describe the regional efforts that will eventually be linked together to form the NHII.

LOCK: To mark a computer file as unchangeable.

LOCKING A DISK: The process of setting a disk or data storage element (Syquest cartridge, optical disk, diskette) into a mode that will prevent computers from writing on to, or deleting from the media, the files that are saved onto the disk (write protect).

LOCKOUT: To deny computer access to a health, medical, or other information database system or file.

LOGICAL DRIVE: The subdivision of a large physical drive, such as a hard drive, into smaller sectors or component drives; B and D drives partitioned from C drive.

LOGICAL OBSERVATION IDENTIFIERS NAMES AND CODES (LOINC®): A database to facilitate the exchange and pooling of laboratory results, such as blood hemoglobin, serum potassium, or vital signs, for clinical care, outcomes management, and research; most laboratories and other diagnostic services use HL7 to send their results electronically from their disparate reporting systems to their care systems; LOINC codes are universal identifiers for laboratory and other clinical observations that solve this problem; the Regenstrief Institute maintains the database and its supporting documentation.

LOGICAL THREAT: Software destruction or alteration uncertainty activated by a normal but unknown input process; logic bomb.

LOGICAL UNIT (LU): A CPU with ALU coordination architecture.

LOGIC BOMB: A software program written to release an unexpected result upon activation of a certain usually previously unknown condition or input; keystroke, virus, worm, or time bomb.

LOGIN: To achieve successful computer, server, network, or online access via some sort of triage or security clearance measure; jack-in.

LOGIN CONTROL: The specific switch or conditions for a successful computer login.

LOGIN MONITOR: Provides user education in the importance of monitoring log-in success or failure and how to report discrepancies.

LOGOFF: Terminating or closing a server, computer, or open online network session; jack out.

LOGON: Opening or commencing a server, computer, or open online network session.

LOGON PROCESS: The process or methodology to commence or open a server, computer, or open online network session.

LOGOUT: To formally exit from a computer system.

LONGHORN: MSFT Windows Vista® OS; code name.

LONGITUDINAL DATA: Linear data function that evolves over time.

LONGITUDINAL HEALTH RECORD: Birth-to-death patient record in chronological order, developed over time; lifetime medical records.

LOONSK, JOHN, MD: ONCHIT Director of Interoperability and Standards.

LOOP: To repeat a computer process or sequence, without end.

LOOPHOLE: Incomplete data, software or hardware control, or computer access program error; a bug; slang term.

LOSSLESS: To compress electronic digital data; slang term.

LOSSLESS COMPRESSION: Condensation or data compression algorithm in a 2:1 ratio.

LOSSY COMPRESSION: Condensation or data compression algorithm in a 100–200:1 ratio; incomplete decompression.

LOST CLUSTER: Disk records that have lost their identification with a file name as when closed improperly, like when the computer is turned off without quitting the application first.

LOTUS 123®: Spreadsheet with early user interface innovation and fast PC clone compatible code; Mitch Kapor 1983; now IBM®.

LOTUS NOTES®: Created by Ray Ozzie of Microsoft as a leading collaborative groupware word processing application; now IBM.

LUDDITE: One who is opposed to health IT, EDI, EHRs, and so forth; technophobe; slang term.

LUMINOSITY: Level of brightness for a computer monitor, plasma screen, LED, and so forth.

LUMPER VOCABULARY: Nondefinitional health lexicon that used codes for combined specific multiple concepts.

LURK: Nonparticipation in an Internet chat room or newsgroup; slang term.

M

M: Megabyte, or 1.024 kilobytes; MB.

MAC: Nickname for the Apple Macintosh PC®; slang term.

MAC BOOK PRO®: A family of laptop computers from Apple, Inc., introduced in 2006 as the first Macintosh portable computer to use Intel CPUs; the first Mac Book Pro included the Core Duo chip running at clock rates from 1.8 to 2.16 GHz.

MACHINE CODE: Basic language of all computer systems, consisting of a series of 0s and 1s.

MACHINE DEPENDENT: Software dependent designed to run on only one computer or family from the same architecture.

MACHINE INDEPENDENT: Software independent designed to run on more than one computer, or family from different architectures.

MACHINE LANGUAGE: Native computer language in binary-coded CPU instructions entirely of numbers, created by assemblers, compilers, and interpreters.

MACHINE READABLE: Health data or other information accessible by a computer regardless of input mechanism.

MACINTOSH: A PC from Apple Computer® Inc., with a GUI and OSX, that was first introduced in 1984; two basic laptop product lines exist; Powerbooks® and iBooks®, while desktop models include Power Macs®, eMacs®, iMacs®, and Mac mini®.

MACINTOSH PORTABLE: An unpopular but portable version of the Macintosh® computer released in 1989; was essentially a fast Mac SE with a floppy disk and optional hard disk; used a 16 MHz Motorola 68000 CPU and monochrome LCD screen.

MAC OS-X®: Operating system that is a UNIX variant for the Apple Macintosh® line of PCs; the tenth (X) version includes minor updates, such as Jaguar v10.2, Panther v10.3, and Tiger v10.4

MAC PRO®: Apple computer with two Intel Xeon® microchips, space for four hard-drives with 2 terabytes of data storage.

MACRO: A variety of keystrokes, commands, or menu selections that can be assigned a name or key combination; an automatic function for an application; user designed utility sequence of instructions for a PC.

MACROMEDIA®: Producer of Internet Web site audiovisual products, such as Flash Freehand® and Dreamweaver®; acquired by Adobe Systems® in 2005.

MACROMEDIA FLASH PLAYER®: A high-performance, lightweight, highly expressive client runtime that delivers powerful and consistent user experiences across major operating systems, browsers, mobile phones, and devices; now Adobe Systems, Inc®.

MACRO RECORDER: A program that converts digital file selections into a macro function.

MACRO VIRUS: Malicious small fragments of a computer program code written in a macro language within a document; potentially very virulent as they can be embedded in traditional word processing software applications and programs.

MAC VIRUS: First widespread Apple Computer® Inc., viruses in 1988; the MacMag and Scores variants.

MAGIC NUMBER: An important number or mathematical formula secretly embedded in software code where users, programmers, and writers are unlikely to find it; slang term.

MAGNETIC DISK: Coated disk used for computer medical information or other data storage.

MAGNETIC STRIPE CARD: A plastic smart card with health or other data contained on an electromagnetic storage strip.

MAGNETIC TAPE: A continuous flexible electronic health data or other storage medium that accepts medical or other information in polarized spots.

MAIL: electronic mail; e-mail; slang term.

MAILBOMB: Sending massive quantities of e-mail often for retaliatory purposes; spam; slang term.

MAILBOT: An auto-responder; automated e-mail message; e-letter bomb.

MAILING LIST: Conducted exclusively through e-mail as a discussion group open to the public; or private; once a user subscribes to a mailing list, all messages they send to the list are copied and sent to all other members of the mailing list; a popular method of engaging in online topic-specific discussions; often referred to as "listservs" or 'majordomos,' named after the types of software used to maintain them.

MAIL MERGE: The integration of a contact information database with a letter template for mass mailings.

MAIL SERVERS: Electronic post office and message facilities for a computer network.

MAIL SLOT: The Windows© NT messaging interface between server and clients.

MAINFRAME: Large scale computer with legacy systems able to support many users and peripheral devices, concurrently; IBM 370 and 3090 series.

MAINFRAME SYSTEMS: Computer configuration that is highly centralized and most applicable to large hospitals and health care systems as this powerful computer performs basically all the information processing for the institution and connects to multiple terminals that communicate with the mainframe to display the information at the user sites; Hospital Information Technology (HIT) departments usually use programmers to modify the core operating systems or applications programs such as billing and scheduling programs.

MAINTENANCE OF RECORD ACCESS AUTHORIZATIONS: Ongoing documentation and review of the levels of IT access granted to a user, program, or procedure accessing health information.

MAINTENANCE OF RECORDS: Documentation of repairs and modifications to the physical and IT components of a health care facility, for example, hardware, software, walls, doors, and locks.

MAJORDOMO: A UNIX Internet list program or free open source software; slang term.

MALICIOUS SOFTWARE: Any virus, worm, Trojan horse, or computer code designed to damage or disrupt a system; malware; slang term.

MALWARE: Malicious computer or network software, such as spyware and adware; slang term.

MANDATORY ACCESS CONTROL (MAC): Any means of restricting computer user access to objects; based on fixed security attributes assigned to users and to files and other objects; cannot be modified by self-users or their programs.

MANDELBROT SET: A famous shape or fractal containing an almost infinite degree of detail; mathematical computer system security equation discovered by Benoit Mandelbrot.

MAN IN THE MIDDLE ATTACK: Occurs when an attacker intercepts messages in a public key exchange and then retransmits them, substituting his own public key for the requested one, so that the two original parties still appear to be communicating with each other; the intruder uses a program that appears to be a valid and secure client/server network.

MAP: To link health data or other information or content from one scheme to another.

MAP DRIVER: Feature that allows quick computer user network navigation.

MARBUGER, JOHN H., III: Director of the White House Office of Science and Technology Policy.

MARCHIBRODA, JANET M.: CEO of the eHI (e Health Initiative and Foundation).

MARIETTI, CHARLENE: Editor of the magazine *Healthcare Informatics*.

MARKETING: To disseminate information about a health product or medical service for the purpose of encouraging patients and recipients to purchase or use the product or service; does not include communications made by a HIPAA-covered health entity.

MARK I: First general purpose digital computer built at Harvard University under the direction of Howard Aiken; used by the Navy for ballistic calculations.

MARK UP LANGUAGE: Any computer language that indicates word processing features such as page breaks, italics, page settings, page footers and headers, and so forth.

MARTIAN: Incorrect computer network routing information.

MASHUP: Hybrid Internet application development approach using Web applications built from many different vendors and sources (blogs, news-feeds, maps, and wikis) but combined into a seamless interface for a new experience; best of breed computer programming to build on-the-spot medical and business applications (for example, Google Maps®, Windows Live®, Office Live®, and so forth); slang term.

MASQERADE: Unauthorized access to a computer, server, Internet, or network under a legitimate user password, ID number, or name.

MASSACHUSETTS HEALTH DATA CONSORTIUM (MHDC): An organization that seeks to improve health care in New England through improved policy development, better information technology planning and implementation, and more informed financial decision making.

MASSIVE PARALLEL PROCESSING (MPP): The independent clustering of multiple computer servers managed by its own operating system for enhanced functionality.

MASS MAILER VIRUS: A fast spreading malicious macro virus; such as the Melissa variant of 1999; and the ILOVE YOU, LOVELETTER, and LOVE BUG social engineering variants of 2000.

MASTER: The control unit in a pair of linked computers, LAN, MAN, or WAN; host; not a slave, thin, or bade device; slang terms.

MASTER BROWSER: Network that archives all servers and computers available on the network.

MASTER FILE: A file of periodically updated semipermanent medical data, health, or other information.

MASTER FILE TABLE (MFT): A list of files in a Net Technology File System volume, which contains the name, size, time, date, and so forth for each file.

MASTER PATIENT (PERSON) INDEX (MPI): Health care facility composite that links and assists in tracking patient, person, or member activity within an organization (or health enterprise) and across patient care settings; hardcopy or electronic identification of all patients treated in a facility or enterprise and lists the medical record or identification number associated with the name; can be maintained manually or as part of a computerized system; typically, those for health care facilities are retained permanently, while those for insurers, registries, or others may have different retention periods; a database of all the patients ever registered (within reason) at a facility; name, demographics, insurance, next of kin, spouse, and so forth.

MATH COPROCESSOR: Integrated auxiliary computer chip addition to the main CPU that performs mathematical functions while the Central Processor Unit (CPU) performs operating system functions.

MAU: A token-ring computer network hub configuration.

MAUCHLY, JOHN (1907–1980): Physicist who attended Johns Hopkins University in Baltimore, Maryland, and collaborated with John Eckert in the construction of the Electronic Integrator and Computer (ENIAC).

MAXIMIZE: To increase or visually enlarge a window on a computer screen/monitor.

MAXIMUM DEFINED DATA SET: All required HIPAA data elements for a particular standard based on a specific implementation specification; a health entity creating a transaction is free to include whatever data any receiver might want or need; the recipient is free to ignore any portion of the data that is not needed to conduct their part of the associated business transaction, unless the inessential data is needed for coordination of benefits; Part II, 45 CFR 162.103.

MB: Megabyte; a measure of computer storage and memory capacity; one MB is equivalent to 1.024 million bytes, 1,024 thousand bytes, or 1.024 kilobytes; the term is also applied to the more rounded term of 1 million bytes.

Mbps: Megabits per second; a measure of bandwidth and rate of data flow in digital transmission; one Mbps is equivalent to one million bits per second.

McAFFE, JOHN: Producer of the commercial anti-virus program Virus Scan in 1987.

McCALLISTER: President and CEO of Humana.

McCLELLAN, MARK, MD, PhD: Former administrator of CMS, and Former Commissioner of the Food and Drug Administration, who resigned in 2006.

McCORMICK, WALTER: CEO of the U.S. Telecommunication Association.

McENERRY, KEVIN, MD: Associate head of informatics for diagnostic imaging at the MD Anderson Cancer Center, Texas.

MCNEALY, SCOTT: Founder and CEO of Sun Microsystems, Inc.®, who was replaced by Jonathan Schwartz as CEO in 2006.

McSLARROW, KYLE: CEO of the National Cable and Telecommunications Association.

MDI-X PORT: Cross-over computer hub configuration that reverses transmissions and receiver wirer pairs to mitigate cross-over cable need.

MEAD, CHARLES N., MD: Member HL7 Board of Directors and senior director, health care strategy, Oracle Corporation.

MEAN TIME BETWEEN FAILURES: Average electronic device operating time between system outages.

MEAT WARE: Portions of a computer or software system made of meat; human user; humorous term.

MEDIA ACCESS CONTROL ADDRESS (MACA): The hardware address for a computer network connection.

MEDIA CENTER PC: A PC equipped with Windows XP® or Vista XP® Media Center Edition for TV, with recording and speaker channels and DVD drive.

MEDIA CONTROLS: Tracks how health media flows in and out of an organization and what is to occur before media is disposed; includes tracking of who can perform various PHI manipulations and tasks, how accountability is tracked, and how hardware and software is disposed.

MEDIA ERROR: Bug or storage unit malfunction.

MEDIA PLAYER: Software used to listen to music or view computer digital videos, such as Windows Media Player®, RealNetworks RealPlayer®, WinAmp®, Macromedia ShockWave®, and Apple QuickTime®.

MEDICAID: A Title 19 Federal program, run and partially funded by individual states to provide medical benefits to certain low-income people; each state under broad federal guidelines, determines what benefits are covered, who is eligible, and how much providers will be paid; historically, all states but Arizona have Medicaid programs.

- MEDICAID 1115 WAIVER: state administration exemption to speed claims processing.
- MEDICAID 1915(b) WAIVER: alternate local, regional, or state managed care model.

MEDICAL ADVANCED TECHNOLOGY MANAGEMENT OFFICE (MATMO): Developed and implemented by the Department of Defense as a medical imaging system that combines PACS and teleradiology networks.

MEDICAL CODE SETS: Computer and hardcopy codes that characterize a medical condition or treatment and are maintained by professional societies and public health organizations; compared to nonclinical administrative code sets.

MEDICAL COGNITION (HEURISTICS): The integrated field of medicine and computer science, which studies human reasoning, logic, decision-making, and problem-solving skills, and applies it to health information system settings.

MEDICAL DATA INTERCHANGE STANDARD (MEDIX): Established by the IEEE as a health and other data communication protocol that is utilized at the applications level.

MEDICAL ECONOMIC VALUE ADDED© (MEVA©): Concept that combines finance and accounting to determine medical practice, clinic, hospital, or other health care business-enterprise entity value as an ongoing concern; medical economic value added; economic medical value added; *i*MBA, Inc®.

MEDICAL EXPERT SYSTEM: Electronic health care clinical decision-making support system or algorithm; clinical path method.

MEDICAL IMAGING: The computerized field of radiological digitalization, storage, retrieval, and transmission of X-rays, MRI, CT and PET scans, and so forth.

MEDICAL INFORMATICS: The use of health care management information, computer systems and digital data capture, storage, and transmission to facilitate medical and clinical patient activities; a system comprised of computer science, information science, and health sciences created to assist in the management and processing of private protected data to support the execution of health care.

MEDICAL INFORMATION BUS (MIB): IEEE open standard for electronic patient monitoring device connectivity.

MEDICAL INVESTMENT POLICY STATEMENT© (MIPS©): A blueprint draft between investment advisors and client (individual medical provider or health organization) that defines the terms of engagement for both parties; defines goals, strategies, asset allocation, risk tolerance, benchmarks reporting duties, fiduciary responsibility, and so forth; especially focused on electronic delivery for the health care industry.

MEDICALLY UNBELIEVABLE EVENT (MUE): Implemented on January 1, 2007, the CMS blockage of payments for medical services that make no sense based on "anatomic considerations" or medical reasonableness when the same patient, date of service, HCPCS code, or provider is involved; unlike other National Correct Coding Initiative (NCCI) edits, MUEs cannot be overridden by a modifier, because there will never be a scenario where the physician had a good reason to submit a claim for removing a second appendix from the same person, and so forth.

MEDICAL NOMENCLATURE: Preferred health care terminology and definitions; health industry lexicon; health ontology index; www.Health DictionarySeries.com.

MEDICAL RECORDS INSTITUTE (MRI): A professional organization that promotes the development and acceptance of electronic health care record systems and PHI integrity.

MEDICAL TRANSCRIPTIONIST: One who converts medical reports into written verbiage; electronic health data and information translator.

MEDICARE: A nationwide, federal health insurance program for those aged 65 and older; covers certain people under 65 who are disabled or have chronic kidney disease; acting CMS Deputy Administrator is Herb Kuhn; Medicare Part A is the hospital insurance program while Part B covers physicians' services; created by the 1965 Title 18 amendment to the Social Security Act:

- MEDICARE PART A: Medicare compulsory hospital compensation program, financed through payroll taxes shared by employers and employees alike. Most folks do not pay a premium because they or a spouse have 40 or more quarters of Medicare-covered employment. It is provided free to anyone who qualifies for Medicare benefits, but the deductible that pays for inpatient hospital, skilled nursing facility, and some home health care was $912 in 2005. The Part A deductible is the beneficiary's only cost for up to 60 days of Medicare-covered inpatient hospital care. However, for extended Medicare-covered hospital stays, beneficiaries paid an additional $228 per day for days 61 through 90 in 2005, and $456 per day for hospital stays beyond the 90th day in a benefit period. For beneficiaries in skilled nursing facilities, the daily co-insurance for days 21 through 100 was $114 in 2005. However, seniors and certain persons under age 65 with disabilities who have fewer than 30 quarters of coverage may obtain Part A coverage by paying a monthly premium set according to a formula in the Medicare statute at $343 for 2004. In addition, seniors with 30 to 39 quarters of coverage, and certain disabled persons with 30 or more quarters of coverage, are entitled to pay a reduced premium of $189. All indexed annually (www.hhs.gov/news/).
  - Coinsurance
    - o $228.00 a day for the 61st–90th day each benefit period.
    - o $456.00 a day for the 91st–150th day for each lifetime reserve day (total of 60 lifetime reserve days—nonrenewable).

- Skilled Nursing Facility Coinsurance: Up to $114 a day for days 21 through 100 in each benefit period (indexed annually).
- MEDICARE PART B: Medicare physician compensation program. This is supplementary medical insurance. It covers most of what isn't covered by Part A and is paid for by the insured individual via an enrollment program. For 2005 the monthly premium was $78.20 and the coverage also involved a $110 annual deductible and a 20% per service coinsurance (indexed annually).

Beneficiary Income Level	Current Premium	2007 Premium
$80,000 or less	$88.50	$93.50
$80–100,000	$88.50	$106.00
$100–150,000	$88.50	$124.70
$150–200,000	$88.50	$143.40
$200,000 and above	$88.50	$162.10

Note: Monthly Medicare premiums per beneficiary; yearly adjusted gross income for individuals; couples filing jointly are allowed approximately double IRS AGI levels of individuals; no monthly premium for those earning less than federal poverty levels. *Source:* CMS.

- MEDICARE PART C: Medicare managed care compensation program, known as *Medicare + Choice* and initiated in 1997. If a beneficiary chooses Part C, it takes the place of Parts A and B. Part C is basically a Medicare HMO plan. In 2000–2004 many carriers ceased offering this type of coverage and those individuals who had elected to go with a Medicare HMO had to backtrack and re-enroll in the original Medicare fee-for-service program (Parts A and B). This may again change beyond 2005 as traditional Medicare premiums continue to increase. Another name for this program is Medicare Advantage.
- MEDICARE PART D: Medicare Prescription Drug Benefits program that began on January 1, 2006; most seniors are eligible to participate, and most drugs are covered; economics benefits, premiums, and deductibles will vary and will be indexed annually:
  - *Premium:* Part D premium is $35 per month ($420 annually). This premium is in addition to the Part B premium (automatically deducted from Social Security checks each month, for most patients).
  - *Annual Deductible:* Patients pay the first $250 of prescription drugs expenses.
  - *Coinsurance:* Medicare pays 75% of costs between $250 and $2,250. Patients pay the other 25% out-of-pocket; or a maximum of $500 for coinsurance.

- *Coverage Gap:* After total prescription drugs expenses reach $2,250, Medicare pays nothing until the patient has spent a total of $3,600 out-of-pocket (hole). *The $3,600 includes the $250 deductible and $500 coinsurance maximum.*
- *Catastrophic Protection:* After spending $3,600, Medicare covers 95 percent of prescription drug expenses for the remainder of the year.
- *Low-Income Assistance:* Patients eligible for both Medicare and Medicaid pay no premium, no deductible, and have no gap in coverage. They pay a $1 copayment per prescription for generic drugs, and a $3 copayment per prescription for brand name drugs.

MEDICARE REMITTANCE ADVICE REMARK CODES: A national administrative code set for providing either claim-level or service-level Medicare-related messages that cannot be expressed with a Claim Adjustment Reason Code and used in the X12 835 Claim Payment & Remittance Advice transactions, and maintained by HCFA (CMS).

MEDISTICK®: A 128-Mbyte USB drive for medical information storage and portable health history information; password protected in multiple languages.

MEDIX: To regulate medical devices throughout the product lifecycle.

MEDLARS: The Medical Literature Analysis and Retrieval System; more than 50 computer databases managed by the U.S. NLM.

MEDLINE: Bibliographic database that is the most used of about 40 MEDLARS medical databases managed by the United States.

MEGABYTE: One million bytes, or 1,048,576 bytes; meg, Mb, Mbyte, and M-byte.

MEGAHERTZ (MHz): Computer processing speed measured in millions of clock-ticks-per second; a gigahertz (GHz) means one billion times; used to refer to a computer's clock to measure the speed of the CPU; for example, a 900 MHz machine processes data internally twice as fast as a 450 MHz machine.

MELANI, KENNETH, MD: President and CEO of Highmark, Inc.

MELISSA: Macro virus of 1999 that attacked MSFT Word® files.

MELTDOWN: Health care organization network system collapse due to computer system information data overload or above normal traffic; slang term.

MEME: Philosophy, idea, skill, habit, or group-think mentality that quickly spreads; sweeping Internet, health care, or computer fad; term coined in 1976 by Richard Dawkins.

MEMEPOOL: An idea and play on the phrase *gene pool;* slang term.

MEMORY: The electronic storage of medical information or digitized data; core; Random Access Memory or Read Only Memory, and so forth.

MEMORY RESIDENT PROGRAM: A loaded program that remains in computer memory and continues to function while other programs run; a terminate-and-stay resident computer program.

MEMORY SPOT: A tiny wireless computer chip from Hewlett-Packard® that can attach data to physical objects.

MEMORY STICK: USB flash or nonvolatile storage device; Sony Compact-Flash®, pen or mini-drive; flash card, smart media, slang terms.

MEMPHIS: MSFT OS Windows 98®; code name.

MENU: A list of computer applications or software programs.

MENU BAR: The pull down applications of a menu list or task bar of computer applications or programs.

MENU INTERACTION: Computerized user interface using pictorial or graphical icons for operator input.

MERCHANT STATUS: A credit, debit, or smart-card authorized health care or business entity.

MERGE: To insert health data or other information into a document within a separate file.

MERON: The mobile version of Intel's© Core 2 Duo microprocessor for note-book computers; code name.

MERRELL, RONALD C., MD: Director of the medical informatics and technology applications consortium for the Virginia Commonwealth University; Co-Editor-in-Chief of *Telemedicine and e-Health* journal.

MeSH: Medical Subject Headings, the controlled vocabulary of about 16,000 terms used for MEDLINE and certain other MEDLARS databases.

MESSAGE: A digital representation of medical or other information.

MESSAGE AUTHENTICATION: Ensuring, typically with a message authentication code, that a message received (usually via a computer network) matches the message sent.

MESSAGE AUTHENTICATION CODE: Data associated with an authenticated message that allows a receiver to verify the integrity of the message.

MESSAGE BOARD: An Internet-based communications forum or discussion group usually in RSS format; electronic bulletin board system (BBS).

MESSAGE DIGEST: The product of a hashing function.

MESSAGE, INSTANT: An instant electronic message; instant, almost live, e-mail.

MESSAGE INTEGRITY: The assurance of unaltered transmission and receipt of health information, medical data, or other message from the sender to the intended recipient.

MESSAGE SWITCHING: A message either in image or text form that is separated into multiple parts that are then transmitted independently to the receiver where they are put back together to form the message.

MESSAGE SYNTAX: Rules and definitions for text arrangements.

MESSAGING: Publishing-scribes and point-to-point health information or other data transmission across a computer network.

MESSAGING SERVICE: A company that creates, parses, serializes, encrypts and decrypts, transforms, delivers, and routes the electronic mass mailings of electronic messages.

META CRAWLER: Utility program that sends search inquires to Internet search engines such as Lycos® or Google® with results summary; crawler; slang term.

META CUSTOMER: Those health care providers, or covered medical entities in need of meta-data access.

META-DATA: The electronic structure of a computer database program; application data; may refer to detailed compilations such as data dictionaries and repositories that provide information about each data element, and may also refer to any descriptive item about data, such as the content of an HTML meta tag or a title field in a media file; commonly spelled as one word, "meta-data" (with the hyphen) is the proper, generic spelling, as the Metadata Company® has trademarked the name, metadata®.

META FILE: An information file that consists of other health or similar data files.

META LANGUAGE: A computer language used to explain or describe another computer language; LISP and Prolog.

META REGISTER: A list of metadata files, usually for some commercial purpose.

METASPLOIT FRAMEWORK: The open source exploit project that created the public tool *Metasploit*, in order to search for data strings within malicious software code; term coined by H. D. Moore.

META STEWARD: One who organizes and maintains a meta-register.

META TAG: A HTML command for Web page or Web site URL information.

META THESAURUS: The integration of several related thesauri into a massive database; a compendium of thesauri.

METERED RATE: A measured or clocked subscription ISP connection.

METROPOLITAN AREA NETWORK (MAN): A network of computers whose reach extends to a metropolitan area; used to link telemedicine applications at a data rate similar to DS1; in some cases may be used by cable companies to offer links to off-network services such as the Internet, airline reservation systems, and commercial information services, in addition to data exchange abilities; compared to a LAN or WAN, it is intermediate.

MEZZANINE BUS: A PC-to-peripheral device connection.

MHz: Megahertz; a measure of bandwidth and rate of information flow for analog transmission; one MHz equals 10^6 cycles per second.

MICHAEL: An 8-bit Message Integrity Code for WPA; MIC slang term.

MICKEY: A minute mouse movement; slang term.

MICROBROWSER: A less memory intense Internet Web browser used for smaller computer devices, laptops, handhelds, palmtops, PDAs, and so forth; Wireless Application Protocol (WAP).

MICROCHANNEL: 32-bit IBM PS/2 multiprocessing computer system.

MICROCHUNK: Surgically precise and removed clip of a digitalized TV program or other broadcast for portable distribution, e-mail, linkage, download, or remix; slang term.

MICROCOMPUTER: A small and usually personalized computer system with I/O device, single microprocessing unit, storage medium, and related peripheral devices; a desktop or laptop PC.

MICROCONTROLLER: A small-task dedicated computer.

MICROPROCESSOR: An integrated circuit with a CPU for a computer; the engine of a PC; Intel© 8080 first launched in 1973.

MICROSITE: An informative but niche specific Web page within a larger generalized Web site.

MICROSOFT© CORPORATION: The world's leading software application, word processor, and visual application producer; ISP, online network, and browser provider; online collaborator and on-demand SAS developer, founded in 1975 by William Gates and Paul Allen who wrote a version of the BASIC language for microcomputers, in Redmond, WA; involved in health care productivity challenges and solutions.

MICROSOFT HEALTHCARE USERS GROUP® (MS-HUG): Mission Statement: "To be the healthcare industry forum for exchanging ideas, promoting learning, and sharing solutions for information systems using Microsoft technologies. MS-HUG will leverage this forum to provide industry leadership, drive appropriate standards and develop associated requirements in support of healthcare solutions. MS-HUG's ability to fulfill this mission is predicated on a broad-based membership which includes CIOs, healthcare end-users, care-givers from provider organizations, and payers; but MS-HUG is primarily focused on information technology professionals and developers from healthcare providers, solution providers, and ISVs. This diverse membership is unified by a shared interest in implementing vendor and user-developed software based on Microsoft technology to improve quality and efficiency in healthcare."

MICROSOFT MALICIOUS SOFTWARE REMOVAL TOOL (MMSRT): A free tool used to scan PC hard disks and remove certain variants of known worms and viruses.

MICROSOFT OFFICE 12: Code-name for the successor to its office business application franchise, which packages together or mash-ups word processing, spreadsheet, presentation, and other programs.

MICROWAVE: High frequency radio waves with spectrum above 2 gigahertz (GHz).

MICROWAVE LINK: A system of communication using high frequency radio signals, exceeding 800 megahertz, for audio, video, and data transmission; require line of sight connection between transmission antennas.

MIDDLEWARE: Software interface or bridge between two computer programs or applications; a common application of middleware is to allow programs written for access to a particular health database to access other databases; slang term.

MIDRANGE: A computer with greater processing power than a PC, but less than a mainframe.

MID-SIZE COMPUTER: Minicomputer or small mainframe computer.

MIGRATE: To replace an older computer legacy system, with a newer system, over time.

MINI COMPUTER: Personal Computer often with dumb terminals or between mainframes and microcomputers; DEC VAX© and IBM 400© series; replaced by LANS, WANs, and MANs.

MINI MAC: Apple computer with 1.66-GHz Core Duo Intel® processor, 8X super drive (DVD = R, DVD+RW/CD-RW), 80-GB hard drive, DVI external display output, optical/digital inputs, infrared Apple remote control, and Mac OSX Tiger®, Front Row®, and Bonjour® software.

MINIMIZE: To shrink or decrease the size of a window or computer screen.

MINIMUM NECESSARY: The amount of protected health information shared among internal or external parties determined to be the smallest amount needed to accomplish its purpose for use or disclosure; the amount of health information or medical data needed to accomplish a purpose varies by job title, CE, or job classification.

MINIMUM NECESSARY RULE: HIPAA regulation that suggests any PHI used to identify a patient, such as a Social Security Number, home address, or phone number, divulge only essential elements for use in transferring information from patient record to anyone else that requires the information; especially important with financial information; changes the way software is written and vendor access is provided. The "Minimum Necessary" Rule states the minimum use of PHI that can be used to identify a person. Only the essential elements are to be used in transferring information from the patient record to anyone else that needs this information. This is especially important when financial information is being addressed. Only the minimum codes necessary to determine the cost should be provided to the financial department. No other information should be accessed by that department. Many institutions have systems where a registration or accounting clerk can pull up as much information as a doctor or nurse, but this is now against HIPAA policy and subject to penalties. The "Minimum Necessary" Rule is also changing the way software is set up and vendor access is provided.

MINIMUM SCOPE OF DISCLOSURE: Suggestion that individually identifiable health information should only be disclosed to the extent needed to support the purpose of the disclosure.

MIRROR(ING): To copy electronic information or make redundant; back-up; mirror site.

MIRROR SET RAID LEVEL 1: A shadow disk in a two-disk array system for instant redundancy.

MIRROR SITE: A secondary physical location identical to the primary health IT site that constantly receives a copy of data from the primary site; a process is typically used to expedite access because the original site resides on another continent; for example, a Web site may be set up in America duplicating an already existing Web site in Europe so that American medical professionals can quickly access the site.

MISCELLANEOUS CODE: National medical supplier submitted identifier for which there is no existing code.

MISFEATURE: An erroneous, buggy, or ill-conceived software feature without benefits; slang term.

MISSION CRITICAL SYSTEM: Health care computer information management system that is considered vital to core medical operations and patient safety and treatment.

MITCHELL, ROBERT: Senior Associate Editor of ADVANCE for Health Information Executives.

MOBILE DEVICE: A portable computing system, or PDA, that is enabled with wireless technology for transmissions and reception; mobile computing; mobile information server.

MODE: To define the present operating state of computer software, hardware, or peripheral equipment.

MODEL: To define a concept or architecture.

MODEM (MODULATOR-DEMODULATOR): A hardware device that converts digital data to analog signals over a regular telephone line for transmission, and analog conversion to digital data for electronic reception; modem ready; modem bank; modem emulator; usually identified by the speed (in bits per second or bps) of communication; the higher the bps, the faster the modem.

MODERATED: Internet electronic communications network subject to censor, review, or editing; live or automated; monitored; used to refer to either mailing lists or newsgroups, a moderated forum is one in which every message sent to the forum is first analyzed by an individual called the 'moderator,' if the message is germane to the forum's topic, and is appropriate, it will be approved and published on that forum; if not acceptable, the message is returned to the author; distinguished from open and closed.

MODIFIER: Two digit codes to indicate an altered CPT code or unusual medical service usually submitted with enhanced code narrative descriptions; modifier key.

MODULARITY: Separate, independent, cohesive computer systems construction pieces.

MODULAR PC: A PC in which upgrading is a simple matter of pulling out old components and dropping in new modular parts.

MODULE: Part of a large electronic ecosystem.

MOIRÉ: The noticeable, unwanted pattern generated by scanning or prescreening a piece of art that already contains a dot pattern; may be caused by the misalignment of screen angles in color work.

MON, DONALD: Vice President, American Health Information Management Association (AHIMA).

MONADIC OPERATION: Manipulating a single piece of health data, medical, or other information.

MONEY MULE: Any fraudster who contacts a victim by computer, persuades him or her to be recruited to receive funds, and then forwards them for a commission; slang term.

MONITOR: Computer screen; cathode ray tube (CRT), light emitting diode, liquid crystal display (thin film display), high-definition, plasma, and so forth.

MONITORING: Active form of health information system or information system surveillance for detection, education, and utilization.

MONOCHROME: A single color; usually refers to a black-and-white or green image.

MONOCHROME MONITOR: A gray-scale monitor for visual display on a computer that presents images as various shades of gray, ranging from black to white.

MONTECITO: Code name for the dual core Itanium® CPU chip series from the Intel Corporation®: Model number: 9050, 9040, 9030, 9020, 9015 and 9010 (cache size: 24, 18, 8, 12, 12 and 6 MB, respectively).

MOORE, GORDON E.: Engineer and cofounder of the Intel Corporation®.

MOORE, H. D.: (In)famous creator of the open-source penetrating test tool *Metasploit*, which disclosed Internet vulnerabilities.

MOORE'S LAW: Empirical observation that integrated circuit complexity doubles in about 18 months; first postulated in 1967; law of transistor density; Gordon Moore.

MORPHING: To transform one digital image into another; morphed; metamorphosing.

MORRIS, THOMAS Q., MD: Professor of Clinical Medicine, College of Physicians and Surgeons of Columbia University, and Past President, Columbia Presbyterian Medical Center, New York, NY.

MOSAIC: An Internet GUI browser created at the University of Illinois Urbana-Champaign in 1993 that was freely distributed and launched the era of browseable content and broad adoption of repurposeable markup computer language; precursor to MSFT Internet Explorer®.

MOTHERBOARD: Main integrated circuit board of a computer that houses its CPU and cooling unit, CMOS, battery, BIOS bus, expansion slots (AGP and PCI), peripheral ports, and so forth.

MOTION PICTURE EXPERTS GROUP (MPEG): Standardized movie/audio format creation, manipulation, storage, and transmissions.

MOTOROLA®: Maker and provider of analog and digital two-way voice and data radio products and systems for conventional as well as wireless communications; cell phone, electronic equipment, and chip maker based in Shaumburg, IL; its microprocessors include the early 6800 and 68000 series for Apple Computer Inc®; subsidiary unit is now Freescale Semi Conductor® Inc., in Austin, Texas.

MOUNT: To make a group of files in a file system structure accessible to a user or user group; a Unix mount command attaches disks, or directories logically rather than physically; a Unix mount command makes a directory accessible by attaching a root directory of one file system to another directory, which makes all the file systems usable as if they were subdirectories of the file system where they are attached; Unix recognizes devices by their location, as compared to Windows®, which recognizes them by their names (D: drive, for example); Unix organizes directories in a tree-like structure, in which directories are attached by mounting them on the branches of the tree. The file system location where the device is attached is called a mount point; may be local or remote; a local mount connects disk drives on one machine so that they behave as one logical system, while a remote mount uses Network File System (NFS) to connect to directories on other machines so that they can be used as if they were all part of the user's file system.

MOUSE: Hardware desktop input device for GUI control execution features; point and click operating system interface with pointer cursor; roller-ball, infrared, remote, mini, and optical types; rubber ball, infrared, or optical control; developed in 1964 by Douglas Engelbart.

MOUSE POTATOE: An Internet user addicted to aimless browsing; slang term.

MOUSE TRAP: JavaScript© Web page with functionless "back" button usually used to compel advertiser viewing; slang term.

MOV: Internet files extension for the QuickTime® movie or file format.

MOZILLA: Netscape© open source free Web browser; Firefox©.

MP3 PLAYER: Digital music format and related generic devices with Internet download capability; Apple iPod®, iPod Photo®, iPod Shuffle®, ZUNE®, v-Pod®, and so forth; connects to a PC by a USB or FireWire port.

MPEG-1 AUDIO LAYER 3: Often referred to as MP3; a popular digital audio encoding and lossy format that reduces the quantity of data required to represent audio; compression technique invented by German engineers who worked in a digital radio research program that became an ISO standard in 1991.

MQ SERIES: IBM compatible software family whose components are used to tie together other software applications so that they can work together; business integration software; middleware.

MS-DOS: Microsoft Operating Systems first developed in the early 1980s for the 8086 series of CPUs from the Intel® Corporation and the IBM PC of 1981:

- 2007: Windows® Vista for Health care
- 2007: Windows® Vista
- 2001: Windows® XP
- 2000: Windows® ME
- 2000: Windows® 2000
- 1998: Windows® 98
- 1996: Windows® NT 4.0
- 1995: Windows® 95
- 1994: Windows® NT 3.5
- 1993: Windows NT 3.1
- 1990: Windows® 3.0
- 1987: Windows® 2.0
- 1985: Windows® 1.0

M-TECHNOLOGY: Write once-run anywhere functionality.

MULTICAST: Networked computer transmission meant for many reception nodes.

MULTICS: Precursor computer language program to UNIIX, with MRDS relational database.

MULTIHOMED HOST: A computer or server physically connected to more than two networks, with multiple IP addresses and interfaces.

MULTIMEDIA: Voice, video, and graphical digital information that requires broad bandwidth for multiple transmissions on one compressed line and much storage capacity.

MULTIPARTITE VIRUS: A worm, trojan, or malicious computer system code that combines types of boot sector and files miscreants; Ghostballs variant.

MULTIPLEXOR: Hardware peripheral device that allows multiple voice-video or graphical data source transmissions; by combining and interweaving low-capacity channels in discrete time or frequency slices, this equipment allows transmission of multiple lines of audio, video, or data information in one high-capacity communications channel.

MULTIPOINT CONTROL UNIT (MCU): A centrally located service offered by switch network providers that allows three or more users to be connected, allowing audio and video teleconferencing.

MULTIPROCESSING: Computer or system with two or more CPUs.

MULTIPROGRAM VIRUS: Macro virus first infecting several MSFT Word©, Excel©, and PowerPoint© files at once; originally appeared in 1999 as the TriState variant.

MULTISITE TEST: An application or program stress beta-review for many geographic locations.

MULTITASK: The ability of an operating system to run multiple computerized tasks or applications simultaneously; for example, Windows NT©.

MUNDIE, CRAIG: Chief Research and Strategy Officer of the Microsoft Corporation.

MUSICAL INSTRUMENT DIGITAL INTERFACE (MIDI): Musical information interchange standardized transmission protocol.

MY COMPUTER: Windows© drive feature; accessed from Start Menu.

MY DOCUMENTS: MSFT Windows© desktop computer file folder.

MY NETWORK PLACE: MSFT Windows© computer folder of available network resources.

MYSQL: Open source database software utility program.

N

NAGIOS®: Open source computer security network host and service application monitoring system; by GroundWork®.

NAG SCREEN: The first page of a shareware computer program listing its maker, credentials, requests for donations, and so forth; nagware; slang term.

NAME: Linguistic expression of an object-file designation.

NAMED PIPES: Used for unidirectional or bidirectional connectionless messaging between clients and computer servers.

NAME RESOLUTION: Mapping, identifying, or connecting a computer machine name to its corresponding IP address.

NAME SPACE: Individual objects that are named in a computer networking environment; XML identifying attributes.

NANDA TAXONOMY: List of nursing diagnostics that identify and code medical problems or life processes; second version.

NANO MEMBRANE: Ultra-thin, flexible semiconductor CPU chip developed at the University of Wisconsin, at Madison.

NANO MEMORY: A single molecule trapped between electrodes that may be switched between conductive states and serves as stored medical data or other information.

NANO SECOND: One billionth of a second.

NAPSTER: Defunct utility provider of P2P music file shareware applications; 1999–2001.

NARROWBAND: Electronic communication transmission rates below 64 Kbps; a telecommunications medium that uses low frequency signals, not exceeding 1.544 Mbps; slow.

NARROWCAST: Electronic transmission to invited individuals.

NASTYGRAM: Malicious e-mail message that targets security poles of a targeted computer system; slang term.

NATIONAL ASSOCIATION OF HEALTH DATA ORGANIZATIONS (NAHDO): A group that promotes the development and improvement of state and national health information systems.

NATIONAL CENTER FOR HEALTH SERVICES RESEARCH (NCHSR): Former name of the Agency for Health Care Policy and Research (AHCPR).

NATIONAL CENTER FOR HEALTH STATISTICS (NCHS): A federal organization within the CDC that collects, analyzes, and distributes health care statistics; maintains ICD-n-CM codes.

NATIONAL COMMITTEE ON VITAL AND HEALTH STATISTICS (NCVHS): A Federal advisory body within HHS that advises the Secretary regarding potential changes to the HIPAA standards.

NATIONAL COUNCIL FOR PRESCRIPTION DRUG PROGRAMS (NCPDP): An ANSI-accredited group that maintains a number of standard formats for use by the retail pharmacy industry, some of which are included in the HIPAA mandates.

NATIONAL DRUG CODE (NDC): A medical code set that identifies prescription drugs and some over-the-counter products, and that has been selected for use in the HIPAA transactions.

NATIONAL EMPLOYER ID: A system for uniquely identifying all sponsors of health care benefits.

NATIONAL HEALTH INFORMATION INFRASTRUCTURE (NHII): A health care–specific lane on the Internet described in the National Information Infrastructure (NII) initiative.

NATIONAL HEALTH INFORMATION NETWORK (NHIN): The technologies, standards, laws, policies, programs, and practices that enable health information to be shared among health decision makers, including consumers and patients, to promote improvements in health and health care; vision for the NHII began more than a decade ago with publication of an Institute of Medicine report, *The Computer-Based Patient Record*. The path to a national network of health care information is through the successful establishment of Regional Health Information Organizations (RHIO).

NATIONAL INFORMATION INFRASTRUCTURE (NII): A U.S. government policy developed by the Clinton Administration that involves the synthesis of hardware, software, and skills that will make it easy and affordable to connect people with each other, with computers, and with a wide variety of services and information resources.

NATIONAL INFORMATION TECHNOLOGY COORDINATOR (NITC): Operates under the Secretary for Health and Human Services (SHHS); Dr. David Brailler helped develop and implement a standardized, secure, comparable electronic health record (EHR) for both the private and public health sectors; even though EHRs are being utilized across the United States in some form or manner and in the government with Veterans Affairs (VA), Department of Defense (DoD) facilities, and Indian Health Services (IHS), modifications, enhancements, and changes constantly occur to provide more consistency and uniform definitions, terminology, and functions for the clinical information tool in order to more effectively share and communicate patient clinical information across various health care spectrums; HIPAA Security and Privacy Regulations have a significant impact on the design, integration, interface, implementation, and management of the system nationwide; Federal, State, and private hospitals as well as vendors and insurers will also have to absorb additional cost to adapt to the architecture, as well as security and privacy requirements.

NATIONAL INSTITUTE OF STANDARDS AND TECHNOLOGY (NIST): A unit of the U.S. Commerce Department formerly known as the National Bureau of Standards (NBS), to promote and maintain measurement standards; it also has active programs for encouraging and assisting industry, medicine, and science to develop and use these standards (Table 7).

Of particular interest to health IT stakeholders are:

- SP 800–36 offers guidance on selecting IT security products. This document provides criteria used to evaluate security products, for the following categories: Identification and Authentication, Access Control, Intrusion Detection, Firewalls, Public Key Infrastructure, Vulnerability Scanners, Malicious Code Protection, and Forensics. This will be especially useful for product consideration.
- SP 800–55 explains the measurement of security performance. This summary provides guidance on how an organization, with metrics, identifies the adequacy of in-place security controls, policies, and procedures.
- SP 800–30 deals with IT risk management. Every organization has a mission. In this digital era, as organizations use automated information technology (IT) systems to process their information for better support of their missions, risk management plays a critical role in protecting an organization's information assets, and therefore its mission, from IT-related risk.

NATIONAL LIBRARY OF MEDICINE (NLM): The computer version of the printed *Index Medicus;* citations for 7.5 million articles published since 1966

Table 7: The NIST SP 800–35 Guide for IT Systems

SP 800-30: Risk Management Guide for Information Technology Systems
SP 800-32: Introduction to Public Key Technology and the Federal PKI Infrastructure
SP 800-33: Underlying Technical Models for Information Technology Security
SP 800-34: Contingency Planning for Information Technology Systems
SP 800-41: An Introduction to Firewalls and Firewall Policy
SP 800-42: Guideline on Network Security Testing
SP 800-48: Wireless Network Security: 802.11, Bluetooth, and Handheld Devices
SP 800-50: Building an Information Technology Security Awareness and Training Program
SP 800-53: Recommended Security Controls for Federal Information Systems
SP 800-55: Security Metrics Guide for Information Technology Systems
SP 800-64: Security Considerations in the Information System Development Life Cycle
SP 800-66: An Introductory Resource Guide for Implementing the Health Insurance Portability and Accountability Act (HIPAA) Security Rules

from about 3,700 health and biomedical journals are compiled in MED-LINE, which is updated at a rate of 6,600 articles every week; about 75% of citations are for English-language articles.

NATIONAL PATIENT ID: A system for uniquely identifying all recipients of health care services and often referred to as the National Individual Identifier (NII), or as a health care ID.

NATIONAL PAYER ID (NPID): A system for uniquely identifying all organizations that pay for health care and medical services.

NATIONAL PROVIDER (PATIENT) FILE (NPF): A database for use in maintaining a national provider registry for doctors and patients.

NATIONAL PROVIDER (PATIENT) ID (NPID): A numerical system for uniquely identifying all providers of health care services; patients, supplies, and equipment.

NATIONAL PROVIDER (PHYSICIAN-PRACTITIONER) IDENTIFIER (NPI): Originally was an eight-digit alphanumeric identifier. However, the health care industry widely criticized this format, claiming that major information systems incompatibilities would make it too expensive and difficult to implement. DHHS therefore revised its recommendation, instead specifying a *10-position numeric identifier with a check digit in the last position to help detect keying errors.* The NPI carries no intelligence; in other words, its characters will not in themselves provide information about the provider. More recently, CMS announced that HIPAA-covered entities, such as providers completing electronic transactions, health care clearinghouses, and large health plans, must use only the NPI to identify covered health care providers in standard transactions by May 23, 2007. Small health plans must use only the NPI by May 23, 2008. The proposal for a Standard Unique National Health Plan (Payer) Identifier was withdrawn on February 2006. (According to CMS, "withdrawn" simply means that there is not a specific publication date at this time. Development of the rule has been delayed; however, when the exact date is determined, the rule will be put back on the agenda.)

NATIONAL PROVIDER REGISTRY (NPR): The organization for assigning National Provider IDs.

NATIONAL PROVIDER SYSTEM (NPS): The administrative system for supporting a national provider registry.

NATIONAL SCIENCE ADVISORY BOARD FOR BIOSECURITY (NSABB): Established in 2004 to advise all federal departments and agencies that conduct or support life sciences research that could fall into the "dual use" category: Its objectives are:

- advise on strategies for local and federal biosecurity oversight for all federally funded or supported life sciences research.
- advise on the development of guidelines for biosecurity oversight of life sciences research and provide ongoing evaluation and modification of these guidelines as needed.
- advise on strategies to work with journal editors and other stakeholders to ensure the development of guidelines for the publication, public presentation, and public communication of potentially sensitive life sciences research.
- advise on the development of guidelines for mandatory programs for education and training in biosecurity issues for all life scientists and laboratory workers at federally funded institutions.
- provide guidance on the development of a code of conduct for life scientists and laboratory workers that can be adopted by federal agencies as well as professional organizations and institutions engaged in the performance of life sciences research domestically and internationally.

NATIONAL SCIENCE FOUNDATION (NSF): Federal U.S. government agency that promotes and funds electronic communications causes and projects.

NATIONAL SOFTWARE TESTING LABORATORY (NSTL): One of the first independent organizations to evaluate computer hardware and software; used controlled testing methods to ensure objective results, and publishes its findings in *Software Digest Ratings Report, PC Digest,* and later generations of same.

NATIONAL STANDARD FORMAT (NSF): Generically applies to any nationally standardized data electronic health transmission format, but it is often used in a more limited way to designate the Professional EMC NSF, a 320-byte flat file record format used to submit professional claims.

NATIONAL TELECOMMUNICATIONS AND INFORMATION ADMINISTRATION (NTIA): The federal agency in the Department of Commerce responsible for the National Information Infrastructure (NII) initiative.

NATIONAL TELEVISION SYSTEM COMMITTEE (NTSC): An independent panel that is involved in setting the standards for broadcast television in the United States; standards are sometimes considered a composite video because all video information is combined into one analog signal.

NATIONAL UNIFORM BILLING COMMITTEE (NUBC): An organization, chaired and hosted by the American Hospital Association, that maintains the UB-92 hardcopy institutional billing form and the data element specifications for both the hardcopy form and the 192-byte UB-92 flat file EMC format.

NATIONAL UNIFORM CLAIM COMMITTEE (NUCC): An organization, chaired and hosted by the American Medical Association, that maintains the HCFA-1500 claim form and a set of data element specifications for professional claims submission via the HCFA-1500 claim form, the Professional EMC NSF, and the X12 837; also maintains the Provider Taxonomy Codes and has a formal consultative role under HIPAA for all transactions affecting nondental, noninstitutional professional health care services.

NATIVE FORMAT: Computer readability by a specific application with translation using bridges or filters.

NATURAL LANGUAGE: Fifth generation computer language using human speech.

NAVIGATION: Interacting with a complex computer system; software applications, programs, and so forth.

NAVIGATION TOOL: A multimedia Web presentation and search utility.

NAVIGATOR: An Internet browser developed by the Netscape® Corporation.

NCPDP BATCH STANDARD: An NCPDP standard designed for use by low-volume dispensers of pharmaceuticals, such as nursing homes.

NCPDP TELECOMMUNICATION STANDARD: An NCPDP standard designed for use by high-volume dispensers of pharmaceuticals, such as retail pharmacies.

NEAMAN, MARK: President and CEO of Evanston Northwestern Healthcare, IL.

NEED-TO-KNOW (NTK): A personal health information security principle stating that a user should have access only to the medical data he or she needs to perform a particular function.

NELSON, IVO: Director of IBM's health care business consulting services group, Armonk, NY.

NERD: One interested in computer engineering and health or other IT systems to the exclusion of human interaction; geek; slang term.

NESSUS: A security scanner for Linux that offered high-end security for the mid-tier computer user; by Tenable Network Security®.

NEST(ING): Document input within the body of another document for nonlinear access.

NET: The www or Internet; slang term.

NETBIOS: The BIOS code for a computer network.

NET CAFÉ: A casual meeting place for Internet access; Internet café; slang term.

NET CAST(ING): Pod casting or Web casting; electronic broadcast clips.

NET CENTRIC: An intra- or Internet-worked focused environment for seamless productivity.

NET FRAMEWORK: An architecture framework and business strategy from Microsoft® and its collection of programming support for Web services or the ability to use the Intent rather than a PC; platform includes servers and building-block services, such as XML Web-based data storage, device software, and MS Passport® (fill-in-the-form-only-once identity verification service); vaguely similar to Java.

NET HEAD: Internet addicted user; Web head; net surfer; and so forth, slang term.

NETIQUETTE: Online manners and propriety; such as not spamming or using CAPITAL letters which is the Internet equivalent of shouting; net speak.

NETIZEN: An upright righteous citizen or proper user of the Internet; slang term.

NETMEETING: Electronic collaborative network conferencing functions with groupware capabilities.

NETNEUTRALITY: The inability of telephone lines carriers such as Verizon® and AT&T® to charge extra for premium delivery of Internet content; *save-the-Internet*.

NET PASSPORT: MSFT® online service to use a password and e-mail identifier to sign on to any .NET participating Web site.

NETPHONE: Commonly referred to as the "Internet telephone" and refers to the equipment used to permit two users to talk to one another using the Internet as the connection; Net-2-Phone®.

NETSCAPE NAVIGATOR®: A Netscape Corporation® Web browser with varying GUI formats, acquired by AOL® in 1998.

NETSPEAK: Ouvre of Internet linguistics; netiquette; slang term.

NETWORK: To connect computers or hubs with wireless or wired connectivity to share and manipulate common information; Cisco Systems®, Juniper Networks®, Lucent Technologies®, Cingular®, and Verizon®.

NETWORK ADDRESS TRANSLATION (NAT): To secure internal health network data by changing, entering, and exiting IP addresses; firewall and router functionality.

NETWORK ADMINISTRATOR: One who manages an electronic computer network with servers and client work stations; expert IT systems manager.

NETWORK APPLICATION: A shared and connected program, software code, or operating utility or development tool for a LAN, MAN, WAN, or the Internet, intranet, and so forth.

NETWORK ATTACHED STORAGE (NAS): Architecture that attaches disk arrays to computers throughout a department, giving multiple computers access to high-capacity storage resources; economical because it relies on older, well-established technologies, such as the hard drive standard of the American Telemedicine Association (ATA) and Internet Protocol (IP) data networking.

NETWORK COMPUTER (NC): A thin client-type personal computer with a CPU but little storage capacity running health applications and medical programs over a connected ring of computers.

NETWORK INTERFACE CARD (NIC): Computer-to-network sharing PCI adapter; Windows XP® allows a wide range of network sharing resources such as pictures and music files to printers, scanners, and hard-drives.

NETWORK LAYER: Internet routing destination layer for data and switching functionality; third layer of an OSI model; Internet layer.

NETWORK PRINTER: A shared printing peripheral device available to connected nodule users.

NETWORK REDIRECTOR: Operating system interception function that transfers input requests to a local or remote computer system or machine for processing.

NETWORK TOPOLOGY: The geometry of networked computers and related devices (usually serial bus or star); pattern of links and modes in an interconnected multiple computer network system.

NETWORK TRAFFIC: Amount of linked computer use, usually excessive, from nodule user, and to user.

NETWORK WEAVING: To enter a computer communications network, avoid detection, and trace-back.

NEURAL NETWORK: Nonlinear predictive model for pattern matching and interactive learning.

NEUTRICIDE: Telephone company destruction of Internet neutrality; slang term.

NEVER EVENT (NE): Incidents, such as surgery on the wrong body part or a mismatched blood transfusion, that cause serious injury or death to beneficiaries and result in increased costs to the Medicare program to treat the consequences of the error; no longer financially reimbursable.

NEWBIE: A first time computer, network, or Internet user; slang term.

NEW MEDIA: Nontraditional electronic health data and other communication methods with features such as low cost, centrality, volatility, and multimedia functions.

NEWSFEED: Automatically updated Web site link; Really Simple Syndication (RSS).

NEWSGROUP: A topic-focused Internet message board or discussion group; sometimes referred to collectively as "Usenet" with discussion groups open to the public, or private, where users can read the information posted and add new messages, or articles; uses a hierarchical topic structure to make it easy for the user to find the information; messages posted to newsgroups are sent to every computer connected to the Internet, where it is stored for a few days to give interested users the chance to read it; individual users have the option whether they would like to subscribe to newsgroups; currently, over 29,000 newsgroups exist and are available for subscription, although most users only subscribe to, read, and respond to a few of them.

NEWSGROUP READER: The software used to access, read, and post to medical or other newsgroups.

NEWSLINE: A collaborative electronic publisher.

NEWSREADER: A utility program to use, read, and post electronic messages to a newsgroup.

NIAGRA: Sun Microsystems UltraSPARC® T1 microprocessor chip; code name.

NIBBLE: Half of an eight-bit byte (four bits); slang term.

NIMDA WORM: Malicious computer system code that slows or delays e-mail messages; first released in 2001 and with more current variants.

NODE: Host computer of a link system or connected network.

NOISE: Any health care, medical data, or other computer system electronic transmission interference; slang term.

NOM-DE-HAQUE: Pseudonym or anonymous name used by a computer, network, or Internet hacker.

NOMENCLATURE: The systematic naming of elements in a system; codified terms and abbreviations; ontology, common language; www.Health Dictionary Series.com.

NONCOMPUTING SECURITY METHODS: Safeguards that do not use the hardware, software, and firmware of a health care information technology infrastructure; include physical security (controlling physical access to computing resources), personnel security, and procedural security.

NONOVERWRITING VIRUS: Software extension code or appendix that moves an original malicious computer code to another location.

NONREPUDIATION: Computer system accountability protocol that depends upon the ability to ensure that senders cannot deny sending medical or other information and that receivers cannot deny receiving it; spans prevention and detection and used as a prevention measure because the mechanisms implemented prevent the ability to successfully deny an action; service typically performed at the point of transmission or reception; public and private key infrastructure; ensures that PHI can not be disputed; third party proof.

NONVOLATILE MEMORY: Storage data that remains when power circuitry is disconnected; stable electronic data memory stick, flash card, and so forth.

NOONAN, THOMAS E.: Former President and Chief Executive Officer of Internet Security Systems® (ISS) in Atlanta; responsible for the overall strategic direction, growth, and management of the company; launched in 1994 with Christopher W. Klaus to a preeminent position in the network security industry; holds a mechanical engineering degree from the Georgia Institute of Technology and a CSS in Business Administration from Harvard University; now part of IBM®.

NORDA, RAYMOND: Deceased cofounder of Novell®, Inc., and developer of NetWare® who acquired WordPerfect® Corporation and the Quattro Pro® spreadsheets business of Borland International; father of network computing who coined the term *coopetition*.

NORMALIZATION: Uniform standards or formats for computer operability or use.

NORMALIZATION SERVICE: A firm that provide normalization processes, such as for EHRs, EMRs, CPOEs, and so forth.

NORRIS, JOHN A.: Corporate Executive Vice President, Hill and Knowlton, Inc., Waltham, MA, and Lecturer in Health Law, Harvard School of Public Health, Boston, MA.

NORTH CAROLINA HEALTHCARE INFORMATION AND COMMUNICATIONS ALLIANCE (NCHICA): A medical organization that promotes the advancement and integration of information technology into the health care industry.

NOTEBOOK: A small portable PC.

NOTEBOOK SAFE: A special safe secured to a wall or the trunk of a car used for storing a notebook computer.

NOTEPAD: A limited Windows® text editor.

NOTICE OF INTENT (NOI): A document that describes a subject area for which the federal government is considering developing regulations; may describe the relevant considerations and invite comments from interested parties and then used in developing an NPRM or a final regulation.

NOTICE OF PRIVACY PRACTICE (NPP): A notice to the individual of the uses and disclosures of protected health information and the individual's rights and the covered entity's legal duties with respect to protected health information covered entity disclosure. In its most visible change, the privacy regulations require covered entities to provide patients with a Notice of Privacy Practices (NPP). The NPP replaces the use of consents, which are now optional, although they are recommended. The NPP outlines how PHI is to be regulated, which gives the patient far-reaching authority and ownership of their PHI, and must describe, in general terms, how organizations will protect health information.

The NPP specifies the patient's right to the following:

- Gain access to and, if desired, obtain a copy of one's own health records;
- Request corrections of errors that the patient finds (or include the patient's statement of disagreement if the institution believes the information is correct);
- Receive an accounting of how their information has been used (including a list of the persons and institutions to whom/which it has been disclosed);
- Request limits on access to, and additional protections for, particularly sensitive information;
- Request confidential communications (by alternative means or at alternative locations) of particularly sensitive information;
- Complain to the facility's privacy officer if there are problems; and
- Pursue the complaint with DHHS's Office of Civil Rights if the problems are not satisfactorily resolved.

A copy of the NPP must be provided the first time a patient sees a direct treatment provider, and any time thereafter when requested or when the NPP is changed. On that first visit, treatment providers must also make a good faith effort to obtain a written acknowledgement, confirming that a copy of the NPP was obtained. Health plans and insurers must also provide periodic notices to their customers, but do not need to secure any acknowledgement. Most health information management departments that oversee the clinical coding of medical records also manage the NPP documentations and deadlines, but this may very from hospital to hospital.

NOTICE OF PROPOSED RULEMAKING (NPRM): A document that describes and explains regulations that the federal government proposes to adopt at some future date, and invites interested parties to submit comments related to them; may be used in developing a final regulation.

NOVICE HACKER: An unskilled computer or network person acting as an electronic miscreant; script kiddies; slang term.

NT FILE SYSTEM: An optional file system for Windows NT®, 2000®, XP®, and later operating systems; a more advanced file system than FAT16, -32, -64.

NTLDR: A program that is loaded from the hard drive boot sector and displays the Microsoft Windows NT® startup menu and helps Windows NT® load; short for NT Loader.

NTLDR'S $DATA ATTRIBUTE: NTLDR attribute that contains actual health or other medical data or information for a file.

NUBC EDI TAG: The NUBC EDI Technical Advisory Group, which coordinates issues affecting both the NUBC and the X12 standards.

NULL MODEM: Modem simulator for direct connection between computers, servers, or nodes.

NULL MODEM CABLE: Serial cable with bidirectional crossed pins for direct connection simulation.

NUMERIC DATA: Continuous and discrete medical, health, or other data.

NURSING INFORMATICS: The use of health care management information computer systems and digital data capture, storage, and transmission to facilitate nursing activities.

O

OBJECT: A passive computer entity that contains or receives medical information or health data; note that access to an object potentially implies access to the information it contains.

OBJECT CODE: Machine computer code generated by source code language processors, assemblers, or compilers; source code.

OBJECT IDENTIFIER: A string of numbers to identify a unique item in computer programming.

OBJECT LINKING EMBEDDING (OLE): Method of combining different information from different computer application programs, such as inserting a spreadsheet, figure, medical, or radiology image, and so forth.

OBJECT ORIENTATED PROGRAMMING (OOP): A software development methodology that combines both health information or other data and procedures into a single packet; rapid and flexible software engineering.

OBJECT REUSE: Existing computer software code objects used to create new-to-the-world code objects.

O'BRIEN, PATRICK: CIO and CFO of Ivinson Memorial Hospital, Laramie, WY.

OCTAL: Base zero to eight numbering system.

OCTET: Eight bits, or one byte, of electronic data information.

ODD PARITY: Odd number of 1-bit data parity technique for each byte or word of information.

OFFICE LIVE: MSFT real-time communications server.

OFFICE SUITE: Integrated programs with several business applications, such as word processing, spreadsheets, databases, and so forth; MSFT Office®, Corel WordPerfect Office®, Sun Star Office®, and Lotus SmartSuite®.

OFFLINE: Not connected or controlled to another computer, server, and Internet or intranet nodule system.

OFFLINE NAVIGATOR: Utility to download e-mail, sort, retrieve, and read messages while not network enabled; offline reader; offline storage.

OFFSITE PROCESSING: Remote hospital contracting with a vendor external to the hospital; the hospital sends data over to the vendor site where the actual processing takes place; upon completion, the vendor sends the data back to the hospital, usually in electronic form.

OGG VORBIS: Digital music encoding format; reportedly superior to MP3.

O'LEARY, DENNIS, MD: Longtime president and CEO for the Joint Commission on the Accreditation of Healthcare Organizations (JCAHO) who retired in 2007.

OLSEN, KENNETH: Cofounder and CEO of Digital Equipment Corporation® (DEC) launched in 1957, faltered in the 1990s and was sold to Compaq® (in turn bought up Hewlett-Packard® in 2002); famously opined in 1977, "there is no reason for any individual to have a computer in his home."

OLSSON, SILAS, MSC: Medical Informaticist for the European Commission and Informatics Society of Brussels, Belgium.

OMNI-DIRECTIONAL ANTENNA: A 360-degree beam-width transmitter in all directions.

ON-CHIP APPLICATION: Programs that reside or are embedded in an integrated circuit microchip.

ON-DEMAND COMPUTING (ODC): A bifid software delivery model similar to SAAS (software-as-a-service). The *hosted application management* (hosted AM) model is similar to ASP in that a provider hosts commercially available software for customers and delivers it over the Web. The *software on demand* model gives customers network-based access to a single copy of an application created specifically for SAAS distribution; benefits include:

- easier administration
- automatic updates
- patch and security management
- compatibility and collaboration
- global accessibility

The traditional model of software distribution, in which software is purchased for and installed on personal computers, is sometimes referred to as *software as a product;* shrink-wrapped software.

ON-DEMAND THREATS: Various online Internet security vulnerabilities, "holes," and security breaches:

- Injection Flaws: Malicious commands embedded in external and internal Web application communications.
- XSS Flaws: Malicious code push from Web applications to PCs; unauthorized local PC controls.
- Unvalidated Input: Untested Web application information sent back to individual PC users.
- Denial of Service (DOS): Web application use prevention, manipulated Web traffic to exhaust bandwidth.

ONLINE: Connected or controlled to another computer, server, the Internet, or intranet nodule system; online medical communities, online games, online health care networks, online services, online information systems, and so forth.

ONLINE IDENTITY: A caller ID service for the Web used to create multiple identities online.

ONLINE SERVICE PROVIDER (OSP): A company that provides Internet-based commercial computer services; dial-up services.

ONTOLOGY: Conceptual knowledge domain standard that describes dictionary elements and vocabulary expressions of a common language or lexicon.

ONYX: On-demand CRM service provider.

OPEN: Refers to a type of mailing list and signifies a system that permits anyone to post a message to it, independent of their member status; different than a closed or moderated system.

OPEN PREPRESS INTERFACE: Image-swapping technology that allows low resolution images inserted into a page layout program to be swapped with the high-resolution version for film or plate setting.

OPEN SOURCE CODE: UNIX or LINUX®-based software code now on desktop computers loaded with collaborative tools such as Google Maps® or Gmail; or the Free Software Foundation's Gnu C Compiler; Make, a C programming utility; or Apache Ant®, an open source code for assembling JAVA® applications; open standards; open systems.

OPEN SOURCE SOFTWARE (OSS): Refers to software developed, tested, or improved through public collaboration and distributed with the idea that it must be shared with others, ensuring an open future collaboration; especially those in the academic environment, in developing various versions of Unix; Richard Stallman's idea of a free software foundation and the desire of users to freely choose among a number of products; LINUX.

OPEN SYSTEM: A vendor independent interconnected computer network.

OPEN SYSTEMS ARCHITECTURE: Generic, usually free, and standardized technology for hardware, software, peripheral and online operating systems, databases, programs, communications, storage, and applications; nonproprietary computer systems; for example, Linux was developed by Finnish engineer Linus Torvalds, and is supported by thousands of programmers worldwide who continually update and prove it.

OPEN SYSTEMS ENVIRONMENT: Software systems that operate on different open hardware platforms, computers, and networks.

OPEN SYSTEMS INTERCONNECTION (OSI): A multilayer ISO data communications standard that is industry specific, and HL7 is responsible for specifying the level seven OSI standards for the health industry; a standard reference model for LANs, MANs, and WANs.

OPEN VMS: An operating system that started out on Digital Equipment Corporation's first produced systems (PDP®); migration through the years was to VAX and Alpha systems; VMS had a file system that supported fairly long names, was hierarchical in directory structure, and supported multiple versions of the same file with the same name.

OPEN VMS ALPHA: A family of RISC-based, 64-bit CPUs and computer systems originally developed by Digital, acquired by Compaq®, and then by Hewlett-Packard®.

OPEN VPN: A virtual private networking application.

OPEN WEB APPLICATION SECURITY PROJECT (OWASP): An organization that provides unbiased and practical, cost-effective information about computer and Internet programs and applications to assist individuals, doctors, nurses, businesses, agencies, and health care organizations in finding and using trustworthy computer systems software. The OWASP Top Ten is a list of the most dangerous Web application security flaws, along with effective methods of dealing with them:

1. Unvalidated input: Information from Web requests is not validated before being used by a Web application; attackers can use these flaws to attack backend components through a Web application.

2. Broken access control: Restrictions on what authenticated users are allowed to do are not properly enforced; attackers can exploit these flaws to access other users' accounts, view sensitive files, or use unauthorized functions.

3. Broken authentication and session management: Account credentials and session tokens are not properly protected; attackers that can compromise passwords, keys, biometrics, session cookies, or other tokens can defeat authentication restrictions and assume other users' identities.

4. Cross-site-scripting (XSS) flaws: Web application can be used as a mechanism to transport an attack to an end user's browsers; a successful attack can disclose the end user's session token, attack the local machine, or spoof content to fool the user.

5. Buffer overflows: Web application components in some languages that do not properly validate input can be crashed and, in some cases, used to take control of a process; components can include CGI, libraries, drivers, and Web application server components.

6. Injection flaws: Web applications pass parameters when they access external systems or the local operating system; an attacker can embed malicious commands in these parameters, and the external system may execute those commands on behalf of the Web application.

7. Improper error handling: Error conditions that occur during normal operation are not handled properly; an attacker can cause errors to occur that the Web application does not handle, they can gain detailed system information, deny service, cause security mechanisms to fail, or crash the server.

8. Insecure storage: Web applications frequently use cryptographic functions to protect information and credentials; such functions and the code to integrate them have proven difficult to code properly, frequently resulting in weak protection.

9. Denial of Service (DOS): Attackers can consume Web application resources to a point where other legitimate users can no longer access or use the application; attackers can also lock users out of their accounts or even cause the entire application to fail.

10. Insecure configuration management: Having a strong server configuration standard is critical to a secure Web application; servers have many configuration options that affect security and are not secure out of the box.

OPERA: A Web browsing program.

OPERATING SYSTEM (OS): The set of basic programs and utilities that make a computer run. At the core of an operating system is the kernel, which allows the computer to start or boot-up and run applications or programs; Linux / Variants, MacOS®, CP/M, MS-DOS®, IBM OS/2 Warp®, UNIX / Variants, Windows CE®, Windows 3.x, Windows 95®, Windows 98®, Windows 98 SE®, Windows ME®, Windows NT®, Windows 2000®, Windows XP®, Vista®, and Solaris Enterprise System, from Sun Microsystems, Inc.®

OPERATING SYSTEM CERTIFICATION: Standard or benchmark of computer kernel functionality and performance efficiency.

OPERATING SYSTEM HARDENING: Steps that can be taken to make a personal computer operating system more secure.

OPERATOR: A character used to limit or broaden a search; characters such as and, or, and not are referred to as a Boolean operator.

OPTICAL CARD: Memory card with updatable laser recorded and read data; laser smart plastic card.

OPTICAL CHARACTER RECOGNITION (OCR): Automatic scanning of the translation of printed characters to computer-based text.

OPTICAL DISK: A laser disk used for computer medical data or other information storage; a disc that uses laser technology to record data; used for large quantities (Gbs) of medical data.

OPTICAL FINGERPRINT SENSOR: The most prevalent and mature biometric format that has a delicate interface surface to read human fingerprints but struggles through dirt, oils, inks, and abrasions on the skin.

OPTICAL IMAGE-BASED SYSTEM: Paper medical record that is scanned and stored in electronic format; usually .PDF.

OPTICAL READER: Device whose special shaped characters is recognized by a reading device.

OPTICAL RESOLUTION: A measure of image detail within a given distance; picture sharpness or crispness meter.

OPTION BUTTON: Two or more circular groups of input dialog boxes.

OPT OUT: To deselect from mass e-mail communications, newsgroups, RSS feeds, and so forth.

ORACLE®: The world's largest enterprise software company that supplies comprehensive business intelligencer products such as database with interactive dashboard, embedded analytic applications, real-time predictive decision-making and monitoring, uniform meta-data and data warehousing as well as a range of proprietary and open-source software to manage, share, and protect health care data and other information; based in Redwood Shores, CA; CEO Larry Ellison.

ORANGE BOOK: Compilation of CD format standards; USG *Trusted Computer Systems Evaluation Criteria;* first published in 1985 and defined computer standards for the industry; slang term.

ORDER ENTRY SYSTEM: Any process for requesting and securing items; such as computerized physician order entry (CPOE).

ORGANIZATION FOR THE ADVANCEMENT OF STRUCTURED INFORMATION STANDARDS (OASIS): A nonprofit, international consortium whose goal is to promote the adoption of product-independent standards for information formats such as Standard Generalized Markup Language, Extensible Markup Language, and Hypertext Markup Language; working to bring together competitors and industry standards groups with conflicting perspectives to discuss using XML as a common Web language that can be shared across applications and platforms for health information transmissions and related technologies.

ORGANIZED HEALTH CARE ARRANGEMENT: A clinically or virtually integrated care setting in which individuals typically receive health care from more than one health care provider or an organized system of health care in which more than one covered entity participates, and in which the participating covered entities hold themselves out to the public as participating in a joint arrangement and participate in joint activities.

ORIGAMI: Mobile PC project from MSFT; device that resides between a PDA and a laptop for enhanced health data, medical, and information connectivity; code name.

ORLOV, OLEG, MD, PHD: CMIO for the Telemedicine Foundation of Russia.

ORYX INITIATIVE: JCAHO program that integrates outcome data with accreditation.

OS/2: IBM 32-bit multitasking GUI function operating system for 80286–80–386 series PCs.

OSBORNE, ADAM: Created the Osborne Computer Corporation® in 1980 to produce the first commercially successful portable personal computer, the Osborne 1; a self-contained unit that included 64K of memory, a monochrome monitor, a keyboard, and a disk drive and sold with bundled software packages; Compaq® inherited the design and produced their first portable machine in 1983.

OTELLINI, PAUL: Intel Corporation® CEO and promoter of *Woodcrest* CPU technology.

OTHER PROVIDER NUMBER (OPN): Medical provider identification number often used by physicians and allied health care providers, such as UPIN, SS, DEA, OSCAR, PIN, Payer, Medicaid State Number, and so forth.

OUTLOOK®: MSFT e-mail calendar software application; Outlook Express®.

OUTPUT: The end product of a computer or network electronic data manipulation process.

OUTPUT DEVICE: Electronic machines that display the end product of computer processed input data and information.

OUTPUT RESOLUTION: The resolution of the device used for the final output of a digital file expressed as dots per inch (dpi).

OVERCLOCKED: A desktop PC in which the processor is set to run faster than the manufacturer's speed rating.

OVER-HAGE, MARC J., MD, PHD: CEO, Indiana Health Information Exchange and Senior Investigator Regenstrief Institute.

OVERLAPPING SECURITY DOMAIN: Key health IT elements include flexibility, tailored protection, domain interrelationships, and the use of multiple perspectives to determine what is important in information technology security, as illustrated in Figure 9.

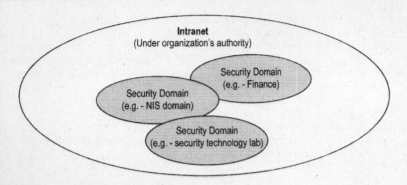

Figure 9: Overlapping health security domains.

OVERWRITE: Top save or write over health data or other information on a floppy disk, CD, memory stick, or other portable storage device; hard-disk, and so forth.

OVERWRITING VIRUS: Malicious computer code that destroys host or server data and replaces source code with viral code.

OZZIE, RAYMOND: One of three chief technical officers for the Microsoft Corporation, Redmond, WA, who is now chief software architect; creator of Lotus Notes®, and the Groove Network®.

P

P2P: Patient to Patient.

P2P: Peer to Peer.

P2P: Patient to Physician.

P2P: Patient to Provider.

P3P: Platform for Privacy Preferences.

P4P: Pay for Performance.

P6: Intel® Corporation name for the 686 Pentium-Pro CPU.

PACKAGE CODE: Manufacturer or private label software or computer code.

PACKET: Small block of digital health information or other data transmitted over a switching network; packet radio; packet monitor; packet filer; packet flood; packet sniffer, packet switch, and so forth; a basic message unit for communications in networks; a short block of data comprised of data, call control signals, and error control information and containing information on its source, content, and destination that is transferred in a packet switched network.

PACKET FILTER FIREWALL: Individual data-block, reviewed by individual data-packet security filtering and screening.

PACKET FORMAT: A digital packet of three standard items: header, information data, and trailer.

PACKET NETWORK: A connected computer system that gives out health data bits in packets.

PACKET SNIFFING: Information pirating, theft, or malicious alteration or data copying.

PACKET SWITCH: Data information sent along multiple destination paths.

PACKET SWITCHING: The procedure of transmitting digital health or other information from addressed packets so that a channel is occupied only during the transmission of the packet.

PACKET SWITCHING NETWORK (PSN): Refers to the transmission of digital health or other information using addressed packets that are transmitted along various routes in a network; more efficient than modem transmission where the channel is occupied throughout the transmission, because the occupation in the channel is limited to packet transmission.

PADLOCK: Computer icon that indicates secure computer network connectivity.

PAGE FILE, PAGING FILE, PAGEFILE.SYS: A Windows swap file.

PAID AS BILLED: Medical invoice, usually electronic, satisfied as submitted without change or adjudication.

PAID CLAIMS: Medical reimbursement that meets contracted terms and conditions; a *clean-claim*.

PAINT: A Windows® image editing and drawing program.

PALM: A PDA the Palm Operating System®.

PALM OS: The operating system for a Palm Pilot® with stylus or mini-keyboard inputting; from PalmSource® of Sunnyvale, CA, since 2003.

PALM PILOT®: A personal digital assistant (handheld computer) with minimal software and hardware complexity, since 1996.

PALM TOP: Generic term for a small computer held in one hand.

PAQUIN, MICHAEL D.: A former MS-HUG chairman.

PARALLEL PORT: PC socket used to connect a parallel port printer or other device.

PARALLEL PROCESSING: Simultaneous use of many individual computers to solve a problem, or run an application, and so forth.

PARAMETER: A symbol, word, or number keyboarded or input into a computer or PDA, after a command, for additional functionality.

PARENT, JAIME B.: CPHIMS Vice President Information Systems and CIO, Maryland General Hospital, Baltimore.

PARITY: A transmission integrity data check; electronic checksum; parity check; parity error; parity bit, and so forth.

PARK, H. K.: Chairman of Biomedical Engineering for the Kyunghee University School of Medicine.

PARKERIAN HEXAD: Six fundamental, atomic, nonoverlapping attributes of medical, health, or other information that are protected by information security measures; defined by Donn B. Parker, they are confidentiality, possession, integrity, authenticity, availability, and utility.

- Confidentiality: Restrictions on the accessibility and dissemination of medical and health information.
- Possession: The ownership or control of medical information, as distinct from confidentiality.
- Data integrity: The quality of correctness, completeness, wholeness, soundness, and compliance with the intention of the creators of the health data. It is achieved by preventing accidental or deliberate but unauthorized insertion, modification, or destruction of data in a database.
- Authenticity: The correct attribution of origin such as the authorship of an e-mail message or the correct description of medical information such as a data field that is properly named.
- Availability: The accessibility of a health system resource in a timely manner; for example, the measurement of a system's uptime.
- Utility: Usefulness; fitness for a particular use. For example, if medical data are encrypted and the decryption key is unavailable, the breach of security is in the lack of utility of the data (they are still confidential, possessed, integral, authentic, and available).

PARSER: An initial step for assembly compilation, interpretation of computer language syntax analysis.

PARTICIPANT: Any employee or former employee of an employer, or any member or former member of an employee health organization, who is or may become eligible to receive a benefit of any type from an employee benefit plan that covers employees of that employer or members of such an organization, or whose beneficiaries may be eligible to receive any of these benefits; includes an individual who is treated as an employee under section 401(c)(1) of the Internal Revenue Code of 1986 (26 U.S.C. 401(c)(1)).

PARTITION: A reserved part of a disk or memory that is set aside for some purpose; for example on a PC, new hard disks must be partitioned using the Fdisk utility before they can be formatted for the operating system; one may create just one partition, creating one drive letter for the entire disk (e.g., "C:"), or several partitions such as drives C:, D:, and E: (all located on the same physical disk, but acting like three separate drives to the operating system and end user).

PASCAL: Computer programming language developed in the 1970s by Nick Wirth; modern version of the ALGOL language.

PASSIVE HUB: A central network connecting device void of processing or regeneration signals; passive node.

PASSIVE THREAT: A potential computer network security breach without the alteration of system status.

PASSPORT: MSFT personally identified online suite of applications, programs, and services; single sign-in functionality.

PASSWORD: String of symbols, characters, or alphanumeric codes for computer, network, or Internet security verification, access, and use; confidential authentication information composed of a string of characters (ISO 7498—2).

PASSWORD CRACK(ER)ING: To breach a security access code, guess, determine, or steal a password; password hacker or cracker; password attack; password protection; password authentication; password(ing); slang term.

PASSWORD MANAGEMENT: Provides user education on creating and changing access keys and on the need to keep such keys confidential; password sniffing.

PASTE: To insert cut data or clipboard information into a document.

PATCH: Internet-based update programs used to fix loopholes in browsers, applications, programs, and so forth (SP1 and SP2); for example, patch Tuesday; slang term.

PATCH MANAGEMENT: Tools, utilities, and processes for keeping computers up to date with new software updates that are developed after a software product is released.

PATENT TROLL: An individual or company that amasses a portfolio of patents with no intention of developing or licensing the involved technology, but makes money by suing companies on the verge of releasing products using legal injunction power to extract monetary settlements; slang term.

PATH: Computer code or input information that names and locates a medical or other electronic file.

PATIENT CARE INFORMATION SYSTEM (PCIS): Clinically focused computer network or Internet-based medical, facility, office, clinic, or integrated hospital electronic information system.

PATIENT IDENTIFIABLE DATA (PID): Personal protected and secure health information, as per HIPAA.

PATIENT (PROVIDER) INFORMATION CONTROL SYSTEM (PICS): An online transaction processing program from IBM® that, together with the programming language COBOL, has formed over the past decades into the most common set of software tools for building patient and provider transaction applications in the world of large enterprise-wide mainframe or hospital legacy computing.

PATIENT RECORD: The entire health care history of an individual patient and their medical encounters.

PATIENT RELATIONSHIP MANAGEMENT (PRM): Modular and integrated software application designed to streamline patient flow, workflow, and cash flow in medical practices; helps providers manage the relationship with patients from initial contact through all clinical stages to billing and collection; seamlessly integrated, combining Practice Management, Electronic Health Records, Electronic Data Interchange, and Mobile PDA Solutions including user-defined dashboard, scheduling, patient prep, e-chart, patient summary, document management, encounter note management, E/M advisor, voice recognition, electronic superbill, order management, e-prescribing, HL7 interfaces to lab and equipment, billing, collections, managed care contract administration, and reporting.

PATIENT SENSITIVE INFORMATION: Clinical information with medical-legal security identity, access, reimbursement, and transmission implications; *bona fide* need to know basis.

PATIENT SPECIFIC DATA: Information that can be traced to an individual; Protected Health Information.

PATIENT TELEMANAGEMENT: Networked or Internet-facilitated clinical and medical personal care, information access or knowledge management.

PATRIOT ACT: Uniting and Strengthening America by Providing Appropriate Tools Required to Intercept and Obstruct Terrorism Act (USA Patriot Act) of October 26, 2001.

PATTERSON, TIMOTHY, PHD: Creator of an operating system for use with Seattle Computer Products' 8086-based computer, a precursor to DOS.

PAYER ID: CMS term for a pre-HIPAA National Payer ID initiative.

PAYLOAD: The harmful content of a worm, virus, or other malware instrument.

PAYMENT: The billing and invoicing activities undertaken by:

- A health plan to obtain premiums or to determine or fulfill its responsibility for coverage and provision of benefits under the health plan; or
- A covered health care provider or health plan to obtain or provide reimbursement for the provision of health care;
- Determinations of eligibility or coverage (including coordination of benefits or the determination of cost sharing amounts), and adjudication or subrogation of health benefit claims;
- Risk adjusting amounts due based on enrollee health status and demographic characteristics;

- Billing, claims management, collection activities, obtaining payment under a contract for reinsurance (including stop-loss insurance and excess of loss insurance), and related health care data processing;
- Review of health care services with respect to medical necessity, coverage under a health plan, appropriateness of care, or justification of charges;
- Utilization review activities, including precertification and preauthorization of services, concurrent and retrospective review of services; and
- Disclosure to consumer reporting agencies of any of the following protected health information relating to collection of premiums or reimbursement.

PAY-PER-CLICK: Advertising models that generate revenue as Web site visitors activate or click on paid Web site icons.

PC CARD: A circuit board of memory chips, fax, modem, network parts, or other peripherals usually used in laptop computers.

PDF/ACROBAT: A platform independent rendering of data content and tools from Adobe Systems, Inc.® that liberated users from paper.

PDF FILE: The electronic facsimile of a paper document (.pdf file extension).

PEACH(Y) VIRUS: Malicious computer code or worm in 2001 that spread through .pdf files.

PEER: A stand-alone computer, hub, node, or network server.

PEER-TO-PEER NETWORK: WAN, MAN, or LAN without a central computer server; a workgroup or network.

PENETRATION: The unauthorized access to protected health care information, medical database, billing statements, insurers, third-parties, and so forth.

PENETRATION TESTING: The security-oriented probing of a computer system or network to seek out vulnerabilities that an attacker could exploit; the testing process involves an exploration of the all-security features of the system in question, followed by an attempt to breech security and penetrate the system; ethical hacking.

PENTIUM©: Intel® performance brand CPU.

PENTIUM II©: Fifth generation IBM compatible Central Processing Unit with 300-bit internal bus, 64-bit external bus, and 64-bit cache system made by the Intel Corporation©.

PENTIUM III®: Intel® CPU released in 1999 with super scale floating point mode.

PENTIUM IV®: Intel® CPU released in 2000 with enhanced RAM bus speed.

PENTIUM 4©: The seventh-generation X86 architecture CPU from Intel© and new CPU NetBurst© design architecture since the Pentium Pro© of 1995. Unlike the P-II, P-III, and Celeron©, the architecture owed little to the

Pentium Pro/P6© design and was new from the ground up; the original Pentium 4©, code-named "Willamette," ran at 1.4 and 1.5 GHz and was released in November 2000. As is traditional with Intel's flagship chips, the Pentium 4© also came in a low-end Celeron© version (often referred to as Celeron 4) and a high-end Xeon© version for SMP configurations. The Pentium 4© line of processors was retired in July 2006, replaced by the Intel Core 2© line, using the "Conroe" core.

PENTIUM CELERON©: Any of several different budget x86 CPUs produced by Intel© as a complement for its higher-performance and more expensive Pentium© family introduced in 1998; the first Celeron was based on a Pentium II© core with later versions on P-III©, P-4, and P-Mobile©.

PENTIUM CENTRINO©: A CPU platform initiative from Intel© that covered a particular combination of P-M©, motherboard chipset, and wireless network functionality for interface in the design of laptop PCs; released March 2003.

PENTIUM M®: Intel CPU®, similar to the PENTIUM III®, with mobile functionality.

PENTIUM PRO©: Sixth-generation IBM compatible Central Processing Unit with 300-bit internal architecture made by the Intel Corporation© with speeds > 150 MHz and optimized for 32-bit software applications and programs; series 686 made by the Intel Corporation©.

PERIODIC SECURITY REMINDER: Provides recollections and memory aides in which employees, agents, and contractors are made aware of security concerns on an ongoing basis (posters, screen savers, oral reminders, and so forth).

PERIPHERAL DEVICE: Any piece of computer hardware distinct from the CPU, central server, or mainframe; scanner, printer, modem, router, and so forth.

PERL: Practical Extraction and Report Language developed by Larry Wall; a dynamic computer language.

PERMISSION: User access ability into a secure health information computer system network, medical, or other database; permission level, permission class, permission log, and so forth.

PERRY, MAURICE: Software and PC visionary, doctor, surgeon, teacher, and cofounder of a privately held firm that created one of the first interactive programs for computer-based physician education.

PERSONAL COMPUTER (PC): Introduced by IBM in 1981, followed in 1983 by the PC/XT built around an 8-bit Intel 8088 microprocessor. The PC/XT used PC-DOS with a hierarchical filing system with hard disk capability; IBM introduced the IBM PC/AT® in 1984, around the Intel® 80286 16-bit microprocessor offering parallel processing but not multitasking or multiuser environments. Compatible PC makers next introduced a

32-bit bus for the 32-bit Intel 80386 to avoid royalties, and a consortium led by Compaq® responded with a 32-bit EISA bus with major compatibility advantages. IBM with Microsoft then produced 16-bit OS/2 for the PS/2 series designed with a GUI to overcome MS-DOS® limitations. Later, the introduction of 80486 CPUs cleared bus bottleneck for graphics adaptors, Windows, and SCSI interfaces used by CD-ROMS, scanners, and hard drives. A number of manufacturers, including Compaq®, Dell®, and Hewlett-Packard developed proprietary local bus systems followed by the 32-bit VESA voluntary standard, which some manufacturers partially implemented for a 64-bit wide data path of the Pentium® CPU and PCI Intel product line. DMA and IRQ configuration troubles ultimately disappeared when Windows dispensed with DOS. Currently, there is a range of different computer disk sizes, graphics adaptors, and hardware add-ons, such as mice, modems, and memory boards available, but the IBM-PC set the standard until 1995; manufacturer's today include Dell®, Gateway®, Hewlett-Packard®, and Lenovo® Group, after the exit of IBM®.

PERSONAL DIGITAL ASSISTANT (PDA): A small wireless mobile and handheld computing system for e-mail, Web surfing, calculator, phone, address book, or calendar functionality, and so forth; such as the first Apple Newton®, Palm Pilot®, or BlackBerry®.

PERSONAL (PROTECTED) HEALTH RECORD (PHR): An electronic application through which individuals can maintain and manage their secure health information (and that of others for whom they are authorized) in a private, secure, and confidential environment.

PERSONAL HOME PAGE (PHP): A script language and interpreter that is freely available and used primarily on LINUX Web servers; originally derived from *PHP: Hypertext Preprocessor,* a "recursive acronym." PHP is often used as an alternative to Microsoft's Active Server Page technology and is embedded within a Web page along with HTML, and before the page is sent to a user, the Web server calls PHP to interpret and perform the operations called for in the PHP script. An HTML page that includes a PHP script is typically given a file name suffix of ".php" ".php3," or ".phtml." Like ASP, PHP can be thought of as "dynamic HTML pages," since content will vary based on the results of interpreting the script. PHP is free and offered under an open-source license.

PERSONAL IDENTIFICATION NUMBER (PIN): A number or code assigned to an individual patient or medical provider and used to provide verification of identity.

PERSONAL INFORMATION (PI): A patient's first name or initial combined with last name plus any one of the following: (1) Social Security Number, (2) driver's license number or California identification card number, or (3) account, credit card, or debit card number in combination with security code or password that enables access to the account; if both the patient's first name and the accompanying identifier are encrypted, the data does not constitute personal information.

PERSONALLY IDENTIFIABLE HEALTH INFORMATION (PIHI): Medical and related business information that includes patient identifiers, such as name, address, telephone number, SS number, and so forth.

PERSONAL REPRESENTATIVE: A person authorized by law to act on behalf of an individual patient; treated as the individual for purposes of disclosure of protected health information.

PERSONAL WEB SERVER: MSFT Web server application functionality for a computer hosting Web sites or Web pages.

PERSONNEL CLEARANCE: Establishes a procedure to ensure that medical personnel are cleared prior to receiving access by using various methods such as criminal background checks, verification of references, and so forth.

PERSONNEL CLEARANCE PROCEDURE: A health information protective measure applied to determine that an individual's access to sensitive unclassified automated information is admissible; the need for and extent of a screening process is normally based on an assessment of risk, cost, benefit, and feasibility as well as other protective measures in place; effective screening processes are applied in such a way as to allow a range of implementation, from minimal procedures to more stringent procedures commensurate with the sensitivity of the data to be accessed and the magnitude of harm or loss that could be caused by the individual (DOE 1360.2A).

PERSONNEL SECURITY: Establishes a procedure to ensure that all health care personnel who have access to sensitive information have the required authority as well as appropriate clearances and supervision; ensures that an authorized knowledgeable person will supervise maintenance personnel when near health information pertaining to individuals (including technical maintenance personnel).

PERVASIVE COMPUTING: The philosophy of ubiquitous access to electronic information, anywhere and anytime.

PHAGE VIRUS: Malicious computer system code that affects the Palm Operating System through doc system or infrared beaming connectivity.

PHANTOM BILLING: Billing for medical services not actually performed; fraudulent medical claim submissions versus CPT *code creep*.

PHARM(ER)(ING): A hacker or cracker who implants hidden software into a computer or network server in order to redirect the user to a fake and malicious copycat site in order to extract private information.

PHARMACY INFORMATION SYSTEM (PIS): Drug tracking and dispensation related health management information system for hospitals and health care organizations.

PHIS(ING): An attempt to fraudulently gather confidential information by masquerading as a trustworthy entity, person, or business in an apparently official e-mail, text message, or Web site; carding or spoofing; video vishing; phis-tank; vish-tank; slang terms.

PHOENIX BIOS: Basic Input Output System; ganglia of the IBM PC that invited clones and compatibility.

PHOSPHOR: The elemental coating on the inside of a cathode ray tube (CRT) or monitor that produces light when hit by an electron beam.

PHP: A dynamic computer language originally designed as a scripting server side software application language.

PHRACK(ER): One of the first computer hacker magazines.

PHREAK(ER): One who defrauds telephone, Internet, or other electronic communications companies; slang term.

PHYSICAL ACCESS: The ability to use any computer hardware, software, or Internet-related electronic or physical health care information system.

PHYSICAL ACCESS CONTROL: Those formal, documented policies and procedures to be followed to limit physical health data access to an entity while ensuring that properly authorized access is allowed.

PHYSICAL ACCESS CONTROL POLICIES: Tracks and records the movement of hardware and software into and out of a cover health care facility; evaluates the information on the equipment and secures the information before the equipment is moved. Ensures that access to health information is allowed only to those authorized.

PHYSICAL LAYER: First layer link between communicating computer devices in an OIS model.

PHYSICAL SAFEGUARDS: Protection of physical computer systems and related buildings and equipment from fire and other natural and environmental hazards, as well as from intrusion; includes the use of locks, keys, and administrative measures used to control access to computer systems and health facilities; physical layer of seven ISO/OSI reference layers used to standardize computer communications; brick and mortar measures, policies, and procedures to protect patient information or a covered medical entity's electronic information systems.

PHYSICAL SECURITY: The process of protecting a computer, itself; all the tangible measures taken to protect clinical data and PHI from inappropriate manipulation, use, theft, or destruction; alarms, cables, screws, enclosures, and plates.

PHYSICIAN DASHBOARD: A GUI that allows doctors to designate information interoperability and construct a personal patient information computer interface.

PHYSICIAN ONLINE DIRECTORY: Electronic yellow pages for doctors and medical professionals.

PICASA: Facial recognition technology by Google®; slang term.

PICOSECOND: One trillionth of a second.

PICT: An image format that contains black and white, color, or grayscale information in a language called QuickDraw® to render the graphic.

PICTURE ARCHIVING AND COMMUNICATIONS SYSTEM (PACS): A system capable of acquiring, transmitting, storing, retrieving, and displaying digital medical images and relevant patient health data from various imaging sources and communicates the information over a network; teleradiology and imaging.

PICTURE DIGITAL FILE FORMATS: Digital imaging formats:

- GIF: Lossless; small files with poor quality
- BMP: Windows standard lossless picture format
- TIFF: Lossy or lossless flexible image format with excellent picture quality
- JPEG: High-quality images

PIGGYBACK: The unauthorized use of a health care management information system's architecture gained through anonymous access when a current legitimate user remains online, but has not logged-off; "hijacking"; slang term.

PING(ING): A test for wireless computer network connectivity by sending an echo data packet request to the target IP address and timing the reaction response.

PING OF DEATH (POD): A DoS attack caused by a deliberate IP packet larger than the 65,536 bytes allowed by the IP protocol, as a feature of TCP/IP is fragmentation to allow a single IP packet to be broken down into smaller segments. In 1996, attackers began to take advantage of that feature when they found that a packet broken down into fragments could add up to more than the allowed 65,536 bytes. Many operating systems didn't know what to do when they received an oversized packet, so they froze, crashed, or rebooted. PODs are very bad because the identity of the attacker sending the oversized packet can be spoofed, and because the attacker didn't need to know anything about the machine they were attacking except for its IPA address. By 1997, operating system vendors made patches available, although many Web sites continue to block Internet Control Message Protocol ping messages at their firewalls to prevent any future variations of this DoS attack. POD is also known as "long ICMP."

PIPELINE: To read computer instructions before executing them in order to enhance electronic transmission speeds.

PIXEL: The smallest unit of electronic imaging data that a CRT is able to display, and is symbolized by a numerical code in the computer; they appear on the monitor as dots of a specific color or intensity; there are many, many pixels in a single image; picture element.

PIXEL SKIP: Image resolution reduction by deleting pixels.

PKZIP®: A software compression utility program; PKUNZIP® is used for reverse decompression; PKWare® Inc.

PLAIN TEXT: Readable or clear original electronic computer text.

PLASMA: Glowing bright gas, as in a plasma computer screen or monitor.

PLATTER: One of the disks in a hard disk drive; each platter provides a top and bottom recording surface.

PLENUM: Common fire resistant wall or area for hardware security and protection.

PLONE®: Content Medical Management System for the UNC School of Medicine, in Chapel Hill, built on the open source application server Zope® and accompanying content management framework.

PLOTTER: A computer device for producing graphics.

PLUG AND PLAY (PNP): Automatic computer recognition and installation of parts, software applications, or peripheral devices with IRQ and DMA resources; slang term.

PLUG-IN: Software utility tool that allows more efficient Web browsing, Internet downloads, videos, audio, and so forth.

PODCAST: A digital audio file usually placed on a Web site to be downloaded later, usually to a stored computer file, PDA, MP3 player, or as a Web-feed; i-podding, broadcast, or Webcasting.

POINTCAST: Personalized Internet news services that deliver preselected medical data, health, or other information or knowledge content to end-user subscribers via push technology.

POINT CLICK: To move the mechanical, optical, or infrared mouse pointer to a specific location of a computer screen, and then activate the right or left mouse buttons or input triggers.

POINTER(ING): To move the mechanical, optical, or infrared mouse pointer to a specific location of a computer screen; hovering.

POINT-TO-POINT TRANSMISSION PROTOCOL (PPTP): Secure health or other data transmission standardized capability for a VPN.

POINT-TO-POINT TUNNELING PROTOCOL (PPTP): Standard secure serial medical or other data transfer with Internet communications between computers.

POLICY GUIDELINE WORK STATION: Documented instructions/procedures delineating the proper functions to be performed, the manner in which those functions are to be performed, and the physical attributes of the surroundings, of a specific computer terminal site or type of site, dependent upon the sensitivity of the health information accessed from that site.

POLYMORPHIC VIRUS: A computer virus capable of change, disguise, or alteration after infestation; 1260/V2P1 variant.

POP: Post Office Protocol for Internet servers and e-mail delivery.

POP3: A type of e-mail server.

POP DOWN BOX: GUI interface that appears after icon selection with various selection options and choices; drop down menu.

POP DOWN MENU: GUI interface that appears after icon selection with various sub-boxes, selection options, and other choices; drop down box.

POP MAIL: Regular e-mail service; POP3.

POP-UNDER: A separate Web program window that instantaneously occurs behind the Web page being viewed; usually an advertisement; pop-up variant.

POP-UP: A separate Web program window that instantaneously occurs when certain Web pages are viewed; usually an advertisement.

POP-UP/DOWN BLOCKER: A software utility program to reduce or prevent unwanted computer pop-up ads; pop-under blocker.

PORT: The plug in connection socket for a peripheral computer device (COM1) or CMO2); printer port (LPT); PS/2 or USB ports; small computer system interface (SCSI) or FireWire (IEEE1394 or Sony iLink®) high-speed connection ports, and so forth.

PORT 80: The port that a server "listens to" or expects to receive from a Web client, assuming that the default was taken when the server was configured or set up; HTP daemon.

PORTABILITY: The ability to run on different computer systems and architectures.

PORTABLE: Mobile, wired, or wireless computer system interconnectivity; medical or other EDI.

PORTABLE DOCUMENT FORMAT (FILE) (.PDF): Adobe® Acrobat Systems Inc., family of electronic document readers and writers; fixed format; permits the user to read a document and print it out using Adobe's Acrobat® reader, a free piece of software; PDF files may only be read or printed using this software.

PORTAL: A Web site consisting of links to other or related information; not a destination Web site.

PORT SCANNING: Sending a flood of information to all of the possible network connections on a computer.

POST: To place an electronic message or response on a newsgroup, e-mail, Web site, social network, BBS, RSS feed, and so forth; post-office protocol; postmaster utility program, and so forth; the process of adding a new message or article to a newsgroup, conference, or mailing list discussion area online.

POSTSCRIPT®: A page description programming language created by Adobe Systems, Inc.® that is a device-independent industry standard for outputting documents and graphics.

POTTER, CHARLES: CIO of Strang Cancer Prevention Center and Associate Computer Scientist in Surgery for the Weill Medical College of Cornell University, Ithaca, NY.

POWERBOOK®: A family of popular laptop computers from Apple, Inc. introduced in 1991; originally used Motorola CPUs and subsequently changed to PowerPC® chips.

POWERPC®: An IBM®, Apple®, and Motorola® conceived, reduced instruction set 32- and 64-bit computer, with microprocessor emulation; G1, G2, G3 series, and so forth released in 1994 for Apple only; non-Windows PC based.

POWERPOINT®: MSFT visual presentation application.

POWER SUPPLY UNIT (PSU): AC to DC voltage conversion unit.

PREDICATE MIGRATION: The conversion of pre-existing health or other data to a computer system of mapable vocabulary.

PRE-EMPTIVE MULTITASKING: Occurs when an operating system controls computer applications.

PREFERRED TERMINOLOGY: The most commonly used description attributed to a concept; SNOMED-CT.

PRESENTATION LAYER: The sixth layer of the OSI model for computer network redirection.

PRESET LOCK: A basic lock that has the lock mechanism embedded in the knob or handle.

PRETEXTING: Illegal impersonation and fraud.

PRETTY GOOD PRIVACY (PGP): Public key encryption process for digital signatures.

PREZIOSI, PETER: Executive Director of the American Association for Medical Transcription (AAMT) in Modesto, CA.

PRIMARY ACCOUNTABILITY SERVICE: The maintenance of health data security for user actions as performed primarily by an audit and nonrepudiation services; access control enforcement is usually included as the primary generator of records of user actions (Figure 10).

PRIMARY ASSURANCE SERVICE: Confidence that health IT security objectives are met and encompass both correct and sufficient capabilities; requires consideration of both "what" is provided and "how" it is provided (the architecture, design, and implementation); most impacted by those services that directly impact the correct, on-going security capabilities of the system; presence of an effective restoration capability can provide significant grounds for confidence and an audit can be of great benefit in achieving assurance if used effectively and with recognition for its weaknesses, as illustrated in Figure 11.

PRIMARY AVAILABILITY SERVICES: Those health data IT functions that directly impact the ability of the system to maintain operational effectiveness; protection from unauthorized changes or deletions by defining authorized

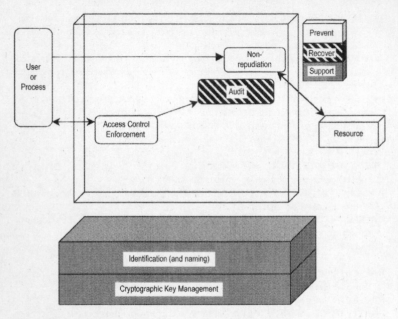

Figure 10: Health system primary accountability IT services.

access and enforcing this definition; mission effectiveness is also maintained by detecting intrusions, detecting a loss of wholeness, and providing the means of returning to a secure state; as illustrated in Figure 12.

PRIMARY CONFIDENTIALITY SERVICE: The protection of health data and communications from disclosure, the enforcement of authorized read accesses, and the capability for privacy provide for confidentiality, as illustrated in Figure 13.

PRIMARY DOMAIN CONTROLLER (PDC): A Windows NT® service that manages security for its local domain; every domain has one PDC, which contains a database of usernames, passwords, and permissions; a domain in a local area network (LAN) is a sub-network comprised of a group of clients and servers under the control of one security database.

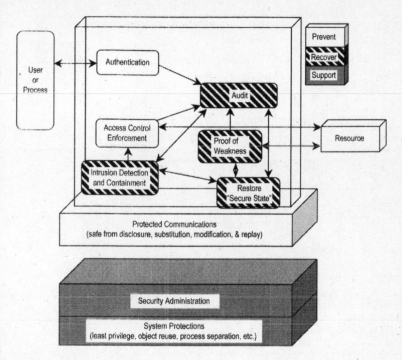

Figure 11:   Health system primary assurance IT services.

PRIMARY INTEGRITY SERVICES: Health IT services that provide for availability and system integrity by maintaining or restoring integrity as an essential part of availability without differentiating between purposes for unauthorized access or between impacts of loss of wholeness, illustrated in Figure 14.

PRIMARY KEY: Primary health data element that identifies a row or value in a database record.

PRIMARY MOUSE BUTTON: Key to select a primary cursor action; a secondary mouse button usually calls up a menu action.

PRIMITIVE: Insufficient defining characteristics to its immediate super-type.

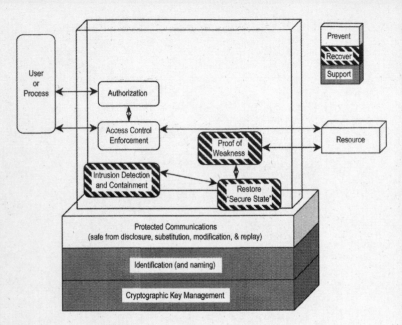

Figure 12: Health system primary availability IT services.

PRINTER: A peripheral device capable of producing hardcopy of computer or networked output material (printout); impact, inkjet, laser (b/w and color).

PRINT SERVER: A computer that manages printer requests from a network in serial queue fashion.

PRIVACY: The quality or state of being hidden, encrypted, obscure, or undisclosed; especially medical data or PHI.

PRIVACY ACT: Federal legislature of 1974 that required giving patients some control over their PHI.

PRIVACY ENHANCED MAIL (PEM): E-mail message standard protocol for enhanced medical, health data, or other security.

PRIVACY OFFICER: A medical entity's protected client information and security officer; required by each covered entity, to be responsible for "the

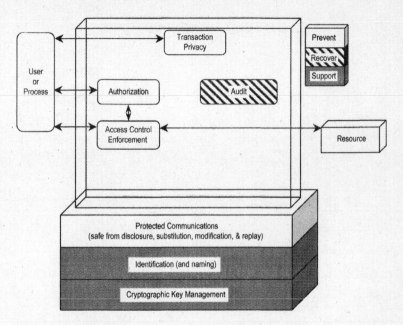

Figure 13: Health system primary confidentiality IT services.

development and implementation of the policies and procedures" necessary for compliance. Covered entities must also designate a "contact person or office" to be responsible for the administration of such tasks such as:

- Creating, posting, and distributing the NPP;
- In facilities with direct treatment providers, securing and recording each patient's acknowledgement of receiving it;
- Processing authorizations for certain kinds of research, marketing, fundraising, and so forth;
- Meeting requests for correction/amendment of health records;
- Considering requests for additional protection for, or confidential communications of, particularly sensitive health information;

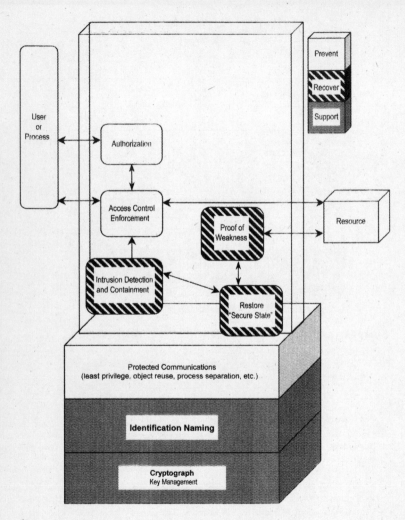

Figure 14:   Health systems primary integrity IT services.

- Providing information to patients (or staff) who have questions about HIPAA or state privacy protections; and
- Handling any complaints from patients (or staff) about possible HIPAA violations.

PRIVACY RULE: The Federal privacy regulations promulgated under the Health Insurance Portability and Accountability Act (HIPAA) of 1996 that created national standards to protect medical records and other protected health information. The Office of Civil Rights (OCR) within the Department of Health and Human Services (DHHS) regulates the privacy rules.

PRIVACY STANDARDS: Any protocol to ensure the confidentiality of PHI.

PRIVATE BRANCH EXCHANGE (PBX): A computerized private telephone switchboard with an extended scope of data and voice services; generally serves one health care organization and is connected to the public telephone network.

PRIVATE KEY: Asymmetric and restricted computer, server, network, or Internet security algorithm used within an organization; secret key.

PRIVATE KEY CRYPTOLOGY: Security measure where the *encryptor* and *decryptor* share the same secure password identifier "key."

PRIVATE KEY SYSTEM: A means of cryptography where the same key is used to both encrypt and decrypt a message.

PRIVILEGE: The right to access secure and confidential PHI.

PRIVILEGED COMMUNICATION: Protected information between clients, patients, supplicants, and others; with attorneys, doctors, the clergy, and others; person-to-professional confidentiality.

PROBLEM DOMAIN: The medical field or specialty under consideration in a computer or other architecture modeling process.

PROBLEM-ORIENTED V-CODE: ICD-9-CM code that notates potential situations that might affect a patient in the future, but are not a current injury or illness.

PROCESS: A series of tasks or operations initiated by an input command.

PROCESSING DEVICE: Machines that conduct the electronic procedures requested; microprocessors; CPU.

PROCESSOR: The CPU of a computer system.

PROCMAIL: UNIX or Linux open source e-mail network transmission standards.

PRODIGY®: Proprietary ISP of Sears® and IBM® that was merged with SBC communications® in 1999.

PRODUCT CODE: Second portion of the National Drug Code (NDC) identifier.

PROFESSIONAL COMPONENT (PC): The portion of a procedure (CPT code) performed by a medical professional or physician.

PROFILE: A statistical and electronic technique used to compare clinical and financial medical provider data.

PROGRAM: A series of electrical statements, structures, or algorithms that informs a computer CPU to operate and perform useful work; software application usually with .exe, .bat, .shs, .com, .vbs, or .scr extension.

PROGRAM FILE: Computer software that runs applications.

PROGRAM LANGUAGE: A code set used by computer software writers to produce applications for work productivity and output:

- artificial intelligence programs: prolog, LISP, and so forth
- business programs: C, RPG, BASIC, COBOL, and so forth
- general purpose small programs: BASIC, VISUAL BASIC, Pascal, and Python
- general purpose large programs: PL/I, C, C++, Pascula, Ada, Modula-2, Java®, and C#
- math and science programs: APL, FORTRAN, Maple, and so forth
- string programs: JavaScript® and VBSCRIPT, SNOBOL, REXX, Awk, Perl, Python®, and so forth

PROGRAM LANGUAGE VIRUS: Macro virus created specifically for applications with their own programming such as the original MS Office Suite®; first seen in 1995.

PROGRAMMER: One who programs and creates line of software codes for a computer.

PROGRAM OFFICE COORDINATOR: A medical office's privacy, client, or patient liaison for protected health information.

PROJECT SENTINEL: National biosurveillance testing program for the collection of de-identified HIPAA compliance data for national benchmarking of bioterror threats.

PROMPT: An input *que* symbol seen on a computer monitor awaiting further instructions or commands.

PROOF OF WHOLENESS: Evidence of health data integrity compromise or the ability to detect a breach when information or system states are potentially corrupted; proven system security and integrity.

PROTECTED COMMUNICATIONS: The ability to accomplish health IT security objectives dependent on trustworthy communications; a protected communications service ensures the integrity, availability, and confidentiality of information while in transit. In most situations all three elements are essential requirements, with confidentiality being needed at least for authentication information.

PROTECTED HEALTH INFORMATION (PHI): § 164.502(j) (1). Any individually identifiable health information held by a HIPAA-covered entity.

Complying with HIPAA's security and privacy regulations requires most covered entities to adopt policies and procedures for handling PHI and to make some hard choices about how these policies will be implemented. For example, HIPAA suggests hiring a health security officer (HSO) to oversee protection of PHI and also eliminate the use of role-based access to the electronic health record (EHR) system (for example, logging into a system as a doctor, as opposed to a patient registrar or nurse). Implementation of the security safeguards as outlined in the final security regulation will not only require information technology (IT) infrastructure changes, but will also require that other database fields be programmed into the software.

PROTECTED HEALTH INFORMATION FLOW CHART: A documented path of patient information as it moves between registration, medical use, accounting, and storage and retrieval; useful in providing a patient with the security policy procedures used by a covered health care entity.

PROTECTED HEALTH INFORMATION PRIVACY ACT (PHIPA): Clinical and related business information that includes patient identifiers, such as name, address, telephone, and SS numbers, and whose privacy must be electronically and traditionally safeguarded, according to HIPAA mandates and the Privacy Act of 1974.

PROTECTED PATIENT: Those individuals with known risk of injury by others must be protected. Their identification will be protected by the assignment of an alias on the Admission/Discharge/Transfer (ADT) system; however, the health record number may remain unchanged and valid for the patient.

PROTOCOL: Rules, definitions, and standards for PC hardware, software, and wired (802.3—Ethernet) or wireless networks, usually by the IEE, ISO, or OSI, that governs the transmission of secure electrical data in a network, intranet, or Internet. The OSI model includes seven layers of related tasks for networking protocols: physical, data, network, transport, session, presentation, and application.

PROTOTYPE: Blocks or lines of software code, programs, or algorithms that enhance speedy application development.

PROVIDER: A supplier of services as defined in section 1861(u) of the HIPAA; a supplier of medical or other services as defined in section 1861(s) of the HIPAA.

PROVIDER TAXONOMY CODES: An administrative code set for identifying the provider type and area of specialization for all health care providers; a provider may have several Provider Taxonomy Codes used in the X12 278; Referral Certification and Authorization and the X12 837 Claim transactions are maintained by the NUCC.

PROXY: A server that acts as an intermediary between a workstation user and the Internet so that the enterprise can ensure security, administrative control, and caching service; associated with or as part of a gateway server that separates the enterprise network from the outside network and a firewall server that protects the health care enterprise network from outside intrusion.

PROXY SERVER: A firewall application that disconnects server and receiver with third party forwarding and porting.

PS/2: The second generation of IBM Micro Channel® computer architecture.

PSEUDO CODE: A computer application written in some programming language as well as English.

PUBLIC DIRECTORY: FTP user addressable and retrievable by anonymous users; public files.

PUBLIC DOMAIN: Noncopyrighted software programs and applications, music, literature, or whose copyright has expired and not been renewed.

PUBLIC INFORMATION: Nonsecure and nonprotected information or data.

PUBLIC KEY: Asymmetric and restricted computer, server, network, or Internet security algorithm that links two or more facilities or nodes outside an organization; digital signatures.

PUBLIC KEY ALGORITHM: Public key encryption with private key decryption security standards.

PUBLIC KEY CERTIFICATE: A digitally signed health data or information document that serves to validate the sender's authorization and name and consists of a specially formatted block of data that contains the name of the certificate holder and the holder's public key and digital certificate for authentication; the certification authority attests that the sender's name is the one associated with the public key in the document; a user ID packet, containing the sender's unique identifier, is sent after the certificate packet and there are different types of public key certificates for different functions, such as authorization for a specific action or delegation of authority. Public key certificates are part of a PKI that deals with digitally signed protected care data documents. The other components are public key encryptions, trusted third parties (such as the certification authority), and mechanisms for certificate publication and issuing.

PUBLIC KEY CRYPTOLOGY: Security measure where a linked pair of *encryptor* and *decryptor* keys share the same secure password identifier; digital signatures.

PUBLIC KEY INFRASTRUCTURE (PKI): Digital certifications and authentications for electronic data and health information transmission that verify both sender and receiver.

PUBLIC KEY SYSTEM: A means of cryptography where two keys are used.

PUBLIC HEALTH AUTHORITY: An agency or authority of the United States, a State, territory, political subdivision of a State or territory, Indian tribe, person, or entity acting under a grant of authority from or contract with such public agency including the employees or agents of such public agency, its contractors or delegated persons that are responsible for public health matters as part of its official mandate.

PUBLIC SWITCHED TELEPHONE NETWORK (PSTN): A public telephone network.

PUCK: A computer GUI icon used for digital drawing; slang term.

PULL: To actively request and/or receive health data or other information from a computer network system as retrieved by the end user.

PULL DOWN: Drop down icon used to access a subgroup of applications, programs, features, and so forth.

PULL DOWN MENU: Hidden list or collection of computer input options or commands.

PULSE CODE MODULATION (PCM): A process of encoding audio signals.

PUNCH CARD: 80-column stiff paper card of IBM® compatibility that can be fed into a mechanical computer and read for data processing purposes.

PURGE: To securely eliminate medical data or delete PHI or other files or data.

PUSH: The active giving or placement of input data, rather than requesting or passively allowing it; to put data on a stack; to passively receive health data or other information from a computer network system that is forced on the end user.

PUSH-INSTALL: A proprietary feature of Executive Software® that eliminates the time and cost of manual installation or uninstalls, keeping a site's technology current with fast, two-click central control; without a learning curve it is easily installed/uninstalled software, updates, upgrades, and patches, which are logo-compliant for Windows 2000®, XP®, and Vista®, or are Microsoft-Installer compliant on selected machines throughout a site from a central location. PushInstaller can be used to install Windows XP® and Vista® itself.

PUSHWARE: Software program automatically delivered at prescribed intervals without request.

PUSKIN, DENA, SCD: CIO for the Advancement of Telemedicine, Rockville, MD.

PYTHON: A dynamic small computer string programming language used in Zope® application servers and Mnet® and BitTorrent® file sharing and embedding systems; resembles Java® and C.

Q

Q-BASIC: A Microsoft compiler program often provided with DOS and Windows©.

QUAD CORE PROCESSOR: A four-core microprocessor made for dual-processor computer servers; essentially eight-processor servers (two processors x four cores each); such core expansion is a dominant theme for Intel© and AMD© with tens of cores possible within a decade; Xeon 5300®, Tigerton, Barcelona, and so forth.

QUADRATURE PHASE SHIFT KEYING: (QPSK): A four-phase state wireless 802.11b radio modulation technique.

QUALIFIED MEDICAL EXPENSE: Defined by IRS Code 213(d) as an expense used to alleviate or prevent a mental defect, illnesses, or physical defects.

QUALITY OF SERVICE (QOS): The concept idea that Internet or network transmission rates, error rates, and other characteristics can be measured, improved, and to some extent, guaranteed in advance; transmitting this kind of content dependably is difficult in public networks using ordinary "best effort" protocols; not suitable for PHI.

QUANT: One who is mathematically inclined to apply various numerical and IT approaches in analyzing or performing health care or other EDI functions; statistician or mathematician; slang term.

QUANTUM COMPUTING: Electromagnetic ion (electrically charged atoms) trap that is ideal for use as bits and qubits; which unlike a standard computer bit represented by a 0 or 1, may be both 0 and 1, simultaneously.

QUANTUM CRYPTOGRAPHY: Health data and medical information security technology using photons and fiber-optic channel transmission.

QUANTUM ENCRYPTION: Encoded server information on an individual photon or electron, sent to a recipient with particle information like size or polarization allowing interpretation.

QUERY: An Internet client request to a Web server, or request for health information or other data; action to ask for additional operations on health care EDI such as medical data insertion, updating, or deletion; languages used to interact with databases are called *query languages*; Structured Query Language (SQL) is the well-known standard.

QUERY LANGUAGE: Computer program that allows selected database or other health records acquisition.

QUERY MANAGEMENT FACILITY (QMF): To retrieve data from a mainframe or legacy health care, or other IT system.

QUERY PROGRAM: Software algorithm that counts sums and retrieves selected records from a health, medical, or other database.

QUEUE: Serial microprocessor waiting system; temporary holding place for health data; electronic prioritized storage concept such as the inventory costing FIFO method.

QUICKEN©: A popular financial management program for computers useful in small to mid-sized medical offices.

QUICKTIME®: Methodology to create, edit, sort, and view digital sound and video on a Macintosh computer.

QUICK TIME VIRTUALITY (QTVR): Panoramic digital computer screen scene image file, with .mov format extension.

QUINN, JOHN: CTO and senior executive for Accenture Health and Life Sciences.

QUIT: To end a computer or network EDI session; clear a program or application from core memory.

QUI-TAM: The method in the Federal False Claims Act that allows lawsuits against health care fraud and medical EDI abuse; wrongdoers in "the name of the king, as for himself, who sues in this matter" (Latin phrase).

QWERTY: The first six letters of an English-language keyboard layout.

R

R/3: A comprehensive set of integrated business applications from SAP, a German company that provides client/server ability to store, retrieve, analyze, and process corporate health, medical, and other data for financial analysis, production, operations, human resource management, billing, and most other business or health care EDI processes.

RACKETEER INFLUENCED AND CORRUPT ORGANIZATION ACT (RICOA): Federal legislation used against individuals accused of health care, billing, or medical fraud.

RADIO BUTTON: A small computer screen icon that can only be activated at a given time; on/off toggle switch.

RADIO FREQUENCY IDENTIFICATION (RFID): Automatic device recognition technology void of physical contact; early adopters in health care include: Beth Israel Hospital for equipment, Aramark Healthcare® for online DME tracking, Purdue Pharma® for OxyContin® bottles, GN Diamond® for data, and Pfizer Pharmaceuticals® for drugs.

RADIO FREQUENCY INTERFACE: Electromagnetic wave interference.

RADIOLOGY INFORMATION SYSTEM (RIS): A synthesized system for the electronic processing, storage, and transmission of radiographic images; allows the remote interpretation of radiographic image-teleradiology and may be connected to a Hospital Information System (HIS) and/or Laboratory Information System (LIS).

RAMBUS®: High-speed computer memory interface manufacturer based in Los Altos, CA.

RANDOM ACCESS MEMORY (RAM): The read-write or operating memory used to execute computers, network programs, or applications; a group of memory chips, typically of the dynamic RAM (DRAM) type, functioning as the computer's primary workspace; RAM chips require power to maintain content, which is why information or heath data must be saved onto a hard disk or other storage device before turning off a computer; DDR-SDRAM (Double Data Rate Synchronous Dynamic Random Access Memory); DDR2-SDRAM (more expensive and better performance), and DDR3-SDRAM (video enabled).

RANKED DATA: Ordinal information listed from lowest to highest, and so forth.

RANUM, MARCUS: Computer security system design and implementation expert recognized as the inventor of the proxy firewall and the implementer of the first commercial firewall products such as the TIS firewall toolkit, the Gauntlet® firewall, and NFR's Network Flight Recorder® intrusion detection system; CSO of Security for Tenable Security, Inc®.

RASTER: The process of rendering an image or a page using the technology that helped create the cathode ray television tube or computer monitor/screen.

RASTER GRAPHICS: Digital images created on a grid with file types such as TIFF, GIF, JPEG, and BMP.

RASTER IMAGE: A horizontal or vertical grid of pixels comprising an electronic picture.

RASTERIZED TYPE: Computer image that has rough or stair-stepped edges because it has been rendered at a resolution that is too low.

RDISK: Command in Windows NT® to create an emergency repair disk (ERD).

READ: The flow of meaningful data (language) from object to subject; to transfer electronic information or health data.

READ CODE: UK CTV 3 code; clinical medical terminology in the United Kingdom.

READER/WRITER: Smart card to-CPU, with CPU-to-smart card functionality.

README: First file to review upon opening a new software program or application; instruction manual updates.

READ ONLY MEMORY (ROM): A memory chip that permanently stores medical instructions, health, or other data and control routines in PCs (ROM BIOS), peripheral controllers, and other electronic equipment.

REALAUDIO®: A popular Internet real-time audio streaming technology protocol of Real Networks®; RealPlayer®.

REALLY SIMPLE SYNDICATION (RSS): Internet technology used to enable syndicated content, which is a popular way to distribute medical information from Web sites using a news site or blog that feeds content to a group of subscribers automatically.

REALLY SIMPLE SYNDICATION READER (RSSR): Software designed with user interfaces that resemble e-mail inboxes instead of browsers; used to collect, update, and display RSS feeds.

REAL MEDIA©: A popular streaming media technology for the Internet.

REALSYSTEM G2®: An open platform protocol for rich and real-time media streaming over the Internet; Real Networks®.

REAL TIME: Online platform of simultaneous input/output systems; it refers to an immediate control response process and embedded systems; for example, surgical robot computers must respond instantly to changing operating conditions; it also refers to fast transaction processing systems as well as any electronic operation fast enough to keep up with its real-world counterpart (such as transmitting live audio or video); real-time protocol; real-time streaming; real-time operating system, real video, and so forth; signals received at rates of 30 frames per second.

REBOT: To reload and restart a computer operating system.

REBUILD: Desktop utility operation for Macintosh® computers.

RECEIPT NOTIFICATION: E-mail sender feedback and automated message confirmation.

RECEIVER OPERATING CHARACTERISTICS (ROCs): A procedure involving statistics used to analyze the ability of a medical diagnostic tool to determine whether an individual is healthy or diseased; linked computer servers are most often used in observer performance evaluations of the feasibility and performance of diagnostic imaging systems.

RECORD: A collection of related information fields, health data, or other information.

RECORDS (MEDICAL): 20 U.S.C. 1232g(a)(4)(B)(iv), all:

- Psychotherapy notes recorded (in any medium) by a health care provider who is a mental health professional documenting or analyzing the contents of conversation during a private counseling session or a group, joint, or family counseling session and that are separated from the rest of the individual's medical record; excludes medication prescription and monitoring, counseling session start and stop times, the modalities and frequencies of treatment furnished, results of clinical tests, and any summary of the following items: diagnosis, functional status, the treatment plan, symptoms, prognosis, and progress to date.

- Public health authority means an agency or authority of the United States, a State, a territory, a political subdivision of a State or territory, or an Indian tribe, or a person or entity acting under a grant of authority from or contract with such public agency, including the employees or agents of such public agency or its contractors or persons or entities to whom it has granted authority, that is responsible for public health matters as part of its official mandate.

- Required by law means a mandate contained in law that compels a covered entity to make a use or disclosure of protected health information and that is enforceable in a court of law; includes but is not limited to, court orders and court-ordered warrants; subpoenas or summons issued by a court, grand jury, a governmental or tribal inspector general, or an administrative body authorized to require the production of information; a civil or an authorized investigative demand; Medicare conditions of participation with respect to health care providers participating in the program; and statutes or regulations that require the production of information, including statutes or regulations that require such information if payment is sought under a government program providing public benefits.

RECORDS PROCESSING: Establishes a method of logging data, transmitting, modifying, storing, and disposing of health records.

RECORDS PURGING (REMOVAL-RETENTION) POLICY: Standards of off-site medical information storage, maintenance, and destruction for PHI and similar patient charts.

RECURSION: Calling and recreating a new copy of a procedure, algorithm, application, or computer program.

RECYCLE BIN: A waste icon used for deleting files in Windows©.

RED BOOK: Audio CD standard from the Philips Corporation®, ISO, and Sony Corporation®; U.S. NSA protocol (A-D) secure to nonsecure, for trusted computer networks.

RED-GREEN-BLUE: Color process used by computer displays, as all three colors light waves are perceived by the eye as white; the absence of light is perceived as black or additive color; amount of color generated by RGB mode is much larger than those generated by CMYK.

RED HAT®: Enterprise Linux is a leading platform for open source computing; sold by subscription and certified by enterprise hardware and software vendors; from the desktop to the data center, Linux couples open source technology with business enterprise stability; based in Raleigh, NC.

RED-HERRING: A deliberately misleading or disingenuous technical term, machination, suggestion, program, icon, code, and so forth; fraudulent technology; slang term.

REDIRECT: To go directly to another URL or Web page without user input or mouse click.

REDmedic®: Launched in October 2004 as a consumer-driven health care service firm providing secure and immediate access to personal health care information in emergencies and other medical situations via the Internet with nation-wide call or fax center.

REDUCED INSTRUCTION SET COMPUTER (RISC): Nonmicrocode computer instructions; IBM Power-PC®, DEC Alpha©, RISC and MIPS machines; computer architecture that reduces chip complexity by using simpler instructions.

REDUNDANCY: The process of computer or network data back up; mirroring; copying.

REDUNDANT ARRAY OF INDEPENDENT DISKS (RAID): A computer storage disk subsystem used to increase performance and/or provide fault tolerance as a set of two or more ordinary hard disks and a specialized disk controller that contains its functionality; during the late 1980s and early 1990s, RAID meant an array of "inexpensive" disks (compared to large computer disks or Single Large Expensive Disks); but as hard disks are now cheaper, the RAID Advisory Board changed the name to mean "independent."

REFACTOR: To reorganize or improve the efficiency of a computer program or application without altering its functionality.

REFERENCE INFORMATION MODEL: The ultimate static model and source for HL7 and RIM 3 protocol specifications and standards.

REFERENCE MODEL: Description of a logical system.

REFERENCE MONITOR: The security engineering term for health care IT functionality that (1) controls all access, (2) cannot be bypassed, (3) is tamper-resistant, and (4) provides confidence that the other three items are true.

REFERENCE TERMINOLOGY: Standard terms and codified definition used throughout a similar industry space, such as health care; www.Health DictionarySeries.com.

REFLECTION: Computer system ability to internally diagnosis and self correct.

REFREEZE: Change integration within a stable computer environment.

REFRESH: To update an URL or Web page; to update health data or other information.

REGENSTRIEF INSTITUTE: A research foundation for improving health care by optimizing the capture, analysis, content, and delivery of health care information; maintains the LOINC coding system for use as portion of the HIPAA claim attachments standard.

REGEX: "Regular expression" is a way for a computer user or programmer to express how a computer program should look for a specified pattern in text and then what the program is to do when each pattern match is found.

REGIONAL BELL OPERATING COMPANY (RBOC): Refers to one of seven regional companies formed by the AT&T divestiture in 1984.

REGIONAL HEALTH INFORMATION ORGANIZATION (RHIO): A multi-stakeholder organization that enables the exchange and use of health information, in a secure manner, for the purpose of promoting the improvement of health quality, safety, and efficiency; the U.S. Department of Health and Human Services see RHIOs as the building blocks for the national health information network (NHIN) that will provide universal access to electronic health records; other experts maintain that RHIOs will help eliminate some administrative costs associated with paper-based patient records, provide quick access to automated test results, and offer a consolidated view of a patient's history.

REGIONAL HEALTH INFORMATION ORGANIZATION ARCHITECTURE: There are three architecture types:

- *Federated architecture* (decentralized): An approach to the coordinated sharing and interchange of electronic health information emphasizing partial, controlled sharing among autonomous databases within an RHIO; independent databases (decentralized) connected to share and exchange health information; components in a federated architecture represent the various users, applications, workstations, main frames, and other stakeholder components in an RHIO; each controls its interactions with other components by means of an export schema and an import schema. The export schema specifies the information that a component will share with other components, while the import schema specifies the nonlocal information that a component wishes to manipulate. The federated architecture provides a means to share data and transactions using messaging services, combine information from several components, and coordinate activities among autonomous components.

- *Centralized architecture:* An approach to RHIO data sharing and interchange of electronic information emphasizing full control over data sharing through a centralized repository; components in a centralized architecture refer to the Central Data Repository (CDR) and the requestor. The CDR authenticates the requestor through a technological means, authorizes the transaction, and records it for audit and reporting purposes.
- *Hybrid architecture:* A combination of the two architecture types where various data transactions occur based on a decentralized or centralized method. For instance, an RHIO may have pharmacy transactions occurring within a federated model while lab data is shared through a centralized database. The providers in hybrid architecture may decide to share patient data through a CDR or peer-to-peer.

REGIONAL SETTING: PC operating settings for a specific user.

REGISTER: A row of flip-flop (on/off) binary toggle-like switches.

REGISTRY: In the Microsoft Windows© operating systems beginning with Windows 95®, it is a single place for keeping such information as what hardware is attached, what system options have been selected, how computer memory is set up, and what application programs are to be present when the operating system is started; somewhat similar to, and a replacement for, the simpler INI (initialization) and configuration files used in earlier Windows© (DOS-based) systems; INI files are still supported, however, for compatibility with the 16-bit applications written for earlier systems; a central hierarchical database.

REGRESSION MODEL: Statistical method of data mining correlated between two independent vectors.

REGRESSION TEST: To hypothetically determine a causal relationship between variables.

REINHARDT, UWE, PhD: Professor, Woodrow Wilson School of Princeton University, Princeton, NJ.

REISCHAUER, ROBERT, PhD: President, Urban Institute.

RELATIONAL DATABASE: A database of columns and rows that are electronically joined.

RELATIONSHIP DATA MODULE: The sharing of common health data or other database.

RELATIVE ADDRESS: An IP or other address in relation to another address; nonabsolute address.

RELATIVE URL: Document locator for the same information directory as a current document location.

RELATIVE VALUE (RV): The economic merit of one health data security measure versus another; computer security ROI; RV is determined by dividing the Vulnerability Index (VI) by the Cost of Protection (CP).

RELEASE: Software application, program edition, or version.

RELEASE CANDIDATE: A prerelease or beta version of software.

RELEASE OF INFORMATION (ROI): The disclosure of PHI, medical, or other health data or information.

RELEASE OF PROTECTED HEALTH INFORMATION POLICY: Standards and protocol schemes for how patients may obtain their own medical data and health information.

RELIABILITY: Measure of consistent and efficient performance.

RELOAD: Multiple use microprocessor; smart card; to obtain or input new health data or other information.

REMAIL: Automatic but anonymous e-mail forwarding messaging service.

REMOTE ACCESS SERVER (RAS): Windows NT© computer dial-in functionality combined with network broadcast ability to enhance IP address resolution.

REMOTE ACCESS SOFTWARE: Mobile user network access pass with functionality.

REMOTE ACCESS TROJAN (RAT): A computer network enabled trojan horse virus.

REMOTE BOOT: Computer server start-up across a WAN or LAN; remote login; MS-DOS, Windows 95©, and Windows NT©.

REMOTE DESKTOP: MSFT Windows 2000/Vista® feature that allows one computer to serves as the screen, mouse, and input keyboard for another remote computer.

REMOTE MONITORING: Patient electronic examination from a remote location; telemedicine.

REMOTE STORAGE: A firm that retains and backs up electronic health information or other data off-site or Internet-based for protection in case of disaster such as fire or flood.

- *hot:* real-time backup
- *cold:* periodic regular backups

REMOVABLE DISK: A transferable module inserted into a disk drive for writing and reading.

REMOVAL FROM ACCESS LIST: The physical termination of a health entity's access and user privileges.

REMOVAL OF USER ACCOUNT(S): The termination or deletion of an individual's access privileges to the health information, services, and resources for which they currently have clearance, authorization, and need-to-know; when such clearance, authorization, and need-to-know no longer exists.

RENDER: To format a print job prior to output device printer delivery.

REPEAT: To re-input a computer command; a repetitive active LAN, MAN, or WAN hub that extends network signal reach.

REPEATER: Device to extend LAN, WAN, or MAN functionality; a bidirectional instrument used to amplify or regenerate signals.

REPEAT RATE: Speed of computer character or command input activation.

REPLICATE: The push duplication of health data or other information from one network to another.

REPLICATION VIRUS: Malicious software designed to capture password, security information, credit card numbers, and so forth, and e-mail them back to its creator; as with the BadTrans variant of 2001.

REPORT PROCEDURE: The documented formal mechanism employed to archive security incidents.

REPOSITORY: To store, access, and retrieve health or other data from a central location.

REPUDIATE: Electronic communication system or e-mail message receipt denial; the denial of a computerized action, especially the sending or receipt of medical data or PHI.

RESEARCH: A systematic investigation, including research development, testing, and evaluation, designed to develop or contribute to medical, health, or IT knowledge.

RESEAT: To remove and reinsert/replace an integrated circuit board from its socket to improve connectivity.

RESIDENT VIRUS: Malicious software code embedded into an operating system.

RESIDUAL RISK: The remaining, potential uncertainty after all health care IT security measures are applied and associated with each threat.

RESOLUTION: Benchmark of graphical picture image sharpness, acuity, density, and pixel count; refers to the ability of a device to distinguish between various factors; for example, spatial resolution is the ability to distinguish between adjacent structures, while contrast resolution is the ability to discriminate between shades of gray.

RESOURCE ACCESS DECISION (RAD): Health data transmissions standards designed by security specialists specifically for health care industry requirements to provide a uniform way for application systems to enforce resource-oriented access control policies and let health organizations define and administer a consistent enterprise-wide security policy; standardizes the interface but leaves implementation details to the vendor who supports the use of various access control policies, provides a framework for diverse policy enforcement engines, and allows the following:

- *Architectural separation* of business and security functionality, creating an access control policy that is manageable and auditable;
- *Identification* of caregivers' privileges using credentials supplied by diverse security mechanisms (e.g., CORBASec®, Secure Socket Layer®, Kerberos, Lightweight Directory Access Protocol);
- *Delivery* of a product specifically for health care, with access control rules shared by all RAD-compliant health care components;
- *A simple interface* for requesting access control decisions;
- *Grouping* of secured resources to define access control rules;
- *Definition* of access control rules to include the relationship between patient and *caregiver;*
- *Consultation* of multiple access control policies and control of how decisions governing access to the same resource are reconciled; and
- *Specific standards* for how secured resources are identified to ensure consistent names among vendors.

RESPONSE PROCEDURE: The documented formal rules/instructions for actions to be taken as a result of the receipt of a medical data or health information security incident report.

RESTORE: To resize a computer Web or application page back to its original size.

RESTORE SECURE STATE: Security breach adjustment back to a known state of integrity.

RETENTION: Acquisition, maintenance, and preservation of electronic data and PHI.

RETRO COMPUTE: To collect, restore, buy, sell, and trade older PC or legacy computers, as a hobby.

RETRO VIRUS: Malicious computer software code that avoids detection by attacking another anti-virus security program; an anti-virus utility program.

REUSE: The ability to store and repeat software code or components for various applications or programs; Java class.

REV DRIVE: Removable media drive from Iomega® with USB, SCSI, or FireWire port connections.

REVENUE CODE: A three to four digit Medicare charge master billing form number.

REVERSE ADDRESS RESOLUTION PROTOCOL (RARP): Internet protocol (IP) address network request locator.

REVERSE ENGINEER: The extraction of legacy software information from its source code; to disassemble and examine a computer system, peripheral device, or product.

REVERT: To reinstall or reload from a backed-up (saved) computer storage disk or other medium.

REVOCATION: To withdraw or remove permission or computer system access authorization.

REXX®: A computer operating system command language.

RIBBON BAR: A computer user command interface.

RIBBON CABLE: A flat, thin, multiconductor used in electronics to connect peripheral devices to an internal computer.

RICH E-MAIL: E-mail annotated with audio and visual images.

RICH TEXT: Text that contains word processing codes for pagination, fonts, and so forth.

RICH TEXT FORMAT (RTF): Interchange standard for text electronic messaging with minimal file formatting; a series of word processing directions that are able to be read by the majority of word processing programs in order to retain the formatting rules of the document.

RIGHT-CLICK MENU: Right-hand mouse button Windows© technique to open a menu with a range of options, such as font, bullets, and paragraphs.

RING NETWORK: Nodule configuration of linked closed looped computers; circular topology.

RIP(PER): To convert an audio file to MP3 or other music format; to burn, copy, or save a CD; analog to digital conversion; slang term.

RISHEL, WES: Member of the Healthcare Informatics editorial board and chairman of HL7; also vice president and research area director, Gartner Healthcare Industry Research and Advisory Services, Alameda, CA.

RISK: Uncertainty in all health care IT applications, programs, labor, computers, servers, networks, and so forth; synonymous with IT uncertainty and probability, to include:

- Unauthorized (malicious, nonmalicious, or accidental) disclosure, modification, or destruction of information;
- Nonmalicious errors and omissions;
- IT disruptions due to natural or man-made disasters and
- Failure to exercise due care and diligence in IT implementation and operation.

RISK ANALYSIS: The process of identifying the uncertainty to health care computer system security and determining the probability of occurrence, the resulting impact, and the additional safeguards that mitigate this impact; part of medical risk management and synonymous with IT uncertainty assessment; a process whereby cost-effective security/control measures may be selected by balancing the costs of various health information security and control measures against the losses that would be expected if these measures were not in place; risk assessment analysis.

RISK ASSUMPTION: To accept the potential risk and continue operating a health IT system, or to implement controls to lower the risk to an acceptable level.

RISK AVOIDANCE: To avoid health system IT risk by eliminating its risk cause and/or consequence (e.g., forgo certain functions of the system or shut down the system when risks are identified).

RISK LIMITATION: To limit IT risk by implementing controls that minimize the adverse impact that a health data threat is exercising vulnerability (e.g., use of supporting, preventive, detective controls).

RISK MANAGEMENT: The total process of identifying and controlling health information technology related risks; includes risk analysis, cost-benefit analysis, and the selection, implementation, test, and security evaluation of safeguards; an overall system security review that considers both effectiveness and efficiency, including impact on the mission/business and constraints due to policy, regulations, and laws such as HIPAA, SARBOX, and the Patriot Act; the mitigation of IT uncertainty from attack by technical means, both internally and externally. In general, the strategies employed include transferring the risk to another party, avoiding the risk, reducing the negative effect of the risk, and accepting some or all of the consequences of a particular risk. Traditional risk management focuses on risks stemming from physical or legal causes (e.g., natural disasters or fires, accidents, death, and lawsuits). Financial risk management, on the other hand, focuses on risks that can be managed using traded financial instruments. Regardless of the type of risk management, all large health care corporations have risk management teams and small groups and corporations practice informal, if not formal, risk management. In ideal IT risk management, a prioritization process is followed whereby the risks with the greatest loss and the greatest probability of occurring are handled first, and risks with lower probability of occurrence and lower loss are handled later. In practice the process can be very difficult, and balancing between risks with a high probability of occurrence but lower loss versus. a risk with high loss but lower probability of occurrence can often be mishandled.

RISK MITIGATION: The neutralization of health care data security attacks, holes, flaws and/or breaches, intentional or nonmalicious; involves prioritizing, evaluating, and implementing the appropriate risk-reducing controls recommended from the risk assessment process. Because the elimination of all risk is usually impractical or close to impossible, it is the responsibility of senior management and functional and business managers to use the *least-cost approach* and implement the *most appropriate controls* to decrease mission risk to an acceptable level, with *minimal adverse impact* on the organization's resources and mission. According to the NIST, risk mitigation is a systematic methodology used by senior management to reduce mission risk. Risk mitigation can be achieved through any of the following risk mitigation options:

- Risk Assumption: To accept the potential risk and continue operating the IT system or to implement controls to lower the risk to an acceptable level.
- Risk Avoidance: To avoid the risk by eliminating the risk cause and/or consequence (e.g., forgo certain functions of the system or shut down the system when risks are identified).
- Risk Limitation: To limit the risk by implementing controls that minimize the adverse impact of a threat's exercising vulnerability (e.g., use of supporting, preventive, detective controls).
- Risk Planning: To manage risk by developing a risk mitigation plan that prioritizes, implements, and maintains controls.
- Research and Acknowledgment: To lower the risk of loss by acknowledging the vulnerability or flaw and researching controls to correct the vulnerability.
- Risk Transference: To transfer the risk by using other options to compensate for the loss, such as purchasing insurance.

  - *Flaw exists*-Remedy: implement assurance techniques to reduce flaw likelihood.
  - *Flaw is exploitable*-Remedy: apply layered protections and architectural designs to prevent exploitability.
  - *Attacker's cost is less than gain*-Remedy: apply protections to increase attacker's economic costs.
  - *Loss is too great*-Remedy: apply design principles, architectural designs, and technical protections to limit extent of attack, and reduce loss.

RISK PLANNING: To manage risk by developing a risk mitigation plan that prioritizes, implements, and maintains controls.

RISK TRANSFERENCE: To transfer health data IT risk by using other options to compensate for the loss; such as leasing a live hot-backup system.

RIVEST, RONALD L., PhD: Andrew and Erna Viterbi Professor of Electrical Engineering and Computer Science at MIT, whose research interests in cryptography, computers and network security, electronic voting, and algorithms provided the basics for HIPAA electronic health data transmissions.

RIVEST, R.; SHAMIR, A.; ADELMAN, L. (RSA): Developers of a leading public key asymmetric algorithm encryption system.

ROADMAP: The technical steps toward achieving a major goal; business, strategy, or transition plan.

ROBINSON, JAMES C., PhD, MPH: Professor, University of California Berkeley, CA, and Kaiser Permanente Distinguished Professor of Health Economics School of Public Health Division of Health Policy and Management; expert in health IT and biotechnology policy and strategy, health insurance, physician payment methods, and health care finance.

ROGUE DIALER: An automated program that changes computer modem settings so that a network connection occurs by an expensive, insecure, or toll location.

ROLE-BASED ACCESS CONTROL (RBAC): An alternative to traditional access control models (e.g., discretionary or nondiscretionary access control policies) that permits the specification and enforcement of enterprise-specific security policies in a way that maps more naturally to an organization's structure and business activities; rather than attempting to map a health organization's security policy to a relatively low-level set of technical controls (typically, access control lists), each user is assigned to one or more predefined roles, each of which has been assigned the various privileges needed to perform that role.

ROLL BACK: To return a malfunctioning computer system back to a time when it was running well.

ROLL UP: To reduce the size of a dialog box or menu but maintain its visibility.

ROMAN, MARK: Health care global IT leader for the EDS Corporation.

ROOT: The highest level in an index; the top level (e.g., C:\ is usually the root of the disk); health or other root account, root name, or root web.

ROOT DIRECTORY: Computer systems base that commands other files and nonroot directories organized as a hierarchy or tree that includes all other directories; for Unix as well as in other operating systems the root directory has no name and is simply represented by the special character that separates directories in a file system as: /. Only a few special users of a shared operating system are given the authority to access all file directories and files under the root directory and in a UNIX environment, the special user is known as an avatar.

ROOT-KIT: A set of software to conceal running processes, files, or system data, thereby helping an intruder to maintain access to a system while avoiding detection and known to exist for a variety of operating systems such as SUN Solaris®, Linux, and Windows®; often modify parts of the operating system or install themselves as drivers or kernel modules; the word "root kit" came to public awareness in the 2005 Sony CD copy protection scandal, where a surreptitiously placed root-kit was placed on MSFT Windows® PCs when a Sony® Music-CD was played without mention, referring only to security rights management measures.

ROOT SERVER: A primary domain registry updated daily by Networks Solutions, Inc®.

ROUNDTABLE: MSFT digital video camera with 360 degrees video zoom capability.

ROUTER: Triage switch and IP address delivery gateway between complex computer networks and around the Internet; electronic switch.

ROUTER SERVICE: Commercial application to sort messages through internal computer system integration channels.

ROUTINE: Sequential instructions to direct computer or network performance.

ROUTING: The assignment of a path of digital communication.

ROUTING TABLE: List of network routing destinations.

rPATH: Linux platform that combines virtualization technology with computer appliances for ISVs, medical, and business platforms.

RSA: A public key, prime number asymmetric algorithm security system developed by engineers Ronald Rivest, Ade Shamir, and Leonard Adelman.

RSS: A collection of really-simple-syndication Internet feed formats in the XML software language and used for Web syndications such as blogs, e-logs, and podcasts with several standards:

- Really Simple Syndication (RSS 2.0)
- Rich Site Summary (RSS 0.91, RSS 1.0)
- RDF Site Summary (RSS 0.9 and 1.0)
- Real-time Simple Syndication (RSS 2.0)

RUBY: A dynamic scripting computer language used with syntax for Perl and its object oriented features; Perl, Python©, and Ruby on Railes©.

RUBY ON RAILES© (ROR): A full-stack framework for developing database-backed Web applications according to a model-view-control pattern; from Ajax in the view, to the request and response in the controller, to the domain model wrapping the database, Rails is a pure-Ruby development environment that can go-live with an added database and a Web server.

RULE-BASED EXPERT SYSTEM: Medical algorithm, critical pathway, or electronic treatment protocol.

RULE-BASED SECURITY POLICY: A health care data security policy based on global rules imposed for all subjects; usually rely on a comparison of the sensitivity of the objects being accessed and the possession of corresponding attributes by the subjects requesting access.

RULES ENGINE: Algorithm and math-based health care decision support system.

RUN: The performance of a computer, network, peripheral device, or the Internet, and so forth; to operate or use a program or application.

RUN CHART: Data points of emerging patterns or health trends.

RUNNING HEADER: Small headline that appears on the bottom footer or top of each Web site page; usually an advertisement or site page placement reminder.

RUN TIME: A running or executable computer program, and in some programming languages certain reusable programs or "routines" are built and packaged as a "runtime library." Some programmers distinguish between what gets embedded in a program when it is a compiler and what gets embedded or used at runtime; sometimes called "compile time."

RURAL AREA NETWORK (RAN): Shared-usage networks designed to include a wide scope of users in rural communities, such as educational, health, medical, and business entities.

RXNORM: FDA nomenclature for HL7 to provide standardized names for drugs and doses.

S

SABOTAGE: Intentionally induced computer system damage.

SABRE: Computer language program that revolutionized the airline reservations industry.

SAD MAC: Macintosh computer emoticon to identify an internal operating error or problem.

SAFE BIOPHARMA ASSOCIATION: Industry initiative launched in 2005 and sponsored by the Pharmaceutical Research and Manufacturers Association (PRMA) to deliver digital identity and signature standards increasingly adopted by drug companies.

SAFE GUARD: Any and all protective mechanisms to promote computer system security.

SAFE MODE: Running Windows® OS with many features disabled as a diagnostic feature for integrity testing purposes.

SALAMI: Incremental theft of computer data, files, programs, information, and so forth; slang term.

SAMBA: A file server network and free software utility that provides print, file sharing, and authorization services.

SAMMY: One of the first Web application worms released in October 2005; followed by an AT&T DSL sales site hack in August 2006.

SANCTION: A formal process of verbal warning or notice of disciplinary action placed in personnel files, removal of system privileges, termination of employment, contract penalties, and so forth.

SANCTION POLICY: Health organization policies and procedures regarding disciplinary actions that are communicated to all employees, agents, and contractors, for example, verbal warning, notice of disciplinary action placed in personnel files, removal of system privileges, termination of employment, and contract penalties; in addition to enterprise sanctions, employees, agents, and contractors must be advised of civil or criminal penalties for misuse or misappropriation of health information; employees, agents, and contractors must be made aware that violations may result in notification to law enforcement officials and regulatory, accreditation, and licensure organizations.

SANDBOX: A computer system security feature to prevent the internal change or modification of system features, memory, disk space, and so forth; JAVA® virtual machine secure area.

SANDERS, JAY H., MD: Partner, the Global Telemedicine Group, McLean, VA.

SANITIZE: The deletion or erasure of electronic passwords, or other identifiers; slang term.

SANTY WORM: Malicious software code that exploited certain Google bulletin board systems in 2004.

SAP: A German developer of electronic business software based in Walldorf, Germany; systems-applications-products.

SARBANES-OXLEY ACT (SARBOX): States that all business records, including electronic medical records, PHI, and electronic messages must be saved for "not less than five years" with consequences for noncompliance as fines, imprisonment, or both; federal act that enforces reporting requirements and internal controls on electronic financial reporting systems.

SATA: Type of ATA hard-drive interface to transfer data to a hard disk.

SATELLITE: An electronic retransmission space instrument serving as a repeater, which is a bidirectional device used to amplify or regenerate signals, placed in orbit around the earth in geostationary orbit for the purpose of receiving and retransmitting electromagnetic signals; typically receives signals from a single source and retransmits them over a wide geographic area, known as the satellite's footprint.

SATELLITE CONNECTIONS: A system of communications that uses radio signals sent to and from a satellite orbiting the earth; benefits of this mode of communication are that it allows connection between points at a great distance from each other on the earth's surface, between which direct transmission is difficult, as well as to remote areas that lack cables for telephone lines.

SAVE: To transfer health data or other information from one storage medium to another; retrieving or leading is the reverse process.

SCALABLE: The ability to change sizes; minimize or maximize.

SCALABLE FONT: Input typeface characteristics that are fluid and changeable.

SCALAR PROCESS: A computer capable of processing only one piece of health data or information at a time.

SCAN: To input into an optical imaging system.

SCANNER: Electronic device used to digitalize a document or image; similar to fax technology: handheld, sheet feed.

SCANNING: The act of locating a computer security breach that can be broken into or exploited.

SCAVENGE: Search through discarded electronic files or hard-copy material in search of personal identifiers or confidential information; dumpster diving; slang term.

SCHADE, SUSAN: CIO, Brigham & Women's Hospital, Boston, MA.

SCHEDULER: The operating system movement of input-ready computer programs.

SCHEMA: Abstract representation of interrelated objects usually defined within a set of XML or HTML tags.

SCHERER, WILLIAM P.: Software and PC visionary, doctor, surgeon, and co-founder of a privately held firm that created one of the first interactive programs for computer-based physician education.

SCHMEIST HEAD: The execution of an executable computer command without knowing its outcome; slang term.

SCHMULAND, DENNIS, MD: Director of Microsoft's health plan industry solutions.

SCHNEIER, BRUCE: Internationally renowned information technologist and author described by *The Economist* as a "security guru" and best known as a candid security critic and commentator.

SCHROEDER, CHRIS: CEO of the HealthCentral Internet portal site.

SCHROTH, WILLIAM C.: Chair, Working Group for Health Information Technology, New York State, Department of Health.

SCHUMACHER, SCOTT: Chief Scientist and Senior VP for Initiate Systems.

SCHWARTZ, JONATHAN: CEO of Sun Microsystems, Inc., who replaced former CEO and Founder Scott McNealy, an innovator of the SunSHINE® concept (Sun Solutions for Healthcare Information, Networking, Education).

SCRAP: A copied file that can be dropped or dragged across a computer screen; a bit of electronic information.

SCRATCH DISK: An erasable or reusable backup disk or tape that does not contain any important health data or other information.

SCREEN: Computer system monitor, LCD, plasma, or display.

SCREEN CAPTURE: A still-shot computer screen image; screen shot.

SCREEN ESTATE: Amount of available space on a computer monitor/screen.

SCREENING ROUTER: A computer network traffic governor configured to reject nonadmissible information packets for security protection; first line of defense against network hacks and attacks.

SCREEN NAME: AOL or other ISP or computer system end-user name tag, identifier, or name.

SCREEN SAVER: The default image on an inactive computer system's monitor/screen.

SCRIPT: A set of Web page instructions invisible on the screen but which helps Internet Explorer® to function; sometimes used to mean a list of OS commands that are stored in a file and performed sequentially by the operating system's command interpreter whenever the list name is entered as a single command; a multimedia development program to mean the sequence of instructions entered to indicate how a sequence of files will be presented; font style.

SCRIPT KIDDIES: Younger and less IT sophisticated users who break into a computer with malicious intent; slang term.

SCRIPT LANGUAGE: A computer program or sequence of instructions that is interpreted or carried out by another program rather than by the computer itself; some languages have been conceived expressly as script languages, as are Rexx® (IBM Mainframes), PERL, or JAVAScript; script languages are easier and faster to code in than the more structured and compiled languages such as C and C++, however, they take longer to run than a compiled program because each instruction is being handled by another program first rather than directly by the basic instruction processor.

SCROLL: To slowly search, or view a computer screen, intranet, or Internet.

SCROLL BAR: Bottom computer screen bar that contains a scrolling input and manipulation feature; scroll lock.

SEAGATE TECHNOLOGY, INC.®: A maker of hard drives and electronic storage, access, and management devices.

SEARCH ENGINE: A software program or algorithm the scours the Internet for specific Web sites, pages, keywords or phrases, or other information needs; Google®, ASK©, Lycos©, Altavista©, Yahoo!, Excite©, and so forth; a Web site that indexes an online resource and makes that index available to other users for searching; typically applied to a site that has indexed Web documents, but search engines also index mailing lists and other online resources; an internal search engine index only includes the documents of that particular Web site, which permits the user to find information on that site more easily and quickly.

SEARCH ENGINE OPTIMIZER: An expert who increases a health care or other firm's Web site traffic by improving its search-engine page rankings; especially important task where many patients first learn of an organization and its services through the Web; most are self-taught, learning the trade by researching trends, attending conferences and seminars, participating in discussion forums, and experimenting with sites; courses and certifications in this specialty are being offered by an increasing number of organizations; however, consensus on the value of these programs does not yet exist.

SEAT LICENSE: A per-user concurrent fee paid to a vendor to supply copies of copyrighted material or software services, programs, applications, and so forth.

SECONDARY DATA: Health data and medical information derived from the patient chart.

SECONDARY MOUSE BUTTON: The clickable action menu call-up or retrieve input button device.

SECONDARY RECORD: Patient record derived from the primary medical chart with selected information for nonclinical assistance.

SECONDARY RELEASE: PHI or medical information disclosure without prior patient authorization.

SECONDARY SOURCE: Summary of original source medical and health information.

SECONDARY STORAGE: Additional electronic memory distinct from a CPU.

SECOND GENERATION: Transistor-based computers of the 1950s and 1960s.

SECOND LEVEL DOMAIN: Any moniker beneath a primary level Internet domain name system.

SECRECY: Purposeful concealment of medical information or health data.

SECRET KEY: A protective symmetric algorithm encryption protocol or identifier to access information or initiate use; log-in password; slang term.

SECTOR: The smallest unit of electronic storage, read or written, on an electronic computer disk.

SECURE CHANNEL: Any electronic means of conveying health information from one entity to another such that an adversary does not have the ability to reorder, delete, insert, or read; secure medical data transmission.

SECURE ELECTRONIC TRANSACTION: An algorithm or cryptographic protocol for protected electronic health data and medical information transmission or monetary transactions across the Internet; SSL protocol.

SECURE LOCKER©: A secure download mechanism from Microsoft.

SECURE MESSAGING: Confidential e-mail with personalized and traceable messages; instant message.

SECURE SITE: Any Web site with protected health care information, medical, or other data integrity measures; secured wide area network (SWAN).

SECURE SOCKET LAYER (SSL): A secure Web server data transmission protocol encryption method; indicated by a padlock icon or https://address.

SECURE VIRTUAL PRIVATE NETWORK (SVPN): Use cryptographic tunneling protocols to provide the necessary health data confidentiality (preventing snooping), sender authentication (preventing identity spoofing), and message integrity (preventing message alteration) to achieve the medical privacy intended. When properly chosen, implemented, and used, such techniques can provide secure communications over unsecured networks.

SECURE WEB SERVER: A WAN, LAN, MAN, Internet program, or security computer hub with algorithm or cryptographic protocol to send protected electronic health data transmissions or monetary transactions across the Internet; SSL protocol.

SECURE WORK STATION LOCATION: Physical safeguards to eliminate or minimize the possibility of unauthorized access to information, for example, locating a terminal used to access sensitive information in a locked room and restricting access to that room to authorized personnel, not placing a terminal used to access patient information in any area of a doctor's office where the screen contents can be viewed from the reception area.

SECURITY: A set of health care information technology system characteristics and mechanisms that span the system both logically and physically; electronic access control against unauthorized intervention, both friendly or malicious; encompasses all of the safeguards in an information system, including hardware, software, personnel policies, information practice policies, disaster preparedness, and the oversight of all these areas; the purpose of health information security is to protect both the system and the information it contains from unauthorized access from without and from misuse from within; through various security measures, a health information system can shield confidential information from unauthorized access, disclosure, and misuse, thus protecting privacy of the individuals who are the subjects of the stored data; security life cycle (Table 8).

Table 8: Six Phases of the IT Security Life Cycle

Phase 1: **Initiation**—the organization determines if it should investigate whether implementing an IT security service might improve the effectiveness of the organization's IT security program. This may occur when a security breach is discovered or when purchasing new IT equipment.

Phase 2: **Assessment**—the organization determines the security posture of the current environment using metrics and identifies the requirements and viable solutions. For example, the review of audit trail logs on secure information access.

Phase 3: **Solution**—decision makers evaluate potential solutions, develop the business case, and specify the attributes of an acceptable service arrangement solution from the set of available options.

Phase 4: **Implementation**—the organization selects and engages the service provider, develops a service arrangement, and implements the solution.

Phase 5: **Operations**—the organization ensures operational success by consistently monitoring service provider and organizational security performance against identified requirements, periodically evaluating changes in risks and threats to the organization, and ensuring the organizational security solution is adjusted as necessary to maintain an acceptable security posture.

Phase 6: **Closeout**—the organization ensures a smooth transition as the service ends or is discontinued.

SECURITY ADMINISTRATION: The physical and electrical protection features of an IT health system needed to be managed in order to meet the needs of a specific installation and to account for changes in the health care entities operational environment.

SECURITY ADMINISTRATOR: One who enforces electronic network security matters.

SECURITY ADMINISTRATOR TOOL FOR ANALYZING NETWORKS (SATAN): A computer network vulnerability scanning tool developed by W. Venema and D. Farmer in 1995.

SECURITY ASSOCIATION (SA): Agreed upon security parameters of conduct for VPNs, key strengths, algorithms, and so forth, for an IPSec tunnel.

SECURITY AWARENESS TRAINING: Customized education programs that focus on issues regarding use of health information and responsibilities regarding medical data confidentiality and security.

SECURITY COMPROMISE: Physical or electronic data, file, program, or transmission error due to malicious miscreants or software interventions; confidentiality breach.

SECURITY CONFIGURATION: Measures, practices, and procedures for the safety of information systems that must be coordinated and integrated with each other and other methods, practices, and procedures of the organization established in order to credential safekeeping policy; provides written security plans, rules, procedures, and instructions concerning all components of a health care entity's security; procedures must give instructions on how to report breaches and how those breaches are to be handled within the organization.

SECURITY CONFIGURATION MANAGEMENT: The measurement of practices and procedures for the security of information systems that is coordinated and integrated with each other and other measures, practices, and procedures of the organization so as to create a coherent system of health data security (NIST Pub 800–14).

SECURITY DOMAIN: A set of subjects, their information objects, and a common security policy; foundation for IT security is the concept of security domains and enforcement of data and process flow restrictions within and between these domains.

SECURITY GOAL: The empowerment of a health care facility or medical IT organization to meet all mission/business objectives by implementing systems with due care consideration of related risks to the organization, its partners, and its patients; the five health IT security goals are integrity, availability, confidentiality, accountability, and assurance.

SECURITY INCIDENT: The attempted or successful unauthorized access, use, disclosure, modification, or destruction of information or interference with system operations in an information system.

SECURITY INCIDENT PROCEDURE: Formal, documented instructions for reporting security breaches; security log; security journal, and so forth.

SECURITY LEVEL: Controlled authorization of specific health care data input users.

SECURITY MANAGEMENT: A process that encompasses the creation, administration, and oversight of policies to ensure the prevention, detection, containment, and correction of health security breaches; involves risk analysis and risk management, including the establishment of accountability, management controls (policies and education), electronic controls, physical security, and penalties for the abuse and misuse of its assets, both physical and electronic (Table 8).

SECURITY OBJECTIVE INTERDEPENDENCY: Integration of health care data security objectives by consideration of all other dependent objectives, as depicted in Figure 15.

SECURITY OBJECTIVES: The five health-care IT and medical information security goals and objectives are integrity, availability, confidentiality, accountability, and assurance:

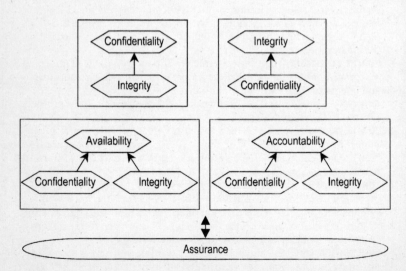

Figure 15: Health data security objective interdependency.

- *Integrity* is dependent on confidentiality, in that if the confidentiality of certain information is lost (e.g., the super-user password), then the integrity mechanisms are likely to be bypassed.
- *Availability* and *Accountability* are dependent on confidentiality and integrity, in that if confidentiality is lost for certain information (e.g., super-user password), the mechanisms implementing these objectives are easily bypassable; and if system integrity is lost, then confidence in the validity of the mechanisms implementing these objectives is also lost.
- *Confidentiality* is dependent on integrity, in that if the integrity of the system is lost, then there is no longer a reasonable expectation that the confidentiality mechanisms are still valid.
- *Assurance* is achieved by defining and meeting functionality requirements in each of the four objectives with sufficient quality; highlights the fact that for systems to be secure, they must not only provide intended functionality, but also ensure undesired actions do not occur.

SECURITY OFFICER: One responsible for enterprise-wide medical and health data information security; chief security officer; CSO, CTO, and so forth.

SECURITY OVERHEAD: Total financial costs of all health care data and information and protection features.

SECURITY POLICY: A statement of the required health care IT protection of information objects such as patient protected health information; the framework within which a health care organization establishes needed levels of information security to achieve the desired confidentiality goals; a policy is a statement of information values, protection responsibilities, and organization commitment for a system (OTA, 1993); the American Health Information Management Association (AHIMA) recommends that security policies apply to all employees, medical staff members, volunteers, students, faculty, independent contractors, and agents.

SECURITY POLICY ENTIRE HEALTH CARE ORGANIZATION: Established enterprise-wide requirements for protecting patients' individually identifiable health information; install supporting technology.

SECURITY POLICY ENTIRE HEALTH CARE ORGANIZATION FOR ELECTRONIC HOSPITAL INFORMATION SYSTEMS (sample):

Mission: The hospital is dedicated to developing and providing the highest quality, compassionate health care to serve the needs of the community. Key to the delivery of quality health care is the design and implementation of programs that support and enhance appropriate access to health information according to HIPAA rules and regulations.

Vision: All information regarding patients and employees is considered confidential and is considered protected health care information (PHI). The hospital will develop consistent approaches to the handling of data across the system that will balance the patient's right to privacy and confidentiality with legitimate uses of data.

Scope: ASP, reverse ASP, electronic medical records (EMRs), and computer-based information systems, or similar, including information and data in any format (for example, paper, electronic, or produced electronically) must be protected from unauthorized access, modification, destruction, or disclosure, whether accidental or intentional. Such protection will be consistent with the sensitivity and the value of the data. Protection can be provided through equipment, software, and procedures that address processing, transmission, and storage of data.

Policies:

1. Accountability and responsibility
   - *Accountability:* It is the responsibility of all hospital employees to consider themselves accountable for the protection of the data, which begins with accessing the database and continues with the use of the information regardless of format. Policies and procedures support the confidentiality and integrity of the information systems within the corporation.
   - *Responsibility:* The information maintained in the computer-based information systems of the hospital is an asset of the corporation. Managers are responsible for the timeliness, security, and integrity of the data maintained within the scope of their position through the use of appropriate control measures and the support of hospital policies.

2. Access
   - ID / password / secure socket layer (SSL) encryption / biometrics
   - Unique identification and password assignments will be made to staff members for access to information on a need-to-know basis, only upon written authority of the owner of the data. Need-to-know is determined by the individual's supervisor. Generally it can be categorized into these areas:
   - access by care providers to individual patient data, for use in patient care or specific hospital operations.
   - access for research, planning, and quality improvement processes within the hospital.
   - access by those employees in the Health Record Department whose role includes record processing-maintenance.
   - use of PKI infrastructure for public and private sectors, as needed, along with SSL technology and biometric encryption.

- individual IDs/passwords may not be shared with another user.
- passwords are changed frequently, as designated by system design.
- users are limited to one log-on at a time, as designated by individual platform design.
- an individual's multiple attempts to sign on with an improper access code will result in a lock-out status of the individual until access privileges are restored by Information Services.
- access of all users is monitored by identification/password assignments. Warning notices are to be displayed on each screen to inform staff of the confidential nature of the information and that their access is being monitored.
- maintenance of the access assignments will be completed with employee change in status (e.g., termination, change of position).
- employee's information.
- each system employee may choose whether his/her personal data will be accessible or restricted for view by medical staff only in the hospital system. The option of requesting restricted access on selected systems and not others will not be available.
- an employee's access to his/her own patient information must follow the process as defined in the release of information policies and procedures.
- pre-employment data will be retained only in the local employee health database.
- sensitive information (psychiatry, substance abuse, VIP, protected patients) is defined in the release of information policies and procedures.
- protected patients: Those patients with known risk of injury by others must be protected. Their identification will be protected by the assignment of an alias on the Admission/Discharge/Transfer (ADT) system. However, the health record number will remain unchanged and valid for the patient.

3. Integrity of database
   - A process must exist for each database by which information is validated within the system.
   - Integrity of data copied and transferred to another system is the responsibility of the receiving system. Responsibility for the correct transfer and validation of data lies with both systems and information services.

4. Security
   - Administration and maintenance
   Appropriate Information Services Departments will monitor and log access to the various systems within the hospital. A description of the methods used is available with each system's documentation. If misuse is suspected, the health information management

specialist and/or department director should be notified. If appropriate, the director of security should be contacted for proper investigation.

- Dissemination

  Secondary disclosure of individual patient information must be in keeping with the process, as defined in the release of information policies and procedures. Internal or external dissemination of data linking patient identifiers with clinical data should be evaluated against the recipient's need to know that information.

5. Compliance with confidentiality and data security policies

- Failure to comply with confidentiality and data security policies, standards, and procedures will result in disciplinary action in accordance with human resources policies, which may include termination or suspension of employment. Compliance means conformity to data security policies and standards as well as the data security procedures developed to meet user needs.
- Improper conduct includes, but is not limited to:
- lack of discretion or unauthorized disclosure of any information concerning patients, visitors, or employees.
- attempting to obtain another person's password or security code or database structure.
- unauthorized access, whether internally or from a remote location.
- unauthorized release of patient information.
- monitoring compliance of security policies and procedures will be through collaboration between the systems administrator and appropriate management staff.
- monitoring compliance of security policies and procedures will be through collaboration between the systems administrator and appropriate management staff.

SECURITY SCANNER: Software or Internet-based data security detection tool identifying potential bugs, viruses, and holes.

SECURITY STANDARDS: HIPAA requirements adopted by HHS or ANSI to preserve and maintain transmitted or stored medical data and PHI.

SECURITY SUPPORTING SERVICES: Health care IT and medical data protection service that is pervasive and interrelated with other services, such as:

- identification (and naming)
- cryptographic key management
- security administration and system protections
- prevention and protected communications

- authentication and authorization
- access control enforcement
- nonrepudiation and transaction privacy
- detection and recovery (contingency)
- audit, intrusion detection, and containment
- proof of wholeness, and
- restoration of secure state

SECURITY SYSTEMS: Any physical, personal, or electrical methodology used to protect health care information and medical data through these five security objectives:

- availability—addressed by physical and technical safeguards of HIPAA regulations;
- integrity—system and data;
- confidentiality—addressed by HIPAA privacy regulations;
- accountability—to the individual level;
- assurance—coordinates security measures both technical and operational and works as intended to protect the system and the information it processes.

SECURITY TESTING: A process used to determine that the security features of a health care system are implemented as designed and that they are adequate for a proposed applications environment; hands-on functional and stress testing, penetration testing, and verification.

SECURITY THREAT: Potential confidential breaches in health care data by users, authorizers, and physical, environmental, or technical failures.

SECURITY TOOL: Software program or algorithm to check, enhance, or monitor a computer security system.

SEERS: Internet users, laymen, medical professionals, and other HIT thought leaders; slang term.

SEGMENT: Related elements in an electronic health data transmission.

SELECT: To activate a computer system object, database, file, and so forth.

SELF-EXTRACTING ARCHIVE: A health or other data file converted into an executable program that decompresses when run.

SELF-EXTRACTION: Software utility program used to decondense (unzip), transport, and archive programs with the file extensions .exe, .hqx, .sea, .sit, .gz, .z, .tar, or .gtar.

SELF-HEALING: Any computing device or system that has the ability to perceive that it is not operating correctly and, without human intervention, make the necessary adjustments to restore itself to normal operation; self-protecting and self-managing.

SEMANTIC DATA MODEL (SDM): To express the structure or scheme of a health care application information model; LOINC.

SEMANTICS: Symbolic meanings within a given computer code; language nuances, terms, or words.

SEMAPHORE: An electronic flag used to indicate computer activity status and/or security.

SEMICONDUCTOR: Any manipulateable material that is neither a good electrical insulator nor conductor; silicone, germanium; diodes, transistors, ICs, CPU devices, and so forth.

SENDMAIL: Type of electronic mail that searches messages for IP addresses in order to embed malicious codes, viruses, worms, and so forth.

SENSITIVE: Data or medical electronic information that is considered potentially harmful, embarrassing, or damaging; protected health information (PHI).

SENSITIVITY LEVEL: Triage level for protected or open electronic data associated with content, input or end-user authority, or information appropriateness.

SEQUENCE DIAGRAM: Interaction scheme between user and health care medical management information system.

SEQUENTIAL PROCESSING: Medical or other health records that are accessed serially.

SERIAL ATA (SATA): The ATA (American Telemedicine Association) standard for disk drives that could be a disruptive technology by bringing manufacturing efficiencies to storage vendors; SATA drives often shuttle data at rates of 150 MB–600 MB per second, or more.

SERIAL DATA: Any method of transmitting health or other electrical information over a wire, one bit at a time.

SERIAL FILE: A medical record or chart with unique identifiers assigned with each subsequent medical encounter.

SERIAL LINE INTERNET PROTOCOL (SLIP): A kind of computer protocol used by modems for online communication.

SERIAL MOUSE: An input device attached to a computer system by a serial port.

SERIAL PORT: A computer information transmission socket used to connect a serial interface peripheral device; usually replaced by USB ports; most PCs have two ports labeled COM1 and COM 2.

SERVER: Centralized WAN, LAN, MAN, computer- or Internet-based hub that provides services to affiliated clients or connected dumb terminals; computer system in a network shared by multiple users; stand-alone PCs and Macs can function as a server to other users on the network, even though they serve as a single workstation to one user ("peer-2-peer" network); this is common in small clinics and medical offices, but servers are usually stand-alone stations; term may refer to both the hardware and software or just the software that performs a particular service. For example,

"Web server" may refer to the Web server software in a computer that also runs other applications, or it may refer to a computer system dedicated only to the Web server application; a large Web site could have several dedicated servers or one very large server; server appliance.

SERVER FARM: Computers connected and housed in a single location; server cluster.

SERVER SIDE APPLICATION: A computer program that uses a LAN, MAN, WAN, or other network rather than a PC.

SERVER SOFTWARE: Computer network server that responds to a dumb or connected terminal request.

SERVICE: A computer program or application that runs unseen by the end user.

SERVICE EVENT: The process or activity of providing a medical service, health care procedure or intervention, diagnosis, or other activity.

SERVICE LINE CODE: One who codes for a particular medical specialty service, such as dental, podiatry, pediatrics, and so forth.

SERVICE PACK (SP): A MSFT or other update program used to fix loopholes in Internet Explorer®; the first SP focused on security while the second SP2, increased functionality with wireless enhancements.

SERVICE SET IDENTIFIER (SSI): A type of health data or information packet identifier for a wireless computer network.

SERVICE V-CODE: ICD-9-CM code for medical examinations, aftercare, or re-imbursable ancillary health care services.

SERVLET: A small Java utility program that runs on a Web server, rather than a Web browser client.

SESSION: A period of medical interaction, as with a patient, or the Internet, and so forth.

SESSION HIJACK: A false traffic computer network transmission connection that overtakes a client TCP session.

SESSION KEY: An encryption/decryption code that is randomly generated to ensure the security of a communication interaction between a user and another computer or between two computers; sometimes called *symmetric keys*, because the same key is used for both encryption and decryption; may be derived from a hash value, using the *CryptDeriveKey* function; transmitted along with each message and is encrypted with the recipient's public key, but because much security relies upon the brevity of use, session keys are changed frequently; a different session key may be used for each message.

SESSION LAYER: OSI model and fifth layer of computer system file management, check points, synchronization, and termination.

SESSION PREDICTION: A method of surreptitiously obtaining data about an authorized visitor to a Web site; normally stored within an URL or cookie.

SEVEN DIMENSIONS OF HIT DATA QUALITY: Accuracy, consistency, currency, granularity, precision, timeliness, and relevancy.

SEVERITY SYSTEM: Statistical probability of disease progression; or information system contamination.

SHAMIR, ADI, PhD: The Paul and Marlene Borman Professor of Applied Mathematics at Weizmann Institute of Science, whose main area of research is making and breaking computer security codes motivated by the explosive growth of computer networks and wireless communication, the Internet, and HIPAA; developer of cryptographic paradigms such as broadcast encryption, ring signatures, and T-functions; new cryptanalytic attacks against block ciphers, stream ciphers, and number theoretic schemes, along with new protective techniques against side channel attacks such as power analysis.

SHARE(D): To make a medical file, health folder, application, or program available for use by others; shared directory, memory folder, medium, memory, resources, machines, and so forth.

SHARED DECISION MAKING (SDM): A style of decision making in health care where the patient is able to take a more active role in decision making, especially by offering them increased control over the choice of treatment, and, as a result, giving them a greater sense of responsibility for their care and health; shared decision medical program.

SHARED ENVIRONMENT: To provide IT health processing for several clients; client-server relationship.

SHARED SERVICES: A full range of health care clinical and medical business organization IT systems that are supplied by a single covered entity.

SHARED SPACE: Computer storage within a network boundary; shared memory and remote storage.

SHAREPOINT®: Microsoft collaborative workgroup software application service.

SHAREWARE: Internet software distributed on an honorary trial basis; computer software that the author gives license to the user to try before buying; users are encouraged to try the software, copy it, and distribute it to other users; if users continue to use the software after the initial sampling, a voluntary payment of a specific sum of money is required; failure to pay the requested fee is a legal violation of the author's copyright.

SHELL: Protection interface used for insulation and protection; a program that accepts OS commands for execution.

SHOCKWAVE®: Nonvolatile, solid-state rewriteable memory file format processing with robust functionality that is durable and low-voltage; Macromedia Flash©.

SHOESHINE: To move a computer or storage tape back and forth to enhance connectivity; slang term.

SHOPPING CART: Icon driven invoicing and billing software used by online merchants.

SHORT CUT: Push-button icon for directly initiating a prearranged computer action or function.

SHORTLIFFE, EDWARD H., MD: Professor of Medicine and Computer Science; Head, Division of General Internal Medicine; and Director, Medical Information Sciences Training Program, Stanford University School of Medicine, Palo Alto, CA.

SHOULDER SURF: To peek over the head and shoulders of a computer system user in order to discern PWs, account numbers, or other confidential information; low tech; slang term.

SHOUT(ING): An uppercase e-mail or text message; slang term.

SHOVELWARE: Bloated excessive software code, program, or application; slang term.

SHRINKWRAP: Retail commercial software sold in premanufactured and plastic covered packages; clear plastic box coating.

SHUGART, ALAN: Codeveloper of the first floppy disk, from IBM in 1971.

SHUT DOWN: The command to save settings, files, or other objects and turn off a computer.

SICONOLFI, FRANCINE: Senior Health care IT Project Manager, Aetna Assurance Company.

SIGNALING SYSTEM 7: A recent development in control systems for the public telephone network enabling faster processing and more efficient telephone service, making more services available to patients and consumers.

SIGNATURE: Computer, network, IM, IRC, or e-mailer identification code; computer miscreant pattern or identifier; digital electronic fingerprints.

SIGNATURE FILE: Automated text file added to an e-mail message typically including contact information; signature block, or file; files that contain updated anti-virus information, and so forth.

SILICONE SUBURBS: Geographic locals where important computer device makers, manufactures, researchers, developers, and universities exist:

- *Alley:* Manhattan, NY
- *Creek:* Atlanta, Dunwoody, and Norcross, GA
- *Fen:* Cambridge, England
- *Glen:* Edinburgh and Glasgow, Scotland
- *Silicorn:* Rural Iowa and the Midwest
- *Valley:* Santa Clara, Cupertino, Sunnyvale, Palo Alta, San Jose, and San Francisco, CA

SIMPLEX: Unidirectional electronic communications channel.

SIMPLY HIRED®: A job and employment search engine; health care IT employment agency.

SIMULATION: Statistical data or information electronic modeling technique; to mimic real life; or to mimic a patient medical session or encounter.

SINGER, SUANNE: Project Director, Maine Health Information Network Technology.

SINGLE AFFILIATED COVERED ENTITY (SACE): Legally separate CEs for purposes of the HIPAA rules and regulations if under common ownership and control, in order to share common consents, and so forth.

SINGLE DOMAIN: WINDOWS© NT system that is independent and void of other domain connections.

SINGLE MASTER DOMAIN: WINDOWS© NT system with other trust and domain connections and resources administered by those domains.

SIPPHONE®: Internet telephone software; VOIP provider.

SIRCAM WORM: Malicious code that sent out personal health information and other data and documents from machines by e-mail.

SITE: An area or location online, typically on the Web, where an organization, medical practice, health care organization, individual, or business stores its information.

SITE LICENSE: Permission for use of a fixed number of copyrighted subscriptions, applications, programs, copies, downloads, and so forth.

SITE MAP: A Web site hierarchal diagram of its pages.

SKIN: To change the share, appearance, fonts, color, and graphics of a Web site, Web page, URL, application, or program.

SKUNK: Dedicated computer engineers or software programmers isolated from peers in order to enhance morale, special project efficiency, and so forth; pirates; slang term.

SLAMECKA, VLADIMIR: Early 1960s computer visionary from The Georgia Institute of Technology, who founded its department of computer science and foresaw the use of digital information for the common good; especially in medical, educational, and urban planning applications.

SLASHDOT: Internet-based company that provides engineering news to computer hobbyists.

SLAVE: Any independent electrical unit; computer, storage device, peripheral or linked machines, and so forth; slang term.

SLIMEWARE: Software that interferes with the end-user experience by changing key computer system settings in order to gain profit; spyware; adware; slang term.

SLOAN, ALEXANDER M., MD: Former Surgeon General USAF and Medical Director for DIANAssociates, University of Maryland Medical Systems.

SLOW-SCAN: The speed of still video image transmission, which is typically over narrow communications channels such as standard telephone lines.

SLOW-SCAN VIDEO: A device that transmits and receives still video images over a narrow communications channel, such as a standard telephone line.

SMALL BUSINESS SERVER (SBS): MSFT Web-based application server for medical, health care, or other small offices using less than about 50 networked PCs.

SMALL COMPUTER SYSTEMS INTERFACE (SCSI): An interface system of rules and procedures used to connect peripherals such as disk drives, scanners, and tape back-up units, to computers; referred to as *skuzzy*.

SMALL FORM FACTOR PC: PC with smaller case compared with an ATX tower in a standard desktop type PC.

SMALL HEALTH PLAN: Traditional or electronic health plan with annual receipts of $5 million or less; Part II, 45 CFR 160.103.

SMART CARD: Plastic card with CPU or magnetic data strip to read, write, and store electronic information, such as patient, financial, insurance, or clinical data; access control for computer systems, servers, or networks; smart device, smart reader, smart phone, and so forth.

SMART MEDIA: A type of medical data or other information storage device for nonvolatile flash memory.

SMART PHONE: A cellular phone with e-mail, mobile Bluetooth©, and/or USB cable and/or docking station; with secure digital memory card, MP3 photo, and video and instant message functionality.

SMART SUITE®: Lotus business application conglomeration of computer programs and business efficiency tools: spreadsheet, word processing, database, graphics, time management, and Internet publishing offerings.

SMILEY: A form of electronic emoticon; a small diagrammatic "face" made out of keyboard characters; for example, ϑ or ;-).

SMOKE TEST: To activate a computer system, software, hardware, or peripheral device for the first time; slang term.

SMURF(FER): To rapidly interrupt, send unwanted data, or otherwise ping a computer maliciously; a denial of service attack; slang term.

SNEAKER: A professional computer systems hacker or crack; security system expert.

SNEAKERWARE: The physical removal and transportation of a secondary computer storage device, such as an external hard or flash drive, instead of using a networked system; slang term.

SNEAKNET: To transfer health disks, memory sticks, floppy disks, CDs, or other stored data across the room, from one computer to another; slang term.

SNIFFER: Network traffic data collection, monitoring, and optimization tool; eavesdropping programs; slang term.

SNIFFING: Listening to the traffic on a computer network and then analyzing it.

SNOOP: Usually a self-contained software program used to monitor other programs, users, or systems without prior knowledge.

SNOWFLAKE TECHNOLOGY: The LUMINETX© format for a type of infrared vein palm-scan viewing for biometric security identification; veins may be used to replace photo IDs, PINs, passwords, signatures, or keys with the following HIT security advantages:

- Access Control and Attendance—Use biometrics for controlling access to facilities and monitoring employee attendance. Biometrics will replace time cards.
- Criminal Identification—Veins offer an additional means to track criminals as they are processed through the criminal justice system.
- Civil Identification—Broad range of applications include activities such as international border control, airport security, authentication of welfare recipients, and voter registration.
- Consumer Identification—From banking to retail, veins can be used to help people securely transact while protecting their identity.
- Device and System Access—Venous recognition can be used to replace passwords for access to computers and other critical devices on which businesses and consumers rely.

SNYDER, DAVID H.: Albany Medical Center, VP of Health Information Systems Technology Management.

SOAP: A Simple, Object, Access Protocol for exchanging XML messages over a computer network using HTTP and providing a basic messaging framework that abstract layers can build upon.

SOBIG.F: Mass e-mailer computer worm that infected PCs through insecure network sharing in 2003.

SOCIAL ENGINEERING: Relying on personal trickery and human deceit to break security and gain access to computers; to goad or manipulate human computer systems users; shoulder surfers (Table 9).

SOCKET: The local address endpoint connections between a communications access point; client server relationship.

SOCKS: A circuit level proxy against a wide range of computer system hack attacks.

SOFT COPY: Electronic data storage files only viewable on a computer screen.

SOFT RETURN: Text document software code inserted to mark the end of a line.

SOFTWARE: Electronic programs used to direct useful computer functions; operating system, programming and application types, and so forth.

SOFTWARE ACCESS: Ability to communicate with an electronic computer program.

SOFTWARE AS A SERVICE (SAAS): A distribution model in which applications are hosted by a vendor or service provider and made available to customers over a network, typically the Internet, and is increasingly prevalent in underlying technologies that support various Web services

Table 9: Human Social Engineering Threats: Threat-Source, Motivation, and Threat Actions

Threat Source	Motivation	Threat Actions
Hacker, Cracker	Challenge	• Hacking
	Ego	• Social engineering
	Rebellion	• System intrusion, break-ins
		• Unauthorized system access
Computer criminal	Destruction of information	• Computer crime (e.g., cyber stalking)
	Illegal information disclosure	• Fraudulent act (e.g., replay, impersonation, interception)
	Monetary gain	• Information bribery
	Unauthorized data alteration	• Spoofing
		• System intrusion
Terrorist	Blackmail	• Bomb/Terrorism
	Destruction	• Information warfare
	Exploitation	• System attack (e.g., distributed denial of service)
	Revenge	• System penetration
		• System tampering
Industrial espionage (companies, foreign governments, other government interests)	Competitive advantage	• Economic exploitation
	Economic espionage	• Information theft
		• Intrusion on personal privacy

Continued

Table 9: Human Social Engineering Threats: Threat-Source, Motivation, and Threat Actions *(Continued)*

Threat Source	Motivation	Threat Actions
		• Social engineering
		• System penetration
		• Unauthorized system access (access to classified, proprietary, and/or technology-related information)
Insiders (poorly trained, disgruntled, malicious, negligent, dishonest, or terminated employees)	Curiosity	• Assault on an employee
	Ego	• Blackmail
	Intelligence	• Browsing of proprietary information
	Monetary gain	• Computer abuse
	Revenge	• Fraud and theft
	Unintentional errors and omissions (e.g., data entry error, programming error)	• Information bribery
		• Input of falsified, corrupted data
		• Interception
		• Malicious code (e.g., virus, logic bomb, Trojan horse)
		• Sale of personal information
		• System bugs
		• System sabotage
		• Unauthorized system access

and service-oriented architectures, as well as mature and new developmental approaches, such as Ajax; closely related to the application service provider and on-demand computing delivery models; the Writely© word processor, Gmail, and Google Spreadsheet are examples of this model; non-prepackaged, shrink-wrapped software.

SOFTWARE BOMB: Malicious software code planted as an inside job; to computer detonate at some predetermined future trigger-time, in order to deliver a destructive load.

SOFTWARE MAINTENANCE: Changes performed on computer software after entering implementation.

SOFTWARE RE-ENGINEERING: Changes performed on an older legacy computer software program in order to update or reconfigure it for increased functionality; PC functionality.

SOFTWARE SECURITY: Hardware devices integrated with software and certified as safe and protected from malicious or accidental access.

SOLARIS©: A UNIX multiprocessing operating system for Sun Microsystems Inc®, SPARC® computers.

SOLE VENDOR: Computer or network applications developed with common design architecture.

SOLID STATE: An electronic component or circuit made of solid materials, such as transistors, chips, and bubble memory without mechanical action, although electromagnetic action takes place within; for health and other data storage, solid state devices are much faster and more reliable than mechanical disks and tapes, but are more expensive.

SOLID STATE FLOPPY DISK CARD (SSFDC): Plastic smart card configured with Flash EEPROM, NOR, and/or NAND memory chips and used as a patient identifier, or in electronic scanners, digital cameras, sound and video recorders, and so forth; Toshiba®, Intel®, and Micron®.

SOUND BLASTER®: PC sound-care from Creative Labs, Inc., of Milpitas, CA.

SOUND CARD: An audio analog to digital converter; this FM Wavetable synthesis is a lower quality sound while newer MIDI (Musical Instrument Digital Interface) is better and more compressed (24-bit).

SOUND FILE FORMAT: The most commonly used audio formats:

- WAVE (.wav): High quality but large size
- MP3 (.mp3): High quality and low size
- Compact Disk Digital Audio (.cda): Used solely for commercial CDs
- WMA (.wma): Windows Media Audio Internet streaming .mp3 analog.
- .midi, .aif, .au, .snd, and so forth.

SOURCE CODE: Refers to the "before" and "after" versions of a computer program that are compiled before it is ready to run in a computer and consist of the programming statements that are created by a programmer with a text editor or a visual programming tool and then saved in a file; programming language (C, C++, Pascal, and so forth).

SOURCE LANGUAGE: Input programming language (C, C++, Pascal, and so forth) for a specific computer process.

SOURCE OF ADMISSION CODE: CMS 1450 form-locator 20.

SOURCE ORIENTATED HEALTH RECORD: Health care data arrangement, medical record, or chart according to patient care department.

SOURCE SYSTEMS: An application system where PHI is collected, extracted, and transformed for use in an EHR feeder system.

SPAGHETTI CODE: Inefficient, incorrect, wrong, poorly written, or disorganized computer code; slang term.

SPAM: The mass electronic mailing of unsolicited messages; junk e-mail; trash mail; slang terms; spam bot.

SPAMDEXIG: Internet algorithm used to fool a search engine indexing program; slang term.

SPAM FILTER: Utility program to reduce or purge e-mail boxes of spam mail; spam blocker.

SPAMMER: One who sends spam or blasts unwanted e-mail messages; key word surfer; spam indexer.

SPARKLE: Microsoft© design tool for creating Windows Vista© and certain Web applications; code name.

SPATIAL RESOLUTION: Characteristic of being able to distinguish two equal-sized adjacent objects in the same place; represents the number of pixels in a specified area of a matrix.

SPAWN: Automated software help application.

SPEECH RECOGNITION: The technology to translate human speech to written text.

SPEECH SERVER: MSFT voice recognition of speech-enabled touch tone applications.

SPIDER: Internet utility search program; Web-crawler, robot, bot, and so forth.

SPINDLE: A rotating shaft on a computer disk drive; with a fixed disk the platters are attached to the spindle, but in a removable disk the spindle remains in the drive.

SPLASH SCREEN: Introductory computer application screen display prior to program launch.

SPLOG: A spammed blog; slang term.

SPLOIT: To exploit or breach a computer security system; slang term.

SPOILATION: Destruction of electronic data, medical, or other information; evidence.

SPOOF: Fake electronic responses used to keep an online computer session active preventing timeouts; type of computer virus.

SPOOL: Overlapping low-speed electronic computer operations.

SPOOLER: A low transmission speed outlet device or buffer service.

SPREAD SHEET: Electronic and manipulateable row and column worksheet for automatic math calculations, accounting, or other data processing determinations.

SPREAD SPECTRUM: Data encryption or encoding technique that disperses radio signals away from interference.

SPRITE: Animated and malleable pixel or moving graphical element.

SPY: A person who has been hired to break into a computer and steal data.

SPYWARE: Programs that collect and transmit unauthorized information from a computer about the user; usually associated with Internet freeware or shareware programs; to capture activity without user knowledge; slang term.

SQL SLAMMER WORM: Code that delivered no malicious payload but overloaded computers, networks, and servers in order to slow Internet connectivity in 2003.

SRINI, JAY: VP of Emerging Technology for the University of Pittsburgh Medical College.

STAAG: One of the original viral programs to infect Linux in 1996.

STACK: A computerized data, file, or health information holding structure that follows the inventory costing concept of LIFO.

STAGES VIRUS: Malicious software code hidden in e-mail attachments that appear to be benign .TXT extensions but are dangerous .EXE executable extensions; first seen in 2000.

STALLMAN, RICHARD: Founder of the GNU project who resigned from the Artificial Intelligence laboratory at MIT to produce and distribute free computer software.

STANDARD DEVIATION: A measure of volatility, risk, or statistical dispersion. It is the positive square root of the variance, calculated by:

- computing the (average) mean of the series,
- then taking the deviation by subtracting the mean from each observation,
- squaring the differences or deviations for each observation,
- dividing the sum of the squared deviations by the number of observations, and
- calculating the positive square root of the sum of squared deviations.

Related terms for computer science include:

- *Standard Normal Distribution* or *Standardized Normal Distribution*: Situation that occurs when the underlying normal distribution is converted by changing its scale. The importance of this is that different normal distributions can now be compared to one another. Otherwise, separate tables of values would have to be generated for each pairing of mean and standard deviation values. This standardized variant term is often expressed as Z is N (0,1), or Z is a normal distribution with a mean value of zero and variance equal to one.

- *Static Analysis:* An approach to study market conditions at a moment in time. It also is a "snapshot view" of the market, corporate financial condition, or other economic time series. It reflects one moment such as the end-of-the-day, end-of-the-month, end-of-the-year, the opening, or any other chronologically defined point.
- *Stationary:* A time series that has a natural mean or tendency toward one. Over time and given larger samples, some economic time series tend to converge toward a natural level with stable volatilities.
- *Statistical Analysis:* A mathematical approach that quantifies securities market action. In its general form, it is reliant on large sample statistics and linear analysis. It assumes independence. Its popular subterms are mean, variance, standard deviation, alpha, and beta.
- *Stochastic:* A condition in computer science, engineering, finance, or economics whereby changes occur on a more abrupt basis than those expected to be "normally" encountered. In some ways stochastic have infinite variance and/or nonconverging means implications.

STANDARD PRESCRIBER IDENTIFICATION NUMBER (SPIN): Medical drug or pharmaceutical provider ID number, or identifier.

STANDARD SETTING: An organization accredited by the American National Standards Institute that develops and maintains standards for medical information transactions or data elements, or any other standard that is necessary for, or will facilitate the implementation of health related data.

STANDARD SETTING ORGANIZATION (SSO): An organization accredited by the American National Standards Institute that develops and maintains standards for health information transactions or other data elements; also set by organizations such as the IEEE, Open Software Foundation, Unix International, OIS, and POSIX.

STANDARD TRANSACTION: HIPAA transaction that complies with applicable standards.

STANDARD TRANSACTION FORMAT COMPLIANCE SYSTEM (STFCS): An EHNAC-sponsored WPC-hosted HIPAA compliance certification service.

STANDARD UNIQUE EMPLOYER IDENTIFIER: Consists of the EIN or employer identification number assigned by the Internal Revenue Service, U.S.

Department of the Treasury; the EIN is the taxpayer identifying number of an individual, covered entity, or other entity (whether or not an employer) assigned under one of the following:

- 26 U.S.C. 6011(b), which is the portion of the Internal Revenue Code dealing with identifying the taxpayer in tax returns and statements, or corresponding provisions of prior law.
- 26 U.S.C. 6109, which is the portion of the Internal Revenue Code dealing with identifying numbers in tax returns, statements, and other required documents.

STAR DOT STAR: *.* characters that symbolize wild card sequences that match DOS and MSFT Windows® file names.

STARK, FORTNEY "PETE": U.S. representative (D-Calif.); ranking member of the Ways and Means health subcommittee.

STARK I: January 1992, from 1989 OBRA (42-USC 1395nn), precludes patient self-referrals by a physician or medical provider to another health care entity of interest; formerly Patient in Ethics Referral Act (PERA).

STARK II: August 1993, strengthens Stark I and further precludes patient referrals to an expanded list of medical services and physician/providers and family members having a financial interest in the entity.

STAR NETWORK: LAN/WAN topology with stellate shape or hub and spoke configuration; smart-server-to-dumb-terminal geography.

STARRED PROCEDURE: Specific surgical procedures listed in a CPT code book; an asterisk-term indicating a special CPT denotation; slang term.

START BUTTON: Activation button to initiate a computer system operation or menu.

START UP MENU: List of computer options, programs, settings, files, peripheral devices, specifications, and so forth initiated with a start button; its six sections include permanent, personal, systems, frequently used folders, all-programs, and on/off button.

STARVE: The lack of necessary computer system resources to complete a task; slang term.

STATE UNIFORM BILLING COMMITTEE (SUBC): A state-specific affiliate of the medical NUBC.

STATIC AUDITING TOOL: A scanner that searches for computer system security breaches, or "holes"; slang term.

STATIC / DYNAMIC: Static means fixed while dynamic usually means capable of action and/or change; both terms can be applied to a number of different types of health IT items such as programming languages, Web pages, and application programs.

STATIC / DYNAMIC IP ADDRESS: A static IP address is a number that is assigned to a computer by an Internet service provider to be its permanent address on the Internet and locate and communicate with each other; but inasmuch as there are not enough IP numbers to go around, many Internet service providers limit the number of static IP addresses they allocate and economize on the remaining number of IP addresses they possess by temporarily assigning an IP address to a requesting Dynamic Host Configuration Protocol computer from a pool of IP addresses; this temporary IP address is called a dynamic IP address. Requesting DHCP computers receive a dynamic IP address for the duration of that Internet session or for some other specified amount of time; once the user disconnects from the Internet, their dynamic IP address goes back into the IP address pool so it can be assigned to another user. Even if the user reconnects immediately, they will not usually be assigned the same IP address from the pool.

STATIC MEMORY: Fast nonpower refreshable computer memory.

STATIC RAM: A memory chip that requires power to maintain data contents.

STATUS LINE: Computer screen activation bar that indicates current settings, systems information, cursor position, and so forth.

STEALTH SIGNAL TRANSMITTER: Software installed on a notebook computer that sends a signal that can be traced.

STEALTH VIRUS: Concealed malicious code embedded in computer files.

STEALTH VIRUS FILE INFECTOR: Malicious computer code released when users take a directory listing of infected systems that illustrate uninfected length.

STEGANOGRAPHY: To embed, hide, or infect computer files in order to steal electronic PHI, medical, or other data.

STEMMING: Lexicology process that determines the morphological root of a word, code set, or IT language.

STOCHASIC: Unpredictable and random; meandering.

STORAGE: A device able to receive, retain, and supply health or other data, on demand; portable or internal floppy, zip, or hard drives, CD/DVD/optical/laser drives, and USB flash drives (key, pen, mini-drive, or memory stick), and so forth.

STORAGE AREA NETWORK (SAN): Computer servers with a fast communications technology, known as fiber channels, to create communications bandwidths of 1 or 2 GB; allows health IT executives to interconnect storage resources across wider physical distances into a shared data pool and still maintain split-second response times for end users; potential to relieve service and logistical problems of separate data repositories in individual departments, or with individual patient files and within enterprise-wide hospital or health care entity data storehouses.

STORAGE MANAGEMENT SOFTWARE (SMS): Computer programs and applications that allow hospitals to acquire and use high-capacity storage hardware as a prime health tool for coping with all data platforms more efficiently.

STORAGE VIRTUALIZATION (SV): A health technology that opens data pooling for widely dispersed storage devices and promises to work across multiple computing platforms and types of storage media; for example, a single computer may access medical image data on a disk array built by one vendor and call up a text file archived in a tape cartridge housed in a different vendor's cabinet, all accomplished without the need for custom interfaces to translate data between two different environments; architecture that uses network-switching hardware to efficiently link end users to far-flung data.

STORE AND FORWARD (SAF): A telemedicine interaction type that creates a multimedia electronic medical record; medical data and images are captured and stored for later transmission, consultation, or downloading; static images or audio-video clips may be transmitted to a remote data storage device, from which they may be retrieved by a medical practitioner for review and physician consultation at any time, obviating the necessity of simultaneous availability of the consulting parties and reducing transmission costs due to low bandwidth requirements.

STORED PROCEDURE: A set of Structured Query Language statements with an assigned name that is stored in the database in compiled form so that it can be shared by a number of programs.

STORED VALUE CARD: Plastic card with magnetic strip or CPU use to store economic value; money funds.

STREAM(ING): Data stored on NTFS in continuous real-time streams with names; a file can have more than one data stream, but exactly one must have no name; continuous flowing medical information, health, or other data; technology to play audio or video files from the Internet; Windows Media Player®, Apple QuickTime® player and RealPlayer®.

STREAM ALGORITHM: A byte by byte data encryption process.

STREAMING SOUND: Real-time audio formats, extension designated as .ra, .ram, or .wma.

STRING: A continuous set of alphanumeric characters that do not contain calculatable numbers.

STRONG ENCRYPTION: A security method using very large numbers such as 128 or 256 bits as its cryptographic key; SSL.

STRONG NAME: Any identifier strengthened by security encryption technology; public key digital signature.

STRUCTURED DATA ENTRY (SDE): A method of medical data collection that constrains the content and format of clinical descriptions for the purpose of ensuring consistent, unambiguous, interchangeable messages.

STRUCTURED QUERY LANGUAGE (SQL): Fourth generation DDM and DDL computer language used for relational databases; although SQL is both an ANSI and an ISOP standard, many database products support SQL with proprietary extensions to the standard language; queries take the form of a command language that allows the user to select, insert, update, locate data, and so forth.

STUB: Spacer for computer code not yet written or incorporated into a program or application.

STUMPF, STEVEN, EDD: Director of project development and management, the Advanced BioTelecommunications and BioInformatics Center, University of Southern California Keck School of Medicine, Los Angeles.

STYLUS: Sharp pen-like pointer or computer keyboard input device.

SUBDIRECTORY: Computer files organization within an existing directory; directory within another directory.

SUBJECT: An active health care entity, generally in the form of a caregiver, patient, process, or device that causes protected information to flow among objects or changes the system state; an active health entity, generally in the form of a person, process, or device that causes information to flow among objects or changes the system state.

SUBJECT / OBJECT SEPARATION: The computer security concept that suggests access to a subject does not guarantee access to the objects associated with that subject.

SUBNET MASK: 32-bit IP network address within a subnetwork computer system.

SUBROUTINE: A function, method, or procedure to instructions with a given name and used by the main program or computer system application.

SUBSCRIPTION SITE: A health information or other information-based e-commerce Web site that requires membership; *Journal of Bone and Joint Surgery;* JAMA, www.HealthCareFinancials.com; and so forth.

SUBSTITUTE CIPHER: Electronic encryption replacement security program.

SUBSTITUTION: Security health data or information cryptology method used by replacing each letter, number, or symbol with another.

SUBSYSTEM UNIX APPLICATION (SUA): Online enterprise functionality designed to allow UNIX applications to run on MSFT Vista® OS machines.

SUITE: Integrated desktop software applications bundled with several business programs from a single vendor, such as word processing, spreadsheets, database, and so forth: MSFT Office®, Corel WordPerfect Office®, Sun Star Office®, Lotus Symphony SmartSuite OpenOffice®; and smaller applications such as Office, ThinkFree®, and AjaxLaunch®, which are Internet-based, as well as GNOME Office, which is installed on the Desktop computer, and AppleWorks® on the Mac OS X®.

SUNDIAL: A type of Internet e-mail.

SUN MICROSYSTEMS, INC®.: Since its inception in 1982 with a singular vision "The Network Is The Computer," SUN is the leading provider of industrial-strength computer hardware, software, and services that make the Internet work in more than 100 countries and on the World Wide Web; makers of SOLAIS® (SunOS) with SPARC-Sun 4 descendent CPUs based in Mountain View, CA.

SUNSHINE: An international community for health care IT innovation created by HIMSS and Sun Microsystems, Inc.

SUN SOLUTIONS FOR HEALTHCARE: Information, Networking, Education (SunSHINE): A Sun Microsystems, Inc., forum created to promote choice and innovation in information technology for health care; a radiant network of professionals committed to looking beyond the obvious for the best solutions to pressing health care IT issues.

SUPERBILL: An invoice form that specifically lists all of the services provided by the physician; cannot be used in place of the standard American Medical Association form.

SUPER COMPUTER: A massive legacy and fast parallel processing computing machine, usually for math calculations, such as the IBM series, Cray vector, and Intel® iPSC series; hard-iron; big-iron.

SUPER TWIST: Liquid crystal display (LCD) screen with increased light wave visibility and polarization.

SUPER USER: One who advocates for a new health information management or other medical data computer system.

SUPER ZAP: The computer security crime of unauthorized utility use to modify existing programs or applications; slang term.

SURF: To search the Internet or intranet for URLs and other data; to browse the Web; to aimlessly view Web pages; slang term.

SURFACE-CONDUCTION ELECTRON-EMITTER DISPLAY (SED): Computer monitor that offers the bright colors of a CRT in a screen for digital radiology.

SURGE PROTECTOR: Suppression device used against unexpected power outs or spikes for computer or electrical device protection.

SURVEILLANCE: The technical observation of electronic equipment for functional utility and security purposes.

SUSE: Software-und System-Entwicklung is a privately owned company founded in 1992 by four German software engineers whose mission was to promote open source software; now owned by Novell®.

SUSPEND: To remove the input/output devices and CPU from a computer system but leave core memory intact for reboot ease; hibernate.

SWAP FILE SPACE: Usually hidden computer operating system space substituted for additional memory.

SWISH®: A flash authoring tool.

SWISH-ENHANCED: A fast, powerful, flexible, free, and easy to use system for indexing collections of Web pages or other text files.

SWITCH: Networked throughput communications device that controls and directs electronic packets; hub; electrical current route; switch box; switch configuration; switch hub, and so forth; mechanical or solid state device that opens or closes circuits, varies operating parameters, or chooses paths or circuits on a space or time division basis.

SWITCHED LINE: Communication link for which the physical path, established through dialing, may change with each use.

SWITCHED NETWORK: A system of telecommunications where each user has a separate address and any two points can be linked directly, using any combination of available routes in the network; throughput electronic communications device where each user controls and directs electronic packets between two or more nodes or points.

SWITCHED SERVICE: A telecommunications service based on telephone technology that switches circuits to connect multiple points.

SYMBOL: Concept or idea designation using letters, numbers, icons, and so forth.

SYMMETRIC KEY: An Internet health data security measure where the sender and receiver of a message share a single, common unit (key) that is used to encrypt and decrypt the message; a public key utilizes two keys—a public key to encrypt messages and a private key to decrypt them; symmetric key systems are simpler and faster, but a major drawback is that the two parties must somehow exchange the key in a safe way; public key encryption avoids the problem because the public key can be distributed in a nonsecure way, and the private key is never transmitted.

SYMMETRIC KEY ALGORITHM: Cryptographic and medical data security method where the same access key is used by sender and receiver.

SYNCHRONOUS DRAM: Dynamic Random Access Memory (DRAM) that runs at higher clock speeds than conventional memory by integrating itself with a computer's CPU bus.

SYNCHRONOUS OPTICAL NETWORK (SONET): A broadband, wide area communications service capable of transmitting extremely high-capacity data, such as interactive medical video or images, at very high speeds ranging from 150 Mbps to 10 Gbps; convenient for real-time digital telemedicine applications.

SYNCHRONOUS TRANSMISSION: Real-time health, medical information, or other data communications in timed intervals; for example, instant messaging; a method by which bits are transmitted at a fixed rate with the transmitter and receiver unified, extinguishing the need for start/stop elements, with the result of providing increased efficiency.

SYNTAX: The conventions in order to validly record medical information, or interpret previously recorded health information, for a specific purpose; X12 transactions, including data-element separators, subelement separators, segment terminators, segment identifiers, loops and loop identifiers, repetition factors, and so forth.

SYSTEM: The methods, procedures, or routines integrated for some form of health or other data integration.

SYSTEM ADMINISTRATOR: One responsible for the functionality and security of a multiuser enterprise-wide health care or other computer system.

SYSTEM ARCHITECTURE: The infrastructure that supports electronic business processes, storage, transmission, and communications.

SYSTEM FILE HIVE / SYSTEM HIVE: A section of registry that is stored in a file on a computer's hard disk located on a specified volume or in the user profiles containing a copy of the entire system branch of the registry, and usually one of the biggest components loaded into memory during boot; because of frequent modification, it can get fragmented and not load correctly.

SYSTEM INFECTOR: Virus that affects the systems of a computer or network; such as hard drives.

SYSTEM INTEGRITY: The quality that a system has when it performs its intended health care IT function in an unimpaired manner, free from unauthorized manipulation of the system, whether intentional or accidental.

SYSTEM MANAGEMENT: Software that manages computer systems in a health care or other business enterprise, which may include any and all of the following functions: software distribution and upgrading, version control, user profile management, backup and recovery, job scheduling, printer spooling, virus protection, and performance and capacity planning.

SYSTEM PROGRAMMER: Expert who writes computer applications, files, programs, compilers, and codes for networked health or other information systems.

SYSTEM PROTECTIONS: A core base of confidence in technical health care IT implementation that represents quality from both the perspective of the design processes used and the manner in which the implementation is accomplished; residual information protection (object reuse), privilege access, process separation, modularity, layering, and minimization of what needs to be trusted.

SYSTEM SECURITY: The result of data integrity safeguards intended for health care IT functions in an unimpaired manner, free from unauthorized manipulation of the system, whether intentional or accidental.

SYSTEM SECURITY ADMINISTRATOR: One who manages physical integrity and electronic data for safe-keeping.

SYSTEM SOURCES: Small memory area located in a window storage facility for tracking and location purposes.

SYSTEMS RESTORE: MSFT Windows® failsafe feature that reconfigures a computer to a previous state or setting.

T

t: time.

T1 LINE: A type of telephone line service offering high-speed data or voice access, with a transmission rate of 1.544 Mbps; also known as D1.

T3 LINE: A digital transmission system for high-volume voice, data, or compressed video traffic, with a transmission rate of 44.736 Mbps; also known as D3.

TABLE: Database structure with roles and columns.

TAGGED IMAGE FILE FORMAT (TIFF): The quality of an image or electronic picture determined by its resolution in grayscale; too low produces a jagged or stair-stepped effect.

TAGS: Web page information formatted with hyperlink capability; material between HTML angled brackets; <>.

TALIGENT®: Company founded in 1992 between IBM® and Apple Computer® to develop a Macintosh microcomputer operating system based on object-oriented technology from the "Pink" project started in 1988; Hewlett-Packard® was partner in 1994, but in 1996 the company became a wholly-owned subsidiary of IBM® that later disbanded in 1998.

TAMPER: To inappropriately modify a computer system, file, program, server, network, or smart card.

TAPE: Flexible plastic magnetized material that stores health or other data.

TAPE DRIVE: An electronic data storage device, or streamer, that writes health or other data stored on a punched or magnetic tape; typically used for archival storage of data stored on hard drives; tape media generally had a favorable unit cost and long archival stability but has been largely replaced by newer data storage methods.

TARGET: The place where health data or other digital information is copied onto and stored in a computer system.

TARIFFS: Pricing guidelines for communication facilities, governed by federal or local governments, intended to permit telephone companies a fair rate of return on their capital investments.

TASKBAR: List of currently running programs or open folders in the Windows® OS.

TASK MANAGER: Provides computer system CPU related information.

TB: Terabyte; a measure of computer memory and the quantity of storage capacity available on a computer; one TB is equivalent to one trillion bytes, or ten to the twelfth power bytes.

TBPS: Terabits per second; a measure of bandwidth and rate of information flow in digital transmission; one Tbps is equivalent to one trillion bits per second.

T-CARRIER: A series of transmission systems using pulse code modulation technology at different channel capacities and bit rates to transmit digital information over telephone lines or other transmission medium.

TECHNICAL SECURITY SERVICES: The processes that are put in place (1) to protect health information and (2) to control and monitor individual access to protected health information.

TECHNOLOGY ADVISORY COMMITTEE: (TAC): A body established to advise senior management on general technology issues (such as selection, evaluation, and performance assessment), and comprised of members from the various medical disciplines that play a part in the life of equipment; a committee present at any level (facility, district, regional, and ministerial) to advise the senior management at that level on such health technology issues.

TECHNOLOGY ASSESSMENT (TA): A process of evaluating the efficiency and efficacy of existing health information technology equipment available on the market and the new and ever-evolving technologies arriving on the market.

TECHNORTI: An Internet blog search engine.

TELECOMMUNICATION: The use of radio waves, wire, laser, ruby, silicone, germanium, optical, magnetic, infrared, or other channels to transmit information; also, the use of a modem to communicate with another computer or network over telephone landlines; telecommute; telematics.

TELECONFERENCE: Interactive communication facilitated by the use of radio, wire, laser, optical, magnetic, infrared, or other transmission channels; electronic medical conference, health care pod cast, and so forth.

TELECONSULTATION: The physical separation between multiple medical providers during a patient consultation.

TELECONSULTING: A medical examination or opinion using interactive electronic communication transmission channels; electronic patient image use as in diagnostic teledermatology; medical teleworker.

TELEDIAGNOSIS: The detection of a disease as a result of evaluating data transmitted to a receiving station from instruments monitoring a remote patient.

TELEHEALTH: Use of electronic communication methods, as well as diagnostic and treatment software algorithms to facilitate medical care and optimal patient well being; use of electronic communications networks for the transmission of information and data focused on health promotion, disease prevention, diagnosis, consultation, education, and/or therapy, and the public's overall health including patient/community education and information, population-based data collection and management, and linkages for health care resources and referrals; sometimes considered broader in scope than telemedicine, there is no clear-cut distinction between the two.

TELEIMAGE: Electronic transmission of photographs, X-rays, MRI, CT or PET scans from one location to another.

TELEMATICS: The use of information processing based on a computer in tele-communications, and the use of telecommunications to permit computers to transfer programs and data to one another.

TELEMEDICINE: Derives from the Greek *tele* meaning *at a distance* and the present word *medicine,* which itself derives from the Latin *mederi* meaning *healing;* first coined and used in the 1970s by Thomas Bird, referring to health care delivery where physicians examine distant patients through the use of telecommunications technologies; prominent medical specialty teleforms include dermatology, internal medicine, neurology, cardiology, radiology, and robotic surgery; the use of audio, video, and other telecommunications and electronic information processing technologies for the transmission of information and data relevant to the diagnosis and treatment of medical conditions, or to provide health services or aid health care personnel at distant sites.

TELEMENTORING: The use of audio, video, and other telecommunications and electronic information processing technologies to provide individual guidance or direction; for example, a physician consultant aids a distant clinician in a new medical procedure.

TELEMETRY: The science and technology of automatic measurement and transmission of data via wires, radios, or another medium from stations based in remote locations to receiving stations for recording and analysis.

TELEMONITORING: The process of using audio, video, and other telecommunications and electronic information processing technologies to monitor the health status of a patient from a distance.

TELENET: Non-GUI supported terminal to terminal computer transmission protocol standard for UNIX.

TELENURSING: Long distance nursing practice through health information system telephony, or any electronic communication methodology available.

TELEPHONE CALLBACK: A method of authenticating the identity of the receiver and sender of information through a series of "questions" and "answers" sent back and forth establishing the identity of each; for example, when the communicating systems exchange a series of identification codes as part of the initiation of a session to exchange information, or when a host computer disconnects the initial session before the authentication is complete, and the host calls the user back to establish a session at a predetermined telephone number.

TELEPHONE HOTLINE: Patient medical demand management system using care paths, medical protocols, or algorithms as an acuity care triage system; usually a medical provider referral system.

TELEPRESENCE: A method of using robotic and other instruments that permit a clinician to perform a procedure at a remote location by manipulating devices and receiving feedback or sensory information that contributes to a sense of being present at the remote site and allows a satisfactory degree of technical achievement; for example, this term could be applied to a surgeon using lasers or dental hand pieces and receiving pressure similar to that created by touching a patient so that it seems as though the patient is actually present, permitting a satisfactory degree of dexterity.

TELETEXT: A broadcasting service utilizing several otherwise unused scanning lines (vertical blanking intervals) between frames of TV pictures to send data from a central database to receiving television sets.

TELMATICS APPLICATIONS SUPPORTING COGNITION (TASC): International health care IT organization in Denmark and Sweden that was an early user of JAVA® applications installed on client-server systems and using large icons to help the cognitively impaired with daily living tasks, while monitoring the location of patients; medical provider software monitor of real-time patient needs and activities with coincident computer information system settings.

TELNET: An application program that permits users to logon to any computer on the Internet for interaction with other users; for example, a telnet program may be used to peruse medical library holdings and receive results.

TEMPORAL KEY INTEGRITY PROTOCOL (TKIP): WPA security element defined by the IEEE for 802.11i wireless encryption; encryption standard that changes and manages encryption keys across a wireless computer network.

TEQUILA VIRUS: One of the first stealth, multipartite, polymorphic, armored, variable encryption viruses with master boot ignition.

TERABYTE: Electronic storage capacity of one trillion bytes; TB.

TERMINAL: A computer keyboard, screen, and storage device allowing smart and dumb data input functions; not a PC; input/output device; terminal server; terminal session.

TERMINAL DIGIT FILE: Health record filing system that uses the last digits to determine final placement.

TERMINAL SERVER: WAN, LAN, MAN, or Internet hub device with peripheral nodule computer connections.

TERMINATION PROCEDURE: Formal, documented instructions, which include appropriate security measures, for the ending of an employee's employment, or an internal/external user's access.

TERRESTRIAL CARRIER: A telecommunication transmission system using land-based facilities such as microwave towers, telephone lines, coaxial cable, or fiber optic cable as differentiated from satellite transmission.

TEST LOG: Computer system examination and follow-up.

TEXAS INSTRUMENTS®️ (TI): Semiconductor manufacturer founded by Jack S. Kilby, developer of the first integrated circuit (IC), in Dallas, Texas.

TEXT BASE: Computer onscreen text using prerecorded fonts or designs.

TEXT BOX: A screened-off area for input messages or commands.

TEXT EDITOR: A text-only file editor.

TEXT FILE: Health information or other data file of text characters.

TEXT MINE: The management of free text data.

THEAD: Most minute data packet retrieved by a CPU scheduler.

THIN CLIENT: A client-terminal that performs little health or other data processing, but operates off a central server as it retains OS functionality on the desktop; little storage capacity.

THIN SERVER: A client-terminal where most health, medical, or other data processing occurs on the client machine.

THIRD GENERATION: Computers originally made with integrated circuits, rather than earlier vacuum tunes, or later CPUs.

THOMPSON, TOMMY: Former Health and Human Services (HHS) secretary and former governor of Wisconsin who joined the pharmacy benefits manager, Medco Health Solutions, Inc., in December 2006.

THRALL, JAMES H., MD: CMIO for the Massachusetts General Hospital, Boston, MA.

THREAD: An online discussion theme or topic; series of messages and responses; threaded discussion; threaded site; threaded newsreader, and so forth.

THREAT: The potential for a source to exploit intentionally, or trigger accidentally, a specific computer, network, or online vulnerability (interruption, alteration, steal or disclose, and destruction).

THREAT ANALYSIS: The examination of threat sources against system vulnerabilities to determine the risks for a particular health care IT system in a particular operational environment.

THREAT MANAGEMENT: Integrated comprehensive approach to health care network security that addresses multiple types of malware, blended threats, and spam, and protects from intrusion at both the gateway and the endpoint levels; components of an integrated threat management system are part of a centrally administered HIT architecture.

THREAT MODEL: A process for optimizing health network security by identifying objectives and vulnerabilities, and then defining countermeasures to prevent, or mitigate the effects of threats to the system, malicious or incidental, that can compromise the assets of the enterprise.

THREAT SOURCE: Either (1) intent and method targeted at the intentional exploitation of a computer, network, or online vulnerability; or (2) the situation and method that may accidentally trigger a vulnerability.

THREAT VULNERABILITY: A flaw or weakness in system security procedures, design, implementation, or internal controls that could be exercised (accidentally triggered or intentionally exploited) and result in a security breach or a violation of a health system's security policy.

THREE FINGER SALUTE: Simultaneously pressing the computer input keys: control-alternate-delete with three manual digits, to terminate DOS and/or Windows® OS; slang term.

THROUGHPUT: Amount of electrical computer system information delivered per given time period; the amount of medical data that is actually transmitted over a network in a given period of time, expressed in bits per second; rates are related to baud rates, but are generally a little lower due to imperfect transmission conditions; usually, higher baud rates will permit higher throughput.

THUMB: An elevated scroll bar box used to navigate a Web page or computer screen image.

THUMBNAIL: A small representation of an image that is expandable upon activation.

THUMBDRIVE®: USB flash drive that was the world's first and smallest portable storage drive, based on Trek's patented technologies, which combines flash memory technologies and encryption technologies with an USB connection to create a self-contained and highly secured drive and media package; plugs directly into the USB port of any computer and can store virtually any digital data from documents and presentations, to music and photos.

THUNK(ING): An electronic 32- to 16-bit code translation; slang term.

TIE LINE: A telephone circuit leased or dedicated to an individual that is provided by common carriers that connect two points together without using the switched telephone network.

TIGER: A security expert charged with discovering computer system flaws, sploits, or bugs in order to correct them; tiger team; slang term.

TILE: A divided computer screen.

TIME BOMB: Logical information release that activates or explodes upon some preset condition or date, usually maliciously; automatic access termination; slang term.

TIME DIVISION MULTIPLEXING: Transmission of more than one line of health information in one high-capacity communications channel using time as the means to separate channels.

TIME-OF-DAY: Access to health data is restricted to certain time fames, for example, Monday through Friday, 9:00 A.M. to 9:00 P.M.

TIME OUT: The end of a response waiting period.

TIME SHARE: The use or sharing of a CPU for two or more operations during the same time period.

TIME SLICE: The brief increment allotted to a multitasking computer system.

TIME STAMP: A notation that indicates, at least, the correct date and time of an action and the identity of the person that created the notation.

TITLE BAR: The top line of a window or screen with identification nomenclature.

T-LINE: High-speed broadband communication telephone line or point-to-point line identified by varying levels of increasing pipe size; T1–T4 lines; T1–T12 are common carrier lines with speeds beyond 274.176 Mbps (megabits per second); T-line carrier, and so forth.

TOGGLE: A simple back and forth; on/off switch.

TOKEN: Physical context authorization or authentication used to provide identity; typically, an electronic device that can be inserted in a door or a computer system to obtain access; special message, token bus, token pass, token ring, and so forth.

TOKEN RING: LAN/WAN network priority transmission protocol system.

TOOKER, JOHN, MD, PHD: CEO, American College of Physicians, and President eHealth Initiative Foundation.

TOP LEVEL DOMAIN (TLD): The terminal portion of an URL or e-mail address, .com, .edu, .gov, and so forth.

TOPOLOGY: The architecture, physical geography, or layout of a computer network.

TOR©: Anonymous Internet communication system for Web browsing and publishing, instant messaging, IRC, SSH, and other applications that use the TCP protocol; also a platform on which software developers can build new applications with built-in anonymity, safety, and privacy features; onion network; TorNetwork®, and Anonymizer©.

TORPARK®: Internet browser designed to disguise an originating IP address, based on Mozilla's Firefox® 1.5 using a worldwide network of encrypted routers to randomly choose a different IP address.

TORRENZA®: AMD technology to connect computer processors to coprocessor devices that handle tasks such as digital video for more realistic radiology images and/or patient-physician simulations; code name.

TORVALDS, LINUS B.: Finnish engineer who initiated the development of the Linux® kernel and now acts as the project's coordinator; inspired by Minix (an operating system developed by Andrew Tanenbaum to develop a capable Unix surrogate operating system that could be run on a PC); Linux now also runs on many other platforms; Red Hat®, Oracle®, and VA Linux® are leading developers of Linux-based software.

TOUCH PAD: A stationary flat surface digital computer pointing device.

TOUCH SCREEN: Interface command, or access control input device induced by physically touching a CRT, LED, or similar activation screen.

TRACER: E-mail attachment that when opened, sends the IP address of the recipient back to the sender.

TRACE ROUTE: A source-to-destination computer path router.

TRACK BACK: The ability of a blog to interact, link, post, and affiliate with another related blog.

TRACK BALL: A round moveable rotating pointing device.

TRACKING COOKIE: Usually malicious and unknown computer utility program that sends Web page and Internet reports back to the main cookie for advertising and sales purposes.

TRAFFIC ANALYSIS: The inference of health care information from observation of traffic flows (presence, absence, amount, direction, and frequency).

TRAFFIC FLOW CONFIDENTIALITY: A security service agreement to protect against online or other traffic analysis.

TRAFFIC SPEED: The rapidity at which a cursor, mouse bar, or other input device moves across a computer screen and activates an input command.

TRANSACTION: The exchange of information between two parties to carry out financial or administrative activities related to health or medical care; the transmission of information between two parties to carry out financial or administrative activities related to health care; includes the following types of information transmissions:

- health care claims or equivalent encounter information,
- health care payment and remittance advice,
- coordination of benefits,
- health care claim status,
- enrollment and disenrollment in a health plan,
- eligibility for a health plan,
- health plan premium payments,
- referral certification and authorization,
- first report of injury, and
- health claims attachments.

TRANSACTION CHANGE REQUEST SYSTEM: A system established under HIPAA for accepting and tracking change requests for any of the HIPAA mandated transactions standards using a single Web site.

TRANSACTION CODE SETS: A set of common HIPAA standards for electronic transmission of clinical health data; in time, standardized data sets may provide building blocks that enable national connectivity among all health care databases.

TRANSACTION PRIVACY: Protects against loss of privacy with respect to transactions being performed by an individual patient or health care system or provider, covered entity, and so forth.

TRANSACTION STANDARD: The set of rules, requirements, or conditions for secure data element and code set HIPAA communications.

TRANSCRIPTIONIST: A medically trained typist or computer input operator.

TRANSISTOR: A type of electrical current switch, amplifier, or logic gate.

TRANSLATION PROGRAM: Software that converts programming language to machine language or binary codes.

TRANSLATOR: A broadband network operation; an instrument located in a central retransmission facility to filter incoming microwave signals and retransmit them in a higher frequency band.

TRANSMISSION: The exchange of electronic data between sender and receiver.

TRANSMISSION CONTROL PROTOCOL (TCP): A common Internet IP standard.

TRANSMISSION CONTROL PROTOCOL/INTERNET PROTOCOL (TCP/IP): The underlying communications rules and procedures that allow computers to interact with each other on the Internet.

TRANSMISSION SPEED: The rate at which information passes over a communications channel; generally given in either bits per second (bps) or baud.

TRANSPONDER: A microwave receiver and transmitter in a satellite that receives signals being transmitted from Earth, amplifies them, and sends them back down to Earth for reception purposes.

TRANSPORT LAYER: The fourth OSI strata between computer hardware and software for correct end-flow processing.

TRANSPOSE: Scrambled character in a message for security purposes.

TRANSPOSITION: Scrambling computer characters, symbols, or language for security encryption purposes.

TRAP DOOR: Unauthorized software or hardware access gate or method; back door; slang term.

TRASH: Storage bin for old deleted computer files; recycle bin.

TRAY: Small icon screen area located to the right of the task bar on Windows® for printer icons, volume control, program icons, clock, and so forth.

TREATMENT: The provision, coordination, or management of health care and related services by one or more health care providers, including the coordination or management of health care by a health care provider with a third party; consultation between health care providers relating to an individual or the referral of an individual for health care from one health care provider to another.

TREE: Data structure linked together in a hierarchical manner; computer system network configuration of resources or topology.

TRI-GATE RESISTOR: Three-dimensional transistors from the Intel Corporation® for health data and other high-volume manufacturing; vPro®, Core Duo®, Centrino®, and V*II*V.

TRIGGER: To induce a computer system action to be launched automatically; automatic virus, worm, or similar activation methodology.

TRIPATHI, MICKY, PHD: CEO, Massachusetts, eHealth Collaborative.

TRIPLE DES: A three-step, 56-bit key, DES encryption/decryption algorithm.

TROJAN HORSE: A non–self-replicating software computer program with a hidden universal malicious function; hidden or covert scam from a known externally delivered function, a Trojan; slang term.

TROLL(ING): Aimless negative Web surfing or online user malicious response baiting; slang term.

TRULIA: A commercial and health care real estate mashup.

TRUNK: Single computer system circuit with many channel switches; a large capacity, long-distance channel that common carriers use to transfer information between its customers.

TRUST: Window© NT-to-Windows© NT domain resource sharing; health information or medical database entry and security rights and mutual administrative permissions; secure two-way electronic relationship.

TRUSTED SYSTEM: A standardized set of security and safeguard attributes; trusted third party (TTP).

TRUSTED USER ACCESS LEVEL: One who requires access to protected health care or other confidential information.

TRUSTWORTHY COMPUTING: Term coined by William H. Gates, CEO of the Microsoft Corporation, to indicate a high level of confidence and assurance in computer software coding and data transmission; a long-term, collaborative effort to provide private and reliable computing experiences; a core company tenet at Microsoft built on four pillars: security, privacy, reliability, and integrity.

TUKEY, JOHN W., PHD (1915–2000): Coined the term "bit" in 1949 and made math and computer science contributions during a long career at Bell Labs and Princeton University.

TULSA: An Intel Xeon® microprocessor platform for multiprocessor server implementation with NetBurst© architecture; code name.

TUNNEL: A private and secure WAN, LAN, or MAN computer system communications link or network; tunneling, tunnel service, and so forth.

TURBO: High-speed computer operations and transmissions mode; slang term.

TURBO PASCAL: A Pascal computer language compiler program with object-oriented extensions, made popular for PCs by Borland International®.

TURING MACHINE: Theoretical "thinking machine" created by mathematician Alan Turing in the 1950s.

TURING TEST: An examination to distinguish a computing machine from a human being; thinking intelligence test.

TURN IN KEYS, TOKEN: Formal, documented procedure to ensure all physical items that allow a terminated employee to access a health care entity, property, building, clinic, or equipment are retrieved from that employee, preferably prior to termination.

TURNKEY SYSTEMS: Vendor provision of a hospital with computer and software systems that are "pre-packaged" so that hospital-based system development is minimal; limited customization using systems analysts or programmers; an integrated method of telecommunications in which all of the installation services and components needed for operational teleconferencing have been provided by a single vendor or contractor.

TURTLE: A cursor that leaves a lighted tail or serves as a pointer for drawing; slang term.

TWEENING: Electronic animation technique; slang term.

TWIDDLE: To make small computer network or operating system changes; without real efficiency improvements; to aimlessly diddle around; slang term.

TWISTED PAIR: The most common type of medium in PSTN's (public switched telephone network) local loops, insulated copper wires are wrapped around each other to void the effects of electrical noise; can transmit voice, data, and low-grade video.

TWO FACTOR AUTHENTICATION: A health data or medical information security process in which the user provides two means of identification, one of which is typically a physical token, such as a card, and the other of which is typically something memorized, such as a security code; two factors involved are sometimes spoken of as *something you have* and *something you know.*

TYPE FACE: The distinctive appearance of letters, symbols, or numbers; Courier, Arial, Times New Roman, and so forth.

TYPE SIZE: The height or size of a particular font style.

TYPO SQUATTER(S): Those who register Web site addresses, either with trademarked terms or common misspellings, in order to benefit from pay-per-click advertising, but place nothing on the Web site pages sans advertisements; cybersquatter, domain name or URL squatter, and so forth.

U

UB-92 UNIFORM BILL 1992: Bill form used to submit hospital insurance claims for payment by third parties. Similar to HCFA (CMS) 1450 and 1500, but reserved for the inpatient component of health services; hardcopy and electronic formats.

UBIQUITOUS COMPUTING: Philosophical concept that patient health care will be improved, more pervasive, and efficient with the universal use of secure and natural language health care information systems and computers, anytime and anywhere; ubicomp; slang term.

UBUNTU®: Linux-based operating system, freely available with both community and professional support; Ubuntu® is suitable for both desktop and server use; current versions support PC (Intel® x86), 64-bit PC (AMD64®), UltraSPARC® T1 (Sun Fire T1000 and T2000), and PowerPC® (Apple iBook® and Powerbook®, G4, and G5) architectures.

UCR: A method of profiling prevailing medical fees in an area and reimbursing medical providers based on that profile; usual, customary, and reasonable.

ULTRAHIGH FREQUENCY (UHF): A radio frequency in the second highest range of the radio spectrum, from 300 to 3,000 MHz.

ULTRAVIOLET LITHOGRAPHY: Technology to help shrink computer chip features even more than the 45–32 nanometer process that Intel launched in 2007.

UNDELETE: Computer file-recovery functionality or utility that provides real-time data protection and instant recovery for PCs, servers, and workstations.

UNDERCODE: Incomplete medical record billing and invoicing documentation usually due to missing information.

UNDERRUN: An abrupt lack of medical information or health data.

UNFREEZE: Health data or information that discontinues current behavior.

UNICODE: 16-bit standard character set with UT-F8 encoding for efficient ASCII characterization.

UNIDIRECTED MESSAGE: Blast e-mail broadcast information without regard to its recipient.

UNIFIED MEDICAL LANGUAGE SYSTEM (UMLS): Protocol lexicon standard, sponsored by the U.S. National Library of Medicine (US-NLM), for clinical medical terms and nomenclature use with electronic health database management functionality.

UNIFIED MESSAGING SYSTEM (UMS): The handling of rich text messages with voice, graphics, audio, and video functionality, in a single e-mail transmission and mailbox.

UNIFORM BILLING CODE OF 1982: UB-82; health care claim form; hardcopy and digital.

UNIFORM BILLING CODE OF 1992: UB-92; health care claim form; hardcopy and digital.

UNIFORM CLAIM FORM: A single claim form and standardized format for electronic medical claims.

UNIFORM CLAIM TASK FORCE (UCTF): An organization that developed the initial HCFA-1500 Professional Claim Form whose responsibilities were assumed by the NUCC.

UNIFORM COMMERCIAL CODE (UCC): A state-wide, not federal, legal codification of commerce involving tangible and intangible health care and other business transactions.

UNIFORM PRACTICE CODE (UPC): A code established and maintained by the National Association of Securities Dealers (NASD) Board of Governors that regulates the mechanics of executing and completing securities trans-actions in the OTC market between members; including publicly traded health care companies.

UNIFORM PRACTICE COMMITTEE: A National Association of Securities Deal-ers district subcommittee that disseminates information and interpretations landed down by the Board of Governors regarding the Uniform Practice Code (UPC).

UNIFORM RESOURCE LOCATOR (URL): Address identification mechanism for Internet surfing and Web browsing; a naming convention, such as http://, ftp://, and so forth; the standard form for an address on the Internet; for example, http://www.base.com/ indicates a Hypertext Transport Proto-col (http) address on the World Wide Web (www) with location "base" and the type of owner (com); other valid guidelines may include ftp and gopher; unlike most e-mail addresses, URLs are always case sensitive, that is, whether a character is upper or lower case does make a difference.

UNINTERRUPTIBLE POWER SUPPLY (UPS): Device to temporarily maintain computer power during a blackout or brownout.

UNION: Data value spacer or electronic computer code place holder; variant.

UNIQUE PHYSICIAN IDENTIFICATION NUMBER (UPIN): The combination name and number assigned and maintained in security procedures for identifying and tracking individual user identity (ASTM).

UNITED NATIONS CENTER FOR FACILITATION OF PROCEDURES AND PRACTICES FOR ADMINISTRATION, COMMERCE, AND TRANSPORT (UN/CEFACT): An international organization dedicated to the elimination or simplification of procedural barriers to international commerce and global health care electronic data information exchange (EDI).

UNITED NATIONS RULES FOR ELECTRONIC DATA INTERCHANGE FOR ADMIN-ISTRATION, COMMERCE, AND TRANSPORT (UN/EDIFACT): An international HIPAA EDI format; interactive X12 transactions use the EDIFACT message.

UNIT FILES SYSTEM: Medical chart that records inpatient and outpatient visit information together.

UNIT NUMBERING: A method for tracking patient records in a medical office or health care facility.

UNIT NUMBER SYSTEM: Medical chart that records the first through last medical encounter with a unique alphanumeric code or other or designation.

UNIT RECORD: A single location for all individual patient health care data or information.

UNIVERSAL CHART ORDER: A similarly formatted medical or health care record for both inpatient and outpatient encounters.

UNIVERSAL CLIENT: A computer or blade-server that can access many net-work applications.

UNIVERSAL DESCRIPTION DISCOVERY AND INTEGRATION (UDDI): An XLM-based registry for businesses worldwide to list themselves on the Internet and whose ultimate goal is to streamline online transactions by enabling companies to find one another on the Web and make their systems interoperable for e-commerce and e-health care, and so forth.

UNIVERSAL IDENTIFIER: A single, secure, and absolute recognition number for protected health information (PHI).

UNIVERSAL MEDICAL DEVICE NOMENCLATURE SYSTEM (UMDNS): Regulatory terms for medical device communications, e-commerce, and procurement.

UNIVERSAL PRODUCT CODE (UPC): Twelve-digit number assigned to retail merchandise, instruments, and durable medical equipment as a bar code numerator.

UNIVERSAL SERIAL BUS (USB): A standard protocol to connect peripheral computer devices, but also commonplace on videogames, PDAs, TVs, home stereo equipment, MP3 players, and other memory devices; spectrum-based USB implementation is known as wireless USB.

UNIX: Machine independent (mini, midi, and microcomputers) modular and extensible open source code computer operating and networking system, developed by Bell Labs in the late 1960s, that supports multitasking and multiuser and networking functionality; replacement for Multics; Solaris® and Linux® are variants; mainframe or legacy computer language.

UNSHIELDED TWISTED PAIR (UTP): Wireless Ethernet cable connection.

UNSTRUCTURED DATA: Human readable and nonbinary health, medical, or other electronic information.

UNSUBSCRIBE: To become removed for a RSS feed, list-service, BBS, newsgroup, and so forth.

UNZIP: To uncompress a compressed or archived data or information file.

UPCODE: CPT codes that represent higher health care provider payment rates than those medical procedures or treatments actually rendered.

UPLEVEL: A later version of a software product or electronic device.

UPLINK: An electronic channel from a satellite to an earth station; referring to a transmitting earth station.

UPLINK PORT: A type of hub or switch for computer network expansion.

UPLOAD: To copy and save files from the Internet or intranet to a computer; the link, or path, from a transmitting earth station to the satellite; transferring files or software from one computer to another.

UPSTREAM: Unidirectional electronic health data or other information transmission from client to server.

UPWARD COMPATIBLE: Compatible with newer product versions; software, hardware, networks, and peripheral computer devices.

URETZ, MICHAEL: Executive Director of the Electronic Health Record Group.

USAGE ANALYSIS: Web site or Web page benchmarking, monitoring, and reporting system.

USA PATRIOT ACT: A federal act designed to broaden the surveillance of law enforcement agencies to enhance the detection and suppression of terrorism.

USB FLASH DRIVE: A small, flash nonvolatile memory stick or similar device with USB computer interface; thumb-drive.

USB HARD DRIVE: Portable hard disk with USB computer port connection.

USE: The sharing, employment, application, utilization, examination, or analysis of PIHI within a covered medical entity that maintains such information.

USENET: A public Internet discussion forum or newsgroup; slang term for user network. Top level topical categories include:

- alternative: alt
- computing: comp
- miscellaneous: misc
- recreation: rec
- science: sci
- social: soc
- discussions: talk
- usenet: news

USER: One who accesses a computer, smart card, server, network, cell phone, fax machine, or other electronic communications device.

USER ACCESS: One authorized to gain entrance and use a computer, smart card, server, network, cell phone, fax machine, or other communications device, and so forth.

USER ACCOUNT: Established end user or identifier in a multiuser medical database or health information computer system.

USER AUTHENTICATION: Security verification for one who uses a computer, smart card, server, network, cell phone, fax machine, or other communications device; optional under the 802.11 standard, but required under WPA.

USER-BASED ACCESS: A health data security mechanism used to grant users of a system access, based upon the identity of the user.

USER DATAGRAM PROTOCOL (UDP): Transmission standard such as TCP used for VOIP or video/audio streaming; connectionless.

USER-DEFINED KEY (UDK): Video terminal keyboard buttons F6–F20 for frequently used video computer commands.

USER EDUCATION CONCERNING VIRUS: Training relative to user awareness of the potential harm that can be caused by a virus or similar miscreant; how to prevent the introduction of a virus to a computer system, and what to do if a virus is detected.

USER EDUCATION IN IMPORTANCE OF MONITORING: Training in user responsibility to ensure the security of health care data or medical information.

USER EDUCATION IN PASSWORD MANAGEMENT: A type of training about the rules to be followed in creating and changing computer system passwords and the need to keep them confidential.

USER FRIENDLY: Computer system that is easy for medical and allied health care providers, and non-IT professionals to implement and use.

USER GROUP: A loose organization of online hobbyists or professionals drawn together by a common interest, such as medicine, health care, economics and finance, and so forth; blog; slang term.

USER IDENTIFICATION: Assurance of the claimed identity of a health care or other covered entity (ASTM E1762 -5); part of a digital signature on the matrix; user name; user profile.

USER INTERFACE: Electronic input device or access methodology; GUI, language, touch-screen, or computer driven menu; design components of a Web page that directs users on how to access the information contained on a Web site.

USUAL, CUSTOMARY, AND REASONABLE (UCR): A physician's full charge if it is reasonable and does not exceed his or her usual charges, and the amount customarily charged for the service by other physicians and medical providers in the area.

UTILITY PROGRAM: Software traditionally used for repetitive tasks such as disk defragmentation, security verification, disk compression, and so forth; includes Internet form filler RoboForm©; USB mini-drive password bookmarker Pass2Go©; conference line provider FreeConferenceService©; data compressor SendThisFile©; pcAnywhere© surrogate Radmin©; Google Desktop; and computer specification reader; Belarc Advisor©, and so forth.

V

V.32 BIS: International standard for data communications using a modem at speeds of up to 14,400 bits per second.

V.34 BIS: International standard for data communications using a modem at speeds of up to 28,800 bits per second.

VACUUM TUBE: Evacuated glass tube that conducts electricity; cathode ray tube.

VALIDATE ACCESS: Verifies work authorizations and entry to workstations and computers before granting physical access, including a procedure to track input, maintenance, and security of health or other business records.

VALIDATION: Specification evaluation, and integrity testing of a computer system.

VALIDATOR: Quality assurance program used to check Hypertext Markup Language for errors; a useful tool for an HTML user who receives health data or other information electronically from a variety of input sources.

VALIDITY: The extent to which medical, health, or other data represents the actual facts and circumstances of a patient encounter or medical intervention.

VALUE ADDED NETWORK (VAN): LAN, WAN, or MAN that offers additional services or utility; medical data; health information; health care RSS feeds, and so forth; VAN reseller.

VANILLA: A software program or computer applications used "as-is," without customization or extra features.

VAPORWARE: Nonexistent software; theoretical or marketing machination; slang term.

VARIANT: Any health data or other information that can act as a spacer or place-holder for other data; union.

VARIANT VIRUS: Modification of an existing computer virus, or malicious code, algorithm, and so forth.

VAX: Virtual address extension for mid-range computer servers from DEC® (now HP), in the late 1970s, using the successor PDP series and a 32-bit operating system known as VMS (virtual memory system); legacy system.

VCARD: An electronic business card with contact information, and so forth.

V-CODE: Descriptors of patient health status and justification for medical encounters other than disease or injury already classified in the ICD-9-CM codes; for fiscal reimbursement.

VECTOR GRAPHICS: Illustrations composed of line and curve segments, created in such programs as Illustrator©, FreeHand©, and CorelDRAW©.

VECTOR PROCESSOR: Any computer capable of executing many calculations in a single step; array computer processor.

VERSION NUMBER: The identification number for released computer software or other applications and programs.

VERY HIGH FREQUENCY (VHF): A radio frequency in the very high range of the radio spectrum, from 30 to 300 MHz.

VERY HIGH LEVEL LANGUAGE: Novice end-user enabling tool used to create software applications.

V-FAST CLASS: Introduced prior to 34; a proprietary modem modulation used for 28.8 Kbps connections; no longer a supported standard.

VIDEO BANDWIDTH: The maximum resolution of a computer screen or monitor.

VIDEO CAPTURE: To secure a digital movie or grab a single pictorial digital frame.

VIDEO CARD: Interface between computer CPU and monitor; two- and three-dimensional types are available for radiologists, radiology imaging, and video-gamers.

VIDEO CHAT: A video conference or network camera conversation in real time.

VIDEO CONFERENCE: An electronic telecommunications meeting driven by broadband Internet connectivity; real-time, two way transmission of digitized video images between multiple locations; uses telecommunications to bring patients and doctors at physically remote locations together for examinations and consultations; each individual location in a video-conferencing system requires a room equipped to send and receive video.

VIDEO EDITING: Software programs used to import raw digital footage and produce, edit, and save video files to a specific format and/or burn a DVD or CD; Adobe Premiere©, Ulead VideoStudio©, Pinacle Studio©, and Sony Vegas©.

VIDEO FORMATS: Digital video file formats:

- AVI (.avi): Supported by WMP, but there are many nonsupported types, too
- MPEG (.mpeg or .mpg): Combined container and codec:
  - MPEG-1: Lowest quality CD/DVDs
  - MPEG-2: Broadcast quality supported by WMP
- QUICKTIME® (.qt and .mov): Apple digital movie format
- RealMedia® (.rm and .ram): Real Networks movie format
- WINDOWS MEDIA®: .asf and .wmv

VIDEO FRAME GRABBER: Device that changes analog video signals into digital.

VIDEO GRAPHICS ARRAY (VGA): A measure of image size, representing the capacity to display 640 x 480 lines, such as on viewing monitors for personal computers.

VIDEO MAIL: Message and video presentations delivered by e-mail services.

VIRTUAL: Electronic sham or computer assisted simulation.

VIRTUAL ADDRESS EXTENSION (VAX): A family of 32-bit computers from HP (DEC and Compaq) first introduced in 1977, with models ranging from desktop units to mainframes, that all ran the same VMS operating system; large VAX multiprocessing clusters served thousands of health care entity users; legacy computers, mid-frame or mainframe; middle iron.

VIRTUAL CARD: Electronic data elements existing without a physical location.

VIRTUAL CIRCUIT: Packet switched network facilities that seem to be an actual end-to-end circuit.

VIRTUAL DISTRIBUTOR: A channel of product delivery where one can purchase books, supplies, software, journals, and educational materials through a Web site; a business-to-business site that uses its services for direct electronic purchases or requests for proposals for medical equipment and supplies; or an auction area where health care agents can buy and sell used equipment and excess inventory; vendors pay a transaction fee to participate in the bidding or purchasing, but buyers usually escape any service fees.

VIRTUAL DOS MACHINE: Computer executing Disk Operating System 16 or WINDOWS© 16-bit applications.

VIRTUAL HEALTH PROGRAM: Integrated and Web-based community health care system with patient empowerment and low cost delivery.

VIRTUAL HOST: An Internet server that contains multiple Web sites.

VIRTUALIZATION: The technical ability to include more servers onto fewer health care computers; suitable for applications, operating systems, and containerization.

VIRTUAL LAN: A software created subgroup that combines user stations and network devices regardless of physical location; virtual MAN, or WAN.

VIRTUAL MACHINE: A nonexistent "computer," such as the VM/ESA OS from IBM that simulates copies of itself; usually using JAVA® applets.

VIRTUAL MEMORY: Hard drive simulation of more RAM than actually exists and thereby allows a computer to run larger or concurrent programs by breaking them into small segments called "pages" and bringing them into memory that fits into a reserved area for that program; if a program's logic points back and forth to opposite ends of the program, excessive disk accesses ("thrashing") can slow down execution.

VIRTUAL NETWORK: A connected group of networks that appear as one unit.

VIRTUAL PC EXPRESS: A Microsoft© online computer network and digital support service.

VIRTUAL PRIVATE NETWORK (VPN): A technical strategy for creating secure connections, or tunnel protocols (IPSec, L2TP or PPTP, and so forth) for encrypted health data or other information, over the Internet; especially in medical care delivery and TPA management; a private communications network usually used within a company, hospital, or by several different companies or health care organizations, to communicate over a public network; VPN message traffic is carried on public networking infrastructure (e.g., the Internet) using standard (often insecure) protocols, or over a service provider's network providing VPN service guarded by a well-defined

Service Level Agreement (SLA) between the VPN customer and the VPN service provider. VPN involves two parts: the protected or "inside" network that provides physical security and administrative security sufficing to protect transmission (sometimes it is not always the case), and a less trustworthy or "outside" network or segment.

VIRTUAL REALITY: Electronic medical mimicry and sensory simulation to assist in the diagnosis and treatment of various medical and mental disorders; for example, agoraphobic virtual reality simulators; a computer-based technology for simulating visual, auditory, and other sensory aspects of complex patient environments to create an illusion of being a three-dimensional world; a teaching world is designed by the computer, and viewed through a special headset that responds to head movements while a glove responds to hand movements; for example, while in a virtual patient exam room, one may move a hand to grasp a stethoscope and auscultate a heart.

VIRTUAL ROUTING: Virtual computer system subgroups independent of physical location but logically treated as a single Internet domain.

VIRTUAL TECHNOLOGY: Engineering protocol that allows the more efficient and transparent use of many computers that are indifferent to their underlying operating systems for enhanced medical or covered entity EDI; Novell Xen©.

VIRUS: Unwanted and usually malicious and externally delivered computer software code that attaches itself to programs and applications for self-replications and mischief; e-mail enhanced electronic miscreants and attachments; stealth; over and nonoverwriting, and variant, and so forth; the *Brain* first released in 1986 was the first self-replicating PC software distributed on a 5.25-inch floppy disk, although the *Elk Cloner* infected Apple IIs in 1982; others include: Lehigh, Jerusalem, Dark Avenger, Integrity Maser, DAME, Michelangelo, Boza, Melissa, ILOVEYOU, Sircam, Nimda, BadTrans, SQL Slammer, Blaster Worm, Sobig.F, Bagle Worm, Santy Worm, Zotob, and so forth; term first coined by Fred Cohen in 1983.

VIRUS CHECK: A computer program that identifies and disables: (1) another "virus" computer program, typically hidden, that attaches itself to other programs and has the ability to replicate; (2) a type of programmed threat or code fragment (not an independent program) that reproduces by attaching to another program and may damage data directly, or it may degrade system performance by taking over system resources which are then not available to authorized users; and (3) code embedded within a program that causes a copy of itself to be inserted in one or more other programs; in addition to propagation, the virus usually performs some unwanted function.

VIRUS CREATION LAB: Set of computer viruses that contained a suite of writing tools in 1991–1992; Dark Avenger Mutation Engine variant.

VIRUS HOAX: A bit of computer code that isn't really a virus at all and may lead unsuspecting users to routinely ignore all virus warning messages leaving them vulnerable to a genuine, destructive virus.

VIRUS PROTECTION: Any method that provides end-user education, including information about the potential harm that can be caused by viruses, how to prevent introduction of a virus to a computer system, and what to do if a virus is detected.

VIRUS SCANNER: An anti-virus software program that searches for signatures or malicious binary patterns that have attached themselves to executable computer programs.

VIRUS SIGNATURE: The machine code and binary pattern of a specific virus; mode of operation; program code look and feel.

VISHING: Use of a phony VOIP number, rather than faux Web link, to fraudulently obtain private information; identity theft scam; similar to text message phishing; slang term.

VISIO©: Software application that produces diagrams, tables, graphs, and other business and medical illustrations.

VISIT: A Web page or Web site view; user eyeballs; also, a request from a Web browser to visit a Web page or Web site; produces multiple "hits."

VISITOR: One who views a Web site or page; user eyeballs.

VISITOR TRACKING: Establishes sign-in procedures to cover the "reception, tracking, and hosting of visitors" at a health care or medical facility; for certain access, "escort" codes or passwords may be provided.

VISTA©: Windows©-based operating system from the Microsoft Corporation®; released in 2007 as the first upgrade since 2001 along with releases for Office 2007 and Exchange Server 2007; health care variant.

VISTA© ID VERIFICATION: Secure fingertip biometric or smart-card reader-ready Windows© operating system.

VISTA© INFOCARD: Windows© operating system enabled Internet Explorer© Web browser with scaleable InfoCard (smart-card) security capabilities.

VISTA© KERNEL: Security features of the Windows operating system, which includes drive signaling requirements to fool online malware, anti-patch technology to reduce kernel manipulation, kernel integrity checks, and restricted user access to physical memory.

VISUAL BASIC©: Modular programming language from the Microsoft Corporation with screen driven programming; released in 1991 to enable the Windows© operating system; NET, VB.NET, C#, C++, Kylix©, JBuilder© for JAVA and Delphi®, Visual Café®, and so forth.

VISUAL HTML EDITOR: Simple Web page designing language or format; WYSIWYG; for example, Adobe Go Live©, MSFT FrontPage©, Macromedia Dreamweaver©, MSFT OfficeLive©, and so forth.

VISUAL STUDIO .NET©: MSFT XML Web page development environment.

VIVOX©: Peer-2-Peer voice technology service.

VLOG: Online data directory filed with video clips, video blogs, and so forth; slang term.

VMWARE: x86: PC-based manageability series that redefined the enterprise health data or other information center.

VOICE GRADE CHANNEL: A telephone circuit of adequate bandwidth to carry signals in the voice frequency range of 300 to 3400 Hertz; the bandwidth of a POTS line.

VOICE MAIL: Computerized telephone messages and audio processing; voice chat; voice message.

VOICE OVER INTERNET PROTOCOL (VOIP): UDP telephone transmission protocol over the Internet; based on Wi-Fi roaming functionality; Google Talk©, Skype©, Vonage©, and so forth.

VOICE RECOGNITION: Natural language computer input interface with vocal commands, and without a pointer, keyboard, stylus, or other physical input device; the ability of a computer to interpret auditory information in the form of spoken words.

VOICE SWITCHING: An electronic method for opening and closing a circuit, such as changing from one microphone to another microphone, or from one video camera to another video camera, responding to the presence or absence of sound.

VOID: Containing no health data, medical, PHI, or other information.

VOKEN: Web site advertisement that appears on an Internet Web page but without a separate open window screen; virtual token; slang term.

VOLATILE: Memory that is erased when computer power is removed; nonpermanent; RAM is volatile; flash sticks are nonvolatile.

VOLUME: Physical computer system storage unit, such as a hard disk, floppy disk, CD-ROM, and so forth, logical storage unit that is a part of one physical drive or one that spans several physical drives.

VOLUME ELEMENT: A voxel is like a pixel in a three-dimensional version and is generated by computer-based imaging systems, such as CT or MRI.

VON-NEUMANN, JOHN, PhD (1903–1957): Mathematician and active member of the Manhattan Project Atomic Energy Commission; later researched and worked on parallel computing processes and networks; has earned the label of the "father of the modern computer."

VORAN, DAVID, MD: Chief Medical Information Officer of Health Midwest, a Kansas City, MO-based health system with 15 acute care facilities and multiple satellites.

vPRO©: Intel© Core 2 Duo microprocessor with integrated technology for enterprise-wide computer systems management, such as remote-heal during power-down, for health information and EDI network management.

VULNERABILITY: A weakness in health care information system security procedures, design, implementation, internal controls, and so forth, that could be accidentally triggered or intentionally exploited and result in a violation of the system's security policy.

VULNERABILITY ASSESSMENT: A process to determine what vulnerabilities exist in the current system against these attacks; vulnerability threat pairs (Table 10).

VULNERABILITY ASSESSMENT MANAGED SERVICES: Agencies that use scanning devices connected to probe a health organization's security to look for vulnerabilities.

VULNERABILITY INDEX (VI): A measure of computer system intrusion or threat magnitude; the product of the cost of compromise (CC) or loss, by the probability of loss or compromise.

VULNERABILITY SCANNER: A program that performs diagnostic phase security analysis and defines, identifies, and classifies security holes

Table 10: Vulnerability Threat Pairs and Assessment

Vulnerability	Threat Source	Threat Action
Terminated employees' system identifiers (ID) are not removed from the system	Terminated employees	Dialing into the company's network and accessing company proprietary data
Company firewall allows inbound telnet, and *guest* ID is enabled on XYZ server	Unauthorized users (e.g., hackers, terminated employees, computer criminals, terrorists)	Using telnet to XYZ server and browsing system files with the *guest* ID
The vendor has identified flaws in the security design of the system; however, new patches have not been applied to the system	Unauthorized users (e.g., hackers, disgruntled employees, computer criminals, terrorists)	Obtaining unauthorized access to sensitive system files based on known system vulnerabilities
Data center uses water sprinklers to suppress fire; tarpaulins to protect hardware and equipment from water damage are not in place	Fire, negligent persons	Water sprinklers being turned on in the data center

(vulnerabilities) in a computer, server, network, or health care or other organization communications infrastructure; can forecast the effectiveness of proposed countermeasures and evaluate how well they work after they are put into use.

VULNERABLE ACCESS LEVEL: Employment, job-driven, or permissible computer security level for those cohorts accessing private patient health information or other sensitive data.

VULNERABLE USER ACCESS: Sensitivity level of individual computer entry within a defined job-space, or security level.

W

W-10: Interhealth agency transfer form.

WAEGEMANN, PETER C.: CEO of the Medical Records Institute.

WAKE-ON-LAN (WOL): A computer network PCI adapter that opens the host from sleep-mode, to make it available to other network users; other PCI features are flow control, full duplex data transfer, and fast 10/100Base-T data transfer.

WALLPAPER: Graphical spread across the background of a computer screen or monitor; screen-saver; slang term.

WAND: A handheld or portable optical reader.

WANG, HAO, PHD: CIO for SAFE Health.

WAR CHALK SYMBOL: Amateur chalk mark or formal identifying logo for a hot spot wireless computer network provider; sidewalk, building, tree IT graffiti; slang term.

WAR DIAL(ER): Using an automatically dialing modem to call out many telephone numbers to breach computer network security and gain unauthorized access to health data or other information.

WAR DRIVE: The processes of driving an automobile around a specific neighborhood in search of a wireless hot spot for an enabled laptop computer with external antenna; slang term.

WAREZ: Usually Peer-2-Peer acquired, or pirated and illegally copied software.

WARM BOOT: Restarting a computer after it has been previously functional.

WARM SITE: An alternative backup site that contains some of the same equipment as the heath organization's actual IT center.

WARP: IBM OS/2 version operating system; or to visually distort a digitized computer image.

WASHER: Spam triage utility software that segregates unwanted spam from wanted e-mail transmissions, based on predetermined ranges.

WASHINGTON PUBLISHING COMPANY (WPC): The firm that publishes the X12N HIPAA Implementation guides and the X12N HIPAA Data

Dictionary; also developed the X12 Data Dictionaries and hosts the EHNAC STFCS testing program.

WATERMARK: Invisible code or ghost pattern on a digital image, used for identification.

WAVE (WAV) FILE: The native digital audio format used in Windows© with a .WAV extension.

WAVELET: Software diagnostic compression pathway; condensed medical decision-making algorithm, radiographic imaging, or other pictorial services.

WEB ADDRESS: Internet protocol or URL identifier with three-part Web server nomenclature:

- www: host name that distinguishes computers
- health dictionary series: owner's name
- com: organization type
- location optional (e.g., uk, fi, and so forth)
- URL: www.HealthDictionarySeries.com

WEB APPLIANCE: A dedicated utility computer with little storage and usually connected to a network.

WEB APPLICATION: Software programs accessed online through the Internet and hosted by a provider such as Google© and Microsoft Office Live©.

WEB AUTHORING: Software used to create Web sites for home, business, or medical practice Internet pages/sites, such as MSFT FrontPage©, Adobe GoLive©, Macromedia Dreamweaver©, and MSFT Office Live© (basic and essentials).

WEB BROWSER: World Wide Web service access software, usually coupled with a GUI interface; Internet Explorer 7®, Mozilla-Firefox©, Opera©, SeaMonkey©, Netscape©, and so forth.

WEB CAM: Wired or wireless digital Internet video camera usually with audio chat functionality.

WEB CAST: A live video program sent to multiple Internet users concurrently; Web short clip; Webby Award©.

WEB CRAWLER: An Internet browser or search engine that identifies, saves, and indexes Web sites and Web pages.

WEB DIRECTORY: Internet search engine or index such as Yahoo!, MSN, Google®, ASK®, Lycos®, Microsoft Live Search®, and so forth.

WEB HEAD: An Internet enthusiast; slang term.

WEBIFY: To maintain the essential components of a PC on its hard-drive, while moving some user files and software that interacts with them to remote ISP type data center servers; to unlock desktop computer health care or other data in favor of an Internet-hosted application suite; slang term.

WEB MASTER: One responsible for maintenance of a Web site; Internet engineer; Web author.

WEB PAGE: Searchable radio channel-like information located on the Internet; information screens or windows; individual component segments of a Web site.

WEB PORTAL: An Internet site entry or access point; homepage.

WEB SEARCH SITE: Internet site that provides search engine functionality.

WEB SECURITY: Protocols to safeguard Web users and related health care organizations or covered entities.

WEB SERVER: Dedicated computer HTTP server that displays Web sites, pages, and services though URL connectivity; machine where Web sites reside; Apache®, Internet Information Server®, Netscape Enterprise Server®, CGI script, and so forth.

WEB SERVICES: The integration of standardized Internet-based applications.

WEB SERVICES DESCRIPTION LANGUAGE (WSDL): An XML language used to describe the services a business offers, and to provide a way for individuals and other businesses to access those services electronically.

WEB SERVICES INTEROPERABILITY (WSI): An association of IT industry companies formed in 2002, including IBM® and Microsoft©, that aim to create Internet specifications that all companies can use.

WEB SERVICES SECURITY (WSS): An IT industry standard that addresses security when data is exchanged as part of a Web service from an industry group that includes IBM®, Microsoft®, and Verisign®.

WEB SITE: GUI Internet location with home page, similar HTTP hyperlinked pages, search index, data, audio, and visual or graphic files of related content; related group of www files.

WEBTOP: A Web browser used as a desktop computer interface.

WEBZINE: An Internet-published magazine; slang term; zine.

WETZELL, STEVEN: Cofounder and health informatist of the Leapfrog Group, Washington, D.C.

WHEEL: A computer systems administrator with increased security privileges; slang term.

WHETSTONE: Computer operating speed benchmarking protocol.

WHIDBEY: Microsoft Visual Studio-2005®; code name.

WHISTLER: Windows XP® and Windows.Net®; code name.

WHITE, JOEL C.: Member of the professional staff of the Subcommittee on Health, House Committee on Ways and Means, who first outlined the issues faced by health care information technology for evolution into the twenty-first century.

WHITEBOARD: Electronic equivalent of a chalk blackboard for networking.

WHITE HAT (WH): One who promotes computer systems security; apostle of health information and data confidentiality; slang term.

WHITE PAPER: An authoritative subject matter technical report.

WHO IS: Reverse software utility service used to search for e-mail addresses; who is client; who is server.

WIDE AREA NETWORK (WAN): A geographical large computer users group, connected to a local server, host, or network hub.

WIDE AREA TELEPHONE SERVICE (WATS): A telephone service with a flat rate for measured bulk-rate, long distance services given on an incoming or outgoing basis; allows a consumer, by use of an access line, to make telephone calls to any telephone number that is able to be dialed in a specific zone for a flat or bulk monthly rate using an 800 number.

WIDEBAND: Electronic transmission rates from 64 Kbps–2 Mbps and beyond.

WI-FI: Wireless fidelity electronic computer transmission standards known as 802.11; two current versions, 802.11a and 802.11b, are protocols that allow data to be transferred wirelessly and enable different devices to communicate; originally 802.11b was the more widely deployed standard, but it operated slowly and has been replaced by 802.11g, which provides a wider range and runs at the same higher speed as 802.11a; but 802.11a continues with certain advantages such as fewer devices running off the 5-GHz band frequency on which it runs; Bluetooth© wireless technology; moving into the next generation with 802.11n, a technology that combines multiple antennas, cleverer encoding, and an optional doubling of spectrum to achieve raw data rates up to 600 Mbps; ratified by IEEE in 2007.

WI-FI PROTECTED ACCESS (WPA): The 802.11i computer network security and encryption standard protocol.

WIKI: Collaborative software or Web site that allows users to add, modify, or delete information, as in a dictionary (www.HealthDictionarySeries.com); the Portland Pattern Repository was the first Wiki, named after the Hawaiian number 7; or "quickie."

WIKIPEDIA: A fluid and free Internet-based and collaborative online dictionary; investopedia; wiki.

WILD CARD: Placement holder character, such as *, used to help define a data field during an Internet search; may be used to ensure a search turns up all forms or derivatives of a word; for example, oz* will turn up both oz and ozone.

WILENSKY, GAIL, PHD: Senior Fellow, Project HOPE.

WIMAX: A more powerful version of Wi-Fi that can provide wireless Internet access over a wider geographic location such as a city. An acronym that stands for Worldwide Interoperability for Microwave Access, and is a certification mark for products that pass conformity and interoperability tests for the IEEE 802.16 standards. IEEE 802.16 is working group number 16 of IEEE 802, specializing in point-to-multipoint broadband wireless access.

WIMAX WILD (WM-W): A fourth-generation wireless data network (4G).

WINCHESTER DRIVE: Hard disk drive originally associated with IBM type AT and XT personal computers using the HFM recording technology; code name.

WINDOW: On-computer screen electronic box or rectangular viewing or input screen; slang term; special purpose computer screen space; one currently views an *active* window.

WINDOWS©: A GUI operating system series for PCs from the Microsoft Corporation® first introduced in 1983; Windows© 3.11 for workgroups; Windows© 95 (Chicago) with a 32-bit graphical multitasking system; Windows XP© was introduced in 2001 and Windows Vista®, in 2007 with six core editions (three for consumers, two for businesses users, and a stripped-down edition for emerging markets); Vista® is designed for advanced 64-bit computing, multimedia, or Tablet PCs. Windows© Vista Home Premium allows one to record and watch high-definition television, burn and author DVDs, and perform multimedia functions; incorporates Tablet PC technology to decipher handwriting and allows physicians or other users to write medical, progress, or similar notes; Vista® Home Premium for the middle market lies between high-end Windows© Vista Ultimate, which includes business-oriented features, and Windows© Vista Home Basic without multimedia capabilities.

WINDOWS 9X: Short for Windows 95® and 98 versions; slang term; replaced by MSFT Home Edition.

WINDOWS 98-SE®: MSFT Operating System with special edition coupled with Internet Explorer in 1999; Windows Millennium Edition®.

WINDOWS 2000®, XP®, AND VISTA®: GUI operating system released by the MSFT Corporation® in 2000, 2001, and 2007 respectively.

WINDOWS ACCELERATOR: A Windows® screen overlay graphics card without the need for CPU input.

WINDOWS CE®: Abbreviated Consumer Electronics operating system from MSFT for PDAs and hand-held computer devices.

WINDOWS© EXECUTABLE FILE VIRUS: Dangerous computer software that overwrites BIOS data rendering the OS inoperable; the CIH (Chernobyl) variant virus of 1998 caused $20–$80M in damage.

WINDOWS FIJI©: MSFT-Windows operating system that followed Vista© with bug fixes, security patches, and enhanced features; code name.

WINDOWS LIVE MESSENGER©: MSFT instant computer messaging service that allows VOIP, telephone calling, videoconferencing, drag-in-drop functionality, text-messaging, folding sharing, two-way address book, alerts and so forth.

WINDOWS© MEDIA PLAYER: MSFT program to view and create digital videos.

WINDOWS NET SERVER©: MSFT Windows© operating system Internet servers.

WINDOWS© NT SERVER: Microsoft 32-bit multitasking and multiprocessing networked GUI operating system.

WINDOWS© NT WORKSTATION: Microsoft 32-bit multitasking and multiprocessing GUI operating system.

WINDOWS® OFFICE 2007: Business productivity software service/package ranging from enterprise to abbreviated basic versions for newer PCs; SKU versions listed most-to-least robust:

- Enterprise [Word®, Excel®, PowerPoint®, One Note®, Publisher®, Access®, InfoPath®, Communicator®, Groove®, and various other integrated options].
- Ultimate [same as above with Business Contact Manager, but sans One-Note mobile 2007].
- Professional Plus [lacks Groove® and OneNote®].
- Professional [highest level on store shelves: sans Communicator, Groove, OneNote, and Communicator].
- Small Business [Word, Excel, Outlook with Business Contact Manager].
- Standard [Word, Excel, Outlook, and PowerPoint].
- Home and Student [Word, Excel, and PowerPoint; replace Outlook and OneNote].
- Basic [PC preloads of Word, Excel, and Outlook].

WINDOWS© SWAP FILE: A disk file used by Windows for virtual memory that temporarily stores segments of the application on a disk when there is not enough memory to hold all the programs used; Windows 95/98® created a temporary swap file (WIN386.SWP), which was dynamically sized and abandoned while NT 4 created a temporary swap file, or paging file (PAGEFILE.SYS) that was generally equal to the size of memory plus 12 MB. It also allowed for one additional swap file to be created on each logical partition on the hard disk.

WINDOWS® VIENA®: MSFT Windows operating system that followed Vista® and interim Fiji® with revamped desktop and the ability to wall off old code from critical parts of the OS for enhanced security and deliver robust features over the Internet using virtual machine technology (VMT).

WINDOWS® VISTA©: MSFT operating system with new upgraded interface that automatically sorts related files into folders, improves engine searches, and contains powerful graphics; with several SKUs: Starter©, Enterprise© with bitlocker, Home Basic©, Home Premium©, Ultimate©, and Business©.

WINDOW WIDTH: The range of the gray scale of the image seen on a screen; the middle value is the "window level."

WIN-FX©: Windows Vista® software development and programming module.

WINKENWERDER, WILLIAM, MD: Assistant Secretary of defense for U.S. Health Affairs.

WINTEL: The Windows®-Intel® (software–hardware) consortium.

WIPE: To format a hard drive in order to erase medical data or other information; slang term.

WIRED EQUIVALENT PRIVACY (WEP): Optional 802.11 encryption security network transmission standard about equal to a wired line.

WIRELESS-A: Electronic radio transmission through the airwaves; 54 Mps and 5 GHz protocol replaced by the Wireless-G standard.

WIRELESS-B: Wi-Fi electronic radio transmission protocol through the airwaves producing 11 Mbps at 2.4 GHz.

WIRELESS-G: Wi-Fi communications protocol 54 Mbps at 2.4 GHz that is compatible with Wireless-B computer systems.

WIRELESS N: Wi-Fi electronic radio transmission protocol through the air-waves producing 100 Mbps at 2.4 GHz; wireless B and G compatible.

WIRELESS ACCESS POINT (WAP): A wireless networks hub with central transmitter.

WIRELESS FIDELITY (WI-FI): Wireless Ethernet Compatibility Association (WECA) specific IEEE 82.11b standard.

WIRELESS HOT SPOT: Specific geographic location in which an access point provides public wireless broadband network services; security is risky for PHI; hotspot.

WIRELESS INTERNET SERVICE PROVIDER (WISP): Unsecured, public Internet access without a reseller that does not use copper wires or standard tele-phone landlines for transmission.

WIRELESS LAN: Computer network with short-distance interconnectivity without wires; uses an ISM band connected to an Ethernet hub or server.

WIRELESS NETWORK ADAPTER: Hardware used to transition from a wired cable network to a wireless one.

WIRELESS TECHNOLOGY: Radio-frequency driven WAN, MAN, or LAN systems for mobility and improved functionality, such as rural access management, remote health care delivery, HIMS, remote medical triage, and so forth.

WITTY WORM: Malicious code that exploited vulnerabilities in security soft-ware produced by Internet Security Systems (NASD-ISSX) of Atlanta, now IBM, that overwrote infected hard disks in 2004.

WIZARD: Windows© operating system assistance or utility help program.

WORD: The number of bits equal to one CPU register and computer type; also, MSFT® word-processing software application; PC and Macintosh versions available.

WORDPAD: A simple Windows® word-processor program.

WORD PROCESSOR(ING): A device to electronically assist in the production of documents or text; dedicated device or multiuse computer.

WORD STAR®: An early word-processing program by MicroPro®.

WORD WRAP: Automatic new text-line initiation while using a word-processing application.

WORK FLOW: The process that defines the linear production of serial effort, electronic, or conscientious industry.

WORK FLOW AUTOMATION: A process that relegates automated responses and decision making to a computer and its minions of decision-supporting and routing applications, such as patient service, inventory management, automated billing and payment, or any number of other tasks that depend upon a consistent set of processes benefit; greatest savings potential is on the paperless transaction side, which accounts for 32% of all health care expenditures.

WORK FORCE: The employees, volunteers, trainees, and other people whose conduct in the performance of work for a covered health entity is under the direct control of such entity, whether or not they are paid by the covered entity.

WORK GROUP: A small collection of networked private computers; intranet.

WORKGROUP FOR ELECTRONIC DATA INTERCHANGE (WEDI): A health care industry group that lobbied for HIPAA and A/S and formed consultative roles under the HIPAA legislation, as well as sponsored SNIP.

WORKING FILES: Files that have been used to generate a graphic file such as an EPS file; software applications such as Macromedia FreeHand©, Adobe Illustrator©, and QuarkXPress© can all generate EPS files.

WORKSTATION: Nodular computer, server, or intelligent terminal hub connected to dumb drones; usually a WAN, MAN, or LAN; a high-performance, single-user computer generally used for medical, architectural, business, enterprise-wide or other graphics, CAD, simulation, and scientific applications; IBM RS/6000; Sun SPARCstation®.

WORKSTATION USE: Defines what functions or activities may be performed at a particular health care or other data workstation; includes instructions and guidelines on screensaver passwords, biometrics, and secure physical placement.

WORLD WIDE WAIT: Time lag for an Internet download file to occur; slang term.

WORLD WIDE WEB (WWW): The Internet collection of electronic information channels or pages using HTTP; the Web; slang term.

WORM: Write once, read many; an optical laser disk.

WORM PROGRAM: Self-replicating and malicious software program, similar to a virus; spreads within a computer system or network host unlike a computer virus; does not have to be attached to an e-mail, for example, Morris Cornell, Mytube, Bagle Worms, and so forth. Worms first eclipsed computer viruses in damage potential in 1999 with the Bubble Boy variant and later by the Sasser worm created by a 17-year-old German college student; electronic tapeworm.

WRAP: Fault tolerant FDDI computer network problem identifier.

WRITABLE CD/DVD DRIVE: Hard drive used to create data, audio, and video disks.

WRITE: To record digital health data or other information on some electronic storage device; disk, tape, CD, flash drive, and so forth.

WRITELY®: Online, free word-processing application by Upstartle, Inc., now Google®.

WRITE ONCE: Electronic storage media that can be written to but not erased.

WRITE PROTECT: A safeguard for the change prevention or copying of an electronic file, application, or program.

X

X12: An ANSI-accredited group that defines EDI standards for many American industries, including health care insurance; most electronic transaction standards are mandated or proposed under HIPAA are X12 standards.

X12 148: The X12 First Report of Injury, Illness, or Incident transaction that was included in HIPAA.

X12 270: The X12 Health Care Eligibility and Benefit Inquiry transaction; version 4010 of this transaction was included in HIPAA.

X12 271: The X12 Health Care Eligibility and Benefit Response transaction; version 4010 was included in HIPAA.

X12 274: The X12 Provider Information transaction.

X12 275: The X12 Patient Information transaction as a part of HIPAA claim attachments standards.

X12 276: The X12 Health Care Claims Status Inquiry transaction; version 4010 was included in HIPAA.

X12 277: The X12 Health Care Claim Status Response transaction; version 4010 was included in HIPAA and claims attachments standard.

X12 278: The X12 Referral Certification and Authorization transaction; version 4010 was included in the HIPAA mandates.

X12 811: The X12 Consolidated Service Invoice and Statement transaction.

X12 820: The X12 Payment Order and Remittance Advice transaction; version 4010 was included in HIPAA.

X12 831: The X12 Application Control Totals transaction.

X12 834: The X12 Benefit Enrollment and Maintenance transaction; version 4010 was included in HIPAA.

X12 835: The X12 Health Care Claim Payment and Remittance Advice transaction; version 4010 was included in HIPAA.

X12 837: The X12 Health Care Claim or Encounter transaction used for institutional, professional, dental, or drug claims; version 4010 was included in HIPAA.

X12 997: The X12 Functional Acknowledgment transaction.

X12F: A subcommittee of X12 that defines EDI standards for the financial industry; maintains the X12 811 [generic] Invoice and the X12 820 [generic] Payment and Remittance Advice transactions, although X12N maintains the associated HIPAA Implementation guides.

X12 IHCEBI & IHCEBR: The X12 Interactive Healthcare Eligibility and Benefits Inquiry (IHCEBI) and Response (IHCEBR) transactions that were combined and converted to UN/EDIFACT version 5 syntax.

X12 IHCLME: The X12 Interactive Healthcare Claim transaction.

X12J: A subcommittee of X12 that reviewed X12 work products for compliance with the X12 design rules.

X12N: A subcommittee of X12 that defined EDI standards for the insurance industry, including health care insurance.

X12N/SPTG4: The HIPAA Liaison Special Task Group of the Insurance Subcommittee (N) of X12 whose responsibilities were assumed by X12N/TG3/WG3.

X12N/TG1: The Property and Casualty Task Group (TG1) of the Insurance Subcommittee (N) of X12.

X12N/TG2: The Health Care Task Group (TG2) of the Insurance Subcommittee (N) of X12.

X12N/TG2/WG1: The Health Care Eligibility Work Group (WG1) of the Health Care Task Group (TG2) of the Insurance Subcommittee (N) of X12; maintains the X12 270 Health Care Eligibility and Benefit Inquiry and the X12 271 Health Care Eligibility & Benefit Response transactions, and is also responsible for maintaining the IHCEBI and IHCEBR transactions.

X12N/TG2/WG2: The Health Care Claims Work Group (WG2) of the Health Care Task Group (TG2) of the Insurance Subcommittee (N) of X12; maintains the X12 837 Health Care Claim or Encounter transaction.

X12N/TG2/WG3: The Health Care Claim Payments Work Group (WG3) of the Health Care Task Group (TG2) of the Insurance Subcommittee (N) of X12; maintains the X12 835 Health Care Claim Payment and Remittance Advice transaction.

X12N/TG2/WG4: The Health Care Enrollments Work Group (WG4) of the Health Care Task Group (TG2) of the Insurance Subcommittee (N) of X12; maintains the X12 834 Benefit Enrollment and Maintenance transaction.

X12N/TG2/WG5: The Health Care Claims Status Work Group (WG5) of the Health Care Task Group (TG2) of the Insurance Subcommittee (N) of X12; maintains the X12 276 Health Care Claims Status Inquiry and the X12 277 Health Care Claim Status Response transactions.

X12N/TG2/WG9: The Health Care Patient Information Work Group (WG9) of the Health Care Task Group (TG2) of the Insurance Subcommittee (N) of X12; maintains the X12 275 Patient Information transaction.

X12N/TG2/WG10: The Health Care Services Review Work Group (WG10) of the Health Care Task Group (TG2) of the Insurance Subcommittee (N) of X12; maintains the X12 278 Referral Certification and Authorization transaction.

X12N/TG2/WG12: The Interactive Health Care Claims Work Group (WG12) of the Health Care Task Group (TG2) of the Insurance Subcommittee (N) of X12; maintains the IHCLME Interactive Claims transaction.

X12N/TG2/WG15: The Health Care Provider Information Work Group (WG15) of the Health Care Task Group (TG2) of the Insurance Subcommittee (N) of X12. This group maintains the X12 274 Provider Information transactions.

X12N/TG2/WG19: The Health Care Implementation Coordination Work Group (WG19) of the Health Care Task Group (TG2) of the Insurance Subcommittee (N) of X12; now X12N/TG3/WG3.

X12N/TG3: The Business Transaction Coordination and Modeling Task Group (TG3) of the Insurance Subcommittee (N) of X12. TG3 maintains the X12N Business and Data Models and the HIPAA Data Dictionary.

X12N/TG3/WG1: The Property and Casualty Work Group (WG1) of the Business Transaction Coordination and Modeling Task Group (TG3) of the Insurance Subcommittee (N) of X12.

X12N/TG3/WG2: The Healthcare Business & Information Modeling Work Group (WG2) of the Business Transaction Coordination and Modeling Task Group (TG3) of the Insurance Subcommittee (N) of X12.

X12N/TG3/WG3: The HIPAA Implementation Coordination Work Group (WG3) of the Business Transaction Coordination and Modeling Task Group (TG3) of the Insurance Subcommittee (N) of X12.

X12N/TG3/WG4: The Object-Oriented Modeling and XML Liaison Work Group (WG4) of the Business Transaction Coordination and Modeling Task Group (TG3) of the Insurance Subcommittee (N) of X12.

X12N/TG4: The Implementation Guide Task Group (TG4) of the Insurance Subcommittee (N) of X12; supports the development and maintenance of X12 Implementation Guides, including the HIPAA X12 IGs.

X12N/TG8: The Architecture Task Group (TG8) of the Insurance Subcommittee (N) of X12.

X12/PRB: The X12 Procedures Review Board.

X12 STANDARD: The term currently used for any X12 standard that has been approved since the most recent release of X12 American National Standards; as a full set of X12 American National Standards is released every five years, it is the X12 standards that are most likely to be in active use; previously called Draft Standards for Trial Use.

X.25: Packet switching network protocol for PVC and SVC assemblers and disassemblers.

XDS: Crossed enterprise clinical document or PHI data sharing.

XEN©: An open source operating system computer language.

XENIX®: Unix-based computer operating system from Microsoft® in the 1980s.

XENSOURCE: Maker of one of the first virtualization search engines with *hypervision,* which can host virtual computers with different operating systems running next to each other; VMware©.

XEON©: Intel's© dual core energy efficient microprocessor released for notebook computers in 2002; Woodcrest; code name.

XOR: High-output gating or filtering technique for a single computer input.

X-ORP: Network application that turns any computer into a router.

X-PATH: A computer language that describes a way to locate and process items in Extensible Markup Language documents by using an addressing syntax based on a path through the document's logic structure, or hierarchy.

X-PATH INJECTION: A hack targeting Web sites that create XPATH queries from health or other intensive user-supplied information.

X-WINDOWS©: Unix-based graphical user interface and operating system developed at MIT.

XSL: Extensible Style sheet Language.

XSS: Cross-site scripting is a security exploit in which the attacker inserts malicious coding into a link that appears to be from a trustworthy source; upon clicking the link, the embedded programming is submitted as part of the client's Web request and can implement on the user's computer, typically allowing the attacker to steal information.

XST: Cross-site tracing is a sophisticated form of cross-site scripting that can bypass health care security measures already put in place to protect against XSS; an attack that allows an intruder to obtain cookies, authentication data using simple client-side scripts.

Y

Y2K: Calendar year 2000.

Y2K COMPLIANT: Computer hardware and software that was PC-based and legacy system sequence compatible between the twentieth and twenty-first centuries.

Y2K PROBLEM: Computer hardware and software that was not PC-based and legacy system sequence-compatible between the twentieth and twenty-first centuries; year-data incongruity.

YAHOO!: A leading Internet search engine, directory, or Web browser.

YASNOFF, WILLIAM, MD, PHD: Senior Advisor for the National Health Information Infrastructure (NHII), Department of Health and Human Services.

YELLOW PAGES: SunSoft© UNIX utility program for Internet resources.

YOUTUBE©: Video sharing Web site and programmable social network founded by Chad Hurley and Steve Chen; sold to Google©.

Z

Z-80: Zilog, Inc. 8-bit CPU that propelled the CP/M OS in the early 1980s.

ZERHOUNI, ELIAS, MD: Director, U.S. National Institute of Health.

ZERO CONFIGURATION: Windows XP® service that enables automatic switching between wireless computer network adapters between ad-hoc and infrastructure modes.

ZERO DAY EXPLOIT: An exploit that takes advantage of security vulnerability on the same day that the vulnerability becomes generally known.

ZILOG PROCESSOR: A 64K RAM Z80 computer microprocessor that ran at 4 MHz with two 5.25-inch floppy drives.

ZIMBRA: An online e-mail application.

ZIMMERMAN, AMY: Director, Rhode Island Health Information Exchange Project.

ZIMMERMANN, PHILIP R.: Creator of *Pretty Good Privacy*, an e-mail encryption software package that was published free on the Internet in 1991 and became the most widely used e-mail encryption program in the world.

ZIP(PING): To condense a large computer file, usually with a utility compression program with .zip extension; an extension for a file name indicating the file is indexed and compressed using Phil Katz's PKZIP compression utilities; a program, called "pkunzip.exe" is needed to decompress and extract the programs within this file.

ZIP DISK: A 3.5-inch removable drive cartridge for mass data storage; password protection capability.

ZIP DRIVE: External removable 100–250 MB storage cartridge device by the Iomega Corporation® of Roy, UT, that connects to a computer by a USB or FireWire port.

ZIP FILE: A file compressed by a PKZIP© utility.

ZOMBIE: A nonterminating UNIX process or loop; a compromised Web site used as an attack point to launch multiple requests toward another attacked site; an old unused Web site (ghost site).

ZONE: A subgroup of LAN, MAN, or WAN users; as in medical or health administration end users; newsgroup members, discussion or use-group, wiki members, and so forth.

ZOO VIRUS: Contained an isolated virus, worm, or malicious code used for further research and study; virus vault; controlled electronic contagion.

ZOOK, ANTHONY P.: President and CEO, AstraZeneca, LP, United States.

ZOPE©: Object-oriented application server written in the Python computer programming language; first used at the UNC School of Medicine, in Chapel Hill, NC, for building medical content management information systems.

Z/OS: The OS for IBM's zSeries 900 (z900) line of larger mainframe servers for e-business initiatives such as health care; a scalable and secure high-performance operating system based on 64-bit architecture; supports Web and JAVA-based mission critical health care and other enterprise applications.

ZUNE©: The name of a project, brand, and MP3 device from MSFT, released in 2007, with music and movies for acquiring and sharing; drive-based media service with WiFi; proprietary and not compatible with Napster, Vongo, Apple iPOD, and so forth.

HEALTH INFORMATION TECHNOLOGY AND SECURITY NUMERICAL TERMS

3COM: Leading maker of Internet systems hardware applications for small and medium businesses.

3-TIER APPLICATION: A computer program organized into three major parts distributed to a different place in a network; workstation, business logic, and database.

4x, 8x, 16x, 32x, 64x, AND SO FORTH: Transfer speeds for CDs or DVDs compared to normal audio or video.

7: Internet Web site that allows users to add, delete, or modify content; really simple syndication (RSS) as in a dictionary (www.HealthDictionarySeries.com); a Wiki is based on the Hawaiian term 7 or 77, meaning "quickie," or informal.

8.3 FILENAME: File moniker with up to eight letters or digits, followed by a dot and up to three more letters or digits, for DOS and Windows© applications, for example, Marcinko.doc.

32: Software applications or program that is void of an owner's copyright.

42 CFR-2: Federal regulations for health data and medical information confidentiality for drug and alcohol abuse and related conditions.

403-FORBIDDEN: HTTP Web address error message.

404-NOT FOUND: HTTP Web address invalid message.

419 SCAM: Usually Nigerian e-mail fraud schemes.

2600: A formalized group of computer hackers or crackers, named after their magazine *(2600 Hacker Quarterly)*; 2600-Hz control tone formerly used in POT systems.

3270: Information Display System from IBM® that was the way the entire corporate world interfaced with a computer before the PC. When first produced (the early 1970s), a 3270 display terminal was considered a vast improvement over its predecessor, the 2260; CRT monitor, black and white screen with green letters; non-GUI.

HEALTH INFORMATION TECHNOLOGY AND SECURITY GREEK LETTERS

APHA: GUI screen/monitor opacity rating system.
BETA: photographic film or digital imaging contrast measure.
MU: micro, a microcomputer, or CPU.
MUC: microcontroller.
MUP: microprocessor, as in CPU.

Acronyms / Abbreviations

The chief merit of language is clearness, and we know that nothing detracts so much from this as do unfamiliar terms.

—Galen (AD 129–199)

AA: Automated Access

AAA: Authentic, Authorized, and Accountable

AAACN: American Academy of Ambulatory Care Nursing

AAAHC: Accreditation Association for Ambulatory Health Care

AAAI: American Association for Artificial Intelligence

AACE: Association for the Advancement of Computers in Education

AAFP: American Academy of Family Physicians

AAFPCHIT: American Academy of Family Physicians Center for Health Information Technology

AAH: American Association of Homecare

AAHAM: American Association of Healthcare Administrative Management

AAHC: American Association of Healthcare Consultants

AAHE: Association for the Advancement of Health Education

AAHP: American Association of Health Plans

AAMA: American Academy of Medical Administration

AAMC: American Association of Medical Colleges

AAMI: Association for the Advancement of Medical Instrumentation

AAMRL: American Association of Medical Records Librarians

AAMT: American Association of Medical Transcription

AAPC: American Academy of Professional Coders

AAPPO: American Association of Preferred Provider Organization

AARP: Apple Talk Address Resolution Protocol

ABBC: Advanced Biotelecommunications and Bioinformatics Center

ABHES: Accrediting Bureau of Health Education Schools

ABN: Advanced Beneficiary Notice

ABR: Auto Baud Rate

ABR: Available Bit Rate

AC: Access Control

ACAHO: Association of Canadian Academic Healthcare Organizations

ACATS: Automated Customer Account Transfer Service

ACC: Attendant Console Controller

ACCE: American College of Clinical Engineering

ACD: Automatic Call Distribution

ACE: Access Control Entry (Enforcement)

ACE: Aetna Claims Exchange

ACG: Access Control Grid

ACH: Automated Clearing House

ACHCA: American College of Health Care Administrators

ACHE: American College of Healthcare Executives

ACHIA: American College of Healthcare Information Administrators

ACI: Audit Controls Integrity
ACID: Automatic, Consistent, Isolated, Durable
ACIG: Academy of Colleges Information Group
ACIS: Ambulatory Care Information System
ACK: Acknowledgment
ACL: Access Control List
ACM: Association for Computer Machinery
ACME: American College of Medical Executives
ACMI: American College of Medical Informatics
ACP: Accelerated Claims Process
ACP: Access Control Policy
ACPE: American College of Physician Executives
ACPI: Advanced Configuration and Power Interface
ACPS: Advanced Claims Processing System
ACR: American College of Radiology
ACR-NEMA: American College of Radiology National Electrical Manufacturers Association
ACS: Access Control System
ACS: Administrative Code Set
ACS: Asynchronous Communications Service
ACT: Automated Confirmation Transaction
ACTION: Accelerating Change and Transformation in Organizations and Networks
AD: Active Directory
AD: Addendum
ADA: American Dental Association
ADB: Apple Desktop Bus
ADC: Advanced Diagnostic Card
ADC: Application Delivery Control

ADCCP: Advanced Data Communication Control Protocol
ADG: Ambulatory Diagnostic Group
ADL: Assertion Definition Language
ADN: Advanced Digital Network
ADN: Application Delivery Network
ADP: Automatic Data Processing
ADPAC: Automatic Data Processing Application Coordinator
ADS: Advanced Detection System
ADSL: Asymmetric Digital Subscriber Line
ADT: Admission, Discharge, Transfer
ADW: Active Data Warehouse
AE: Account Executive
AEA: American Electronics Association
AECHO: Aetna Electronic Claim Home Office
AERS: Adverse Event Reporting System
AES: Advanced Encryption Standard
AFAIK: As Far As I Know
AFE: Apple File Exchange
AFEHCT: Association for Electronic Health Care Transactions
AFH: Adaptive Frequency Hopping
AFP: Apple File Protocol
AFTP: Anonymous File Transfer Protocol
AFUD: Agent Facing Universal Desktop
AG: Application Generator
AGNIS: A Gnomic Nursing Information System
AGP: Accelerated (Advanced) Graphics Port
AGPA: American Group Practice Association
AGPAM: American Guild of Patient Account Managers
AGPS: Assisted Global Positioning System

AH: Authentication Header

AHA: American Hospital Association

AHCA: American Health Care Association

AHCPR: Agency for Health Care Policy and Research

AHIC: American Health Information Community

AHIC: Association for Health Information Connectivity

AHIMA: American Health Information Management Association

AHIP: American Health Insurance Plans

AHLTA: Armed Forces Health Longitudinal Technology Application

AHRMM: American Health Resource and Materials Management

AHRQ: Agency for Healthcare Research and Quality

AHSR: Association for Health Services Research

AHT: Average Handling Time

AI: Accountable Information

AI: Artificial (Applied) Intelligence

AIM: Advanced Informatics in Medicine

AIM: American Institute of Management

AIM: Association for Automatic Identification and Mobility

AIME: European Society for Artificial Intelligence in Medicine

AIMTSH: Association for Information Management and Technology Staff in Health

AIPLA: American Intellectual Property Law Association

AIS: Automatic Information System

AITP: Association of Information Technology Professionals

AJAX: Asynchronous JavaScript and XML

AL: Access Level

ALA: Access Level Authorization

ALE: Ajax Linking and Embedding

ALM: Application Lifecycle Management

ALT Association for Learning Technology

ALU: Arithmetic Logic Unit

AM: Access Measures

AM: Amplitude Modulation

AMA: American Management Association

AMA: American Medical Association

AMCP: Academy of Managed Care Pharmacy

AMD: Advanced Micro Devices

AMDIS: Association of Medical Directors of Information Systems

AMEE: Association for Medical Education in Europe

AMGA: American Medical Group Association

AMI: American Megatrends Incorporated

AMIA: American Medical Informatics Association

AMP: Applied Measurement Professionals

AMP: Automated Medical Payment

AMQP: Advanced Messaging Queuing Protocol

AMRA: American Medical Records Association

ANC: AmeriNet Central

AND: Allowed Natural Death

ANI: Automatic Number Identification

ANIA: American Nursing Informatics Association

ANN: Artificial Neural Network

ANS: American National Standards

ANSI: American National Standards Institute

ANSI-HISB: American National Standards Institute's Healthcare Informatics Standards Board

ANTLR: Another Tool for Language Recognition

AOA: American Osteopathic Association

AOL: America OnLine

AOMRC: Academy of Medical Royal Colleges

AONE: American Organization of Nurse Executives

AORN: Association of Perioperative Registered Nurses

AP: Access Point

APACS: Association for Payment Clearing Services

APC: Ambulatory Payment Class

APCUG: Association of Personal Computer User Groups

APEL: Accreditation of Prior Experiential Learning

APG: Ambulatory Patient Groups

APHA: American Pharmaceutical Association

APHA: American Public Health Association

API: Application Program Interface

API: Association for Pathology Informatics

APIPA: Automatic Private Internet Protocol Address

APL: Accreditation of Prior Learning

APL: Application Program Language

APMA: American Podiatric Medical Association

APN: Appendix

APPAM: Association for Public Policy Analysis and Management

APPC: Advanced Program to Program Communication

APPN: Advanced Patient to Patient Network

APPN: Advanced Peer to Peer Network

APPN: Advanced Physician to Patient Network

APPN: Advanced Physician to Physician Network

AR: Access Rights

ARC: Advanced RISC Computing

ARCNET: Attached Resource Computer Network

ARD: Assessment Reference Date

ARDEN: Arden Syntax Medical Logic Modules

ARI: Access to Radiology Information

ARIN: American Registry for Internet Numbers

ARM: Associate in Risk Management

ARO: Annual Rate of Occurrence

ARP: Address Resolution Protocol

ARPA: Advanced Research Projects Agency of DOD

ARPANET: Advanced Research Projects Agency of DOD Network

ARQ: Automatic Repeat Quest

AS: Administrative Simplification

ASA: Average Speed to Answer

ASAE: American Society of Association Executives

ASC: Accredited Standards Committee

ASC: Administrative Simplification Compliance

ASCII: American Standard Code for Information Interchange

ASCS: Admission Scheduling and Control System

ASC X12: Accredited Standards Committee

ASCX12N: American Standard Committee standard for claims and reimbursement

ASF: Active Streaming Format

ASF: Advanced Streaming Format

ASHE: American Society for Healthcare Engineering

ASHP: American Society of Health Systems Pharmacists

ASHRM: American Society for Healthcare Risk Management

ASME: Association for the Study of Medical Education

ASMOP: A Simple Matter of Programming

ASO: Administrative Services Only

ASP: Application Service Provider

ASP: Association of Shareware Professionals

ASPIRE: Administrative Simplification Print Image Research Efforts

ASS: Administrative Simplification Section

ASS: Administrative Simplification Standards

ASSIMTSH: Association for Information Management and Technology Staff in Health

ASTM: American Society for Testing and Materials

ASTMC-31: American Society for Testing and Materials Committee—Healthcare Informatics

ASTMC-E1384: American Society for Testing and Materials Committee—Automated Primary Care Record

ASTME-31.28: ASTM Proposed National ID System

AT: Advanced Technology

AT: Application Training

AT: Attachment

ATA: American Telemedicine Association

ATM: Adobe Type Manager

ATM: Asynchronous Transfer Mode

ATM: Authentic Trusted Exchange

ATM: Automated Teller Machine

ATNA: Audit Trail and Node Authentication

ATS: Applicant Tracking System

ATSP: Association of TeleHealth Service Providers

ATX: Advanced Technology Extended

AUI: Attached User Interface

AUI: Attachment User Interface

AUIC: Attached User Interface Cable

AUP: Acceptable Use Policy

AUPHA: Association of University Programs in Health Administration

AVERT: Anti-Virus Emergency Response Team

AVI: Audio Video Interleaved

AVVP: Anti-Virus, Virus Program

AYT: Are You There

B/W: Between

B1: DOD computer system security level

B2B: Business to Business

B2C: Business to Consumer (Client)

B2M: Business to Member

B2P: Business to Patient (Provider)

B4: Before

BA: Business Associate

BAA: Business Agency Announcement

BAA: Business Associate Agreement

BAMM: British Association of Medical Managers

BAR: Billing, Accounts Receivable

BASIC: Beginner's All-Purpose Symbolic Instruction Code
BBA: Balanced Budget Act
BBNS: Broadband Network System
BBRA: Balanced Budget Refinement Act
BBS: Bulletin Board System (Service)
BCBSA: Blue Cross Blue Shield of America
BCC: Blind Carbon Copy
BCD: Binary Code Decimal
BCMM: Bar Coded Medical Management
BCP: Best Current Practices
BCS: Biomedical Cognitive Science
BDC: Backup Domain Controller
BDD: Business Desktop Deployment
BEDO RAM: Burst Extended Data Output Random Access Memory
BER: Basic Encoding Rule
BER: Bit Error Rate
BES: BlackBerry Enterprise Server
BFD: Binary File Description
BFT: Binary File Transfer
BGI: Binary Gateway Interface
BGP: Border Gateway Protocol
BH: Black Hat
BHO: Browser Helper Object
BI: Biometric Identifier
BI: Business Intelligence
BIA: Business Impact Assessment
BIDSS: Business Intelligence Decision Support System
BIFF: Binary Interchange File Format
BIND: Berkeley Internet Domain
BIO: Bioinformatics
BIOIT: Biological Information Technology
BIOS: Basic Input/Output System
BIS: Business Intelligence System
BM: Business Model

BNAIC: Binary Automatic Integrated Computer
BNC: Bayonet Nut Connector
BP: Business Partner
BP: Business Process
BPEL: Business Process Execution Language
BPELWS: Business Process Execution Language for Web Services
BPI: Bits Per Inch
BPL: Broadband over Power Lines
BPM: Business Process Management
BPMS: Business Process Management System
BPMT: Business Process Management Technology
BPO: Business Process Outsourcing
BPOC: Bedside Point Of Care
BPR: Business Process Re-engineering
BPS: Bits Per Seconds
BPSK: Binary Phase Shift Keying
BRB: Be Right Back
BRI: Boot Record Infector
BRI: Boot Root Infector
BSC: Binary Synchronous Communication
BSOD: Blue Screen of Death
BTAM: Basic Telecommunication Access Method
BTE: Binary Table
BTE: Bridge to Excellence
BTO: Business Technology Optimization
BTW: By The Way

CA: Certificate Authority
CA: Claim Attachment
CA: Claims Authorizer
CA: Control Access
CABIG: Cancer Biomedical Informatics Grid
CAC: Citizen Advocacy Center

CAC: Computer Assisted Coding

CAD: Computer Assisted (Aided) Design

CAD: Computer Assisted Detection

CAES: Computer Assisted Executions System

CAH: Computer Assisted (Aided) Healthcare

CAI: Computer (Aided) Assisted Instructions

CAL: Client Access License

CAL: Computer Assisted (Aided) Learning

CAM: Component Alignment Model

CAM: Computer Assisted (Aided) Medicine

CAO: Chief Accounting Officer

CAP: Conformance Assessment Process

CAPS: Claims Adjusted Processing System

CAPTCHA: Completely Automated Public Turing Test Tell Computers and Humans Apart

CARC: Claim Adjustment Reasons Code

CARING: Capital Area Roundtable on Informatics in Nursing

CARME: Center for the Advancement of Risk Management Education

CARO: Computer Anti-Virus Research Organization

CAS: Computer Aided (Assisted) Surgery

CAS: Content Addressed Storage

CASE: Computer Aided Software Engineering

CAT 1–5: UTP Categories

CAUCE: Coalition Against Unsolicited Commercial E-mail

CBE: Computer Based Education

CBK: Common Body of Knowledge

CBL: Computer Based Learning

CBME: Computer Based Medical Education

CBMR: Computer Based Medical Records

CBO: Congressional Budget Office

CBO: Cost Budget Office

CBPR: Computer Based Patient Records

CBPRI: Computer Based Patient Records Institute

CBR: Case Based Reasoning

CBR: Computer Based Reference

CBT: Character Based Terminal

CBT: Computer Based Training

CC: Common Criteria for IT Security Evaluation (ISO/IEC 15408)

CC: Credit Card

CCA: Certified Coding Associate

CCBH: Connecting Communities for Better Health

CCC: Clinical Care Classification

CCCA: Claims Adjustment and Analysis

CCD-RAM: Cached-Compact Disk-Random Access Memory

CCEVS: Common Criteria Evaluation and Validation Scheme

CCG: Check Claim Group

CCH: Commercial Clearing House

CCHIT: Certification Commission for Health Information Technology

CCI: Correct Coding Initiative

CCIA: Computer and Communications Industry Association

CCIE: Cisco Certified Internetwork Expert

CCIP: Chronic Care Improvement Program

CCIS: Common Channel Interoffice Signal

CCIT: Coordinating Committee on International Telephony

CCITT: Consultative Committee on International Telephone and Telegraph

CCK: Complementary Code Keying

CCL: Cardiac Care Link

CCO: Chief Compliance Officer

CCOM: Clinical Context Management

CCOW: Clinical Context Object Workgroup

CCR: Continuity of Care Record

CCRA: Certified Review Appraiser

CCS: Certified Coding Specialist

CCS: Clinical Code Sets

CCS: Common Communication Support

CCSP: Certified Coding Specialist Physician

CCT: Coding, Classification, Terminology

CD: Committee Draft

CD: Compact Disc

CDA: Clinical (Decision) Document Architecture

CDAC: Clinical Data Abstraction Center

CDC: Centers for Disease Control

CDCP: Centers for Disease Control and Prevention

CDDL: Common Development and Distribution License

CDF: Channel Definition Format

CDFS: Compact Disc File System

CDFS: CD-ROM File System

CDG: Compact Disc plus Graphics

CDHP: Consumer Directed (Driven) Health Plan

CDI: Compact Disc—Interactive

CDIS: Clinical Data Information Systems

CDIS: Clinical Decision Intelligent System

CDM: Card Dispensing Machine

CDM: Charge Description Master

CDMA: Code Division Multiple Access

CDO: Care Delivery Organization

CDP: Code of Dental Procedures

CDP: Continuous Data Protection

CDPD: Cellular Digital Packet Data

CDPM: Clinical Data Project Manager

CDR: Clinical Data Repository

CDR: Compact Disc—Recordable

CD-ROM: Compact Disc—Read Only Memory

CD-RW: Compact Disc—ReWriteable

CDS: Clinical Documentation System

CDS: Computerized Decision Support

CDSS: Clinical Decision Support System

CDT: Center for Democracy and Technology

CDT: Current Dental Terminology-2

CD-UDF: Compact Disc—Universal Data Format

CD-V: Compact Disc—Video

CDV: Compressed Digital Video

CE: Coded Element

CE: Covered Entity

CEA: Cost Effectiveness Analysis

CEA: Criminal Extortion Activity

CEFACT: Center for Facilitation of Procedures and Practices for Administration, Commerce, and Transport

CEG: Continuous Edge Graphics

CEN: Central European Nations

CEN: *Comité Européen de Normalisation* (Center for European Standardization)

CEN: European Technical Committee for Normalization

CERCLA: Comprehensive Environmental Response Compensation and Liability Act

CERN: *Conseil Européen pour la Recherche Nucléaire* (European Council for Nuclear Research)

CERT: Computer Emergency Response Team

CF: Coded Format

CF: Covered Facility

CF: Covered Function

CFAA: Computer Fraud and Abuse Act

CFE: Coded Format Element

CFML: Cold Fusion Markup Language

CFR: Code of Federal Regulation

CGA: Color Graphics Adapter

CGI: Common Gateway Interface

CGL: Computerized Clinic Guidelines

CGM: Computer Graphics Metafile

CHAP: Challenge Handshake Authentication Protocol

CHC: Connecting for Health Collaborative

CHCS I-II: Composite Health Care System I and II

CHDM: Conceptual Health Data Model

CHECCS: Clearing House Electronic Check Clearing System

CHF: Common Healthcare Framework

CHFE: Certified Health Fraud Examiner

CHFP: Certified Healthcare Financial Professional

CHI: Citizen Health Initiative

CHI: Confidential Health Information

CHI: Consolidated Health Informatics

CHI: Consumer Health Informatics

CHIDS: Center for Health Information and Decision Systems

CHIE: Community Health Information Exchange

CHIM: Center for Health Information Management

CHIME: College of Health Information Management Executives

CHIME: Community Health Information Management Enterprise

CHIN: Community Health Information Network

CHIN: Computer Health Information Network

CHINS: Computer Health Information Network Systems

CHIO: Chief Health Informatics Officer

CHIP: Coalition for Health Information Policy

CHIPP: Canada Health Infostructure Partnerships Program

CHIS: Clinical Hospital Information System

CHITA: Community Health Information Technology Alliance

CHITTA: Canadian Health Information Technology Trade Association

CHMIS: Community Health Management Information Systems

CHN: Canadian Health Network

CHP: Certified in Healthcare Privacy

CHR: Computerized Health Record

CHRIS: Computerized Human Resource Information System

CHS: Center for Healthcare Strategies

CHS: Certified in Healthcare Security

CHS: Community Health Solution

CHS: Cylinder/Head/Sector

CHT: Center for Health and Technology

CI: Clinical Informatics

CI: Clinical Information

CI: Clinical Integration

CI: Coding Institute

CIA: Chief Information (Informatics) Officer

CIAO: Critical Infrastructure Assurance Office

CIC: Customer Information Center

CICS: Customer (Client/Patient) Information Controlled System

CIDR: Classless Inter-Domain Route

CIF: Common Intermediate Format

CIFS: Common Internet File System

CIHI: Canadian Institute for Health Information

CIM: Clinical Information Management

CIMIP: Center for Identity Management and Information Protection

CIO: Chief Information Officer

CIR: Committed Information Rate

CIS: Card Information Structure

CIS: Clinical Information System

CIS: Computer Information System

CISA: Certified Information Systems Auditor

CISC: Complex Instruction Set Computer

CISM®: Certified Information Security Manager®

CISN: Community Integrated Service Network

CISO: Chief Information Security Officer

CISSP: Certified Information Systems Security Professional

CITL: Center for Information Technology Leadership

CIW: Center for Information Work

CKO: Chief Knowledge Officer

CLA: Cross-License Agreement

CLEC: Competitive Local Exchange Carrier

CLIA: Clinical Laboratory Improvement Amendments

CLIS: Clinical Laboratory Information System

CLM: Certificate Lifecycle Manager

CLMA: Clinical Laboratory Management Association

CLR: Common Language Runtime

CM: Clinical Modification

CM: Composite Message

CM: Configuration Management

CMDB: Change Management Data Base

CMDS: Chiropractic Minimum Data Set

CME: Common Message Element

CMET: Common Message Element Type

CMIO: Chief Medical Informatics Officer

CMIP: Common Management Information Protocol

CMIS: Case Mix Information System

CMIS: Common Management Information Service

CMMI-ACQ: Capability Maturity Module Integration for Acquisition

CMO: Chief Marketing Officer

CMOS: Complimentary Metal-Oxide Semiconductor

CMP©: Certified Medical Planner©

CMP: Change Management Program

CMR: Computerized Medical Record

CMRC: Claim Medicare Remark Codes

CMS: Centers for Medicare and Medicaid Services

CMS: Central Management System

CMS: Conversational Monitoring System

CMS: Cryptographic Message Syntax

CMS-1500: Standard claim form

CMT: Certified Medical Transcriptionist

CMV: Controlled Medical Vocabulary

CMVP: Cryptographic Module Validation Program

CMYK: Cyan, Magenta, Yellow, Black

CNA: Certified Network Administrator

CNC: Center for Nursing Classification

CNCL: Cancelled

CNE: Certified Network Engineer

CNHI: Committee for National Health Insurance

CNI: Certified Network Instructor

CNIO: Chief Nursing Informatics Officer

COA: Certificate of Authority

COA: Compliance Orientated Architecture

COACH: Canadian Health Informatics Association

COAS: Clinical Observation Access Service

COBIT: Control Object for Information Related Technology

COBOL: Common Business Orientated Language

COBRA: Consolidated Omnibus Budget Reconciliation Act

COC: AHIMA's Council on Certification

COD: Certificate of Destruction

CODEC: COmpression/DECompression

COLD/ERM: Computer Output Laser Disk/Enterprise Report Management

COM: Common Object Model

COM: Computer Output Microfilm

COM-B1 FORM: Attending physician (medical provider) statement

COO: Chief Operating Officer

COPPA: Children's Online Privacy Protection Act

COR: Cost of Risk

CORBA: Common Object Request Broker Architecture

CORBAMED: Common Object Request Broker Architecture for Medicine Facility

COS: Clinical Outcomes System

COS: Chip Operating System

COSE: Common Open Software Environment

COSS: Common Object Service Specifications

COSTAR: Computer Stored Ambulatory Record

COSTARS: Computer Stored Ambulatory Record System

COT: Chain of Trust

COTS: Commercial Off-the-Shelf

COW: Computer on Wheels

CP: Charge Posting

CP: Clinical Pathway

CP: Critical Pathway

CPD: Central Processing Department

CPG: Clinical Practice Guidelines

CPHIMS: Certified Professional in Healthcare Information and Management Systems

CPHRM: Certified Professional Health Risk Management

CPI: Characters Per Inch

CPI: Consistent Presentation of Images

CP/M: Control Program/Monitor or Control Program for Microprocessors

CPO: Chief Privacy Officer

CPOE: Computerized (Computer) Physician (Provider, Practitioner) Order Entry

CPOES: Computerized Physician (Provider, Practitioner) Order Entry System

CPP: Computer Platform Planning

CPP: Computer Program Package

CPP: Computer Purchase Program

CPR: Computerized Patient Record

CPR: Customary, Prevailing, and Reasonable

CPRI: Computer-based Patient Record Institute

CPRI-HOST: Computer-Based Patient Record Institute—Healthcare Open Systems Trials

CPRS: Computer-Based Patient Record System

CPS: Characters per second

CPT: *Current Procedural Terminology*

CPT-4: *Current Procedural Terminology,* Fourth Edition

CPU: Central Processing Unit

CR: Computed Radiology

CRA: Corporate Responsibility Act, of 2002

CRC: Computer Readable Card

CRC: Cyclic Redundancy Check

CREN: Corporation for Research and Educational Networking

CRL: Certificate Revocation List

CRM: Customer Resource Management

CRO: Chief Risk Officer

CRT: Cathode Ray Tube

CRUD: Create, Retrieve, Update, and Delete

CS: Channel Service

CS: Code Set

CSA: Canadian Standards Association

CSA: Computer Security Act

CSC: Claim Status Codes

CSCC: Claim Status Category Code

CSDTP: Credit Suisse Disruptive Technology Portfolio

CSHSC: Center for Studying Health Systems Change

CSI: Commission on Systems Interoperability

CSI: Computable Semantic Interoperability

CSID: Call Subscriber ID

CSMA: Carrier Sense Media (Multiple) Access

CSN: Circuit Switch Network

CSNW: Client Server Net Ware

CSO: Chief Security Officer

CSRDA: Cyber Security Research and Development Act

CSTA: Computer Supported Telephony Application

CSU: Channel Sharing Unit

CSV: Comma Separated Values

CT: Computer Telephony

CT: Consistent Time

CTI: Computer Telephony Integration

CTO: Chief Technology Officer

CTP: Community Technology Preview

CTS: Clear to Send

CTS: Common Terminal Service

CTV3: Clinical Terms, Version 3

CU: Channel Unit

CU: Control Unit

CU: See You

CUA: Common User Access

CUI: Character User Interface

CUI: Common User Interface

CUI: Concept Unique Identifier

CUPR: Customary Usual Prevailing Rate

CUPR: Customary Usual Prevailing Reasonable

CUSIP: Committee on Uniform Security Identification Procedures

CVE: Common Vulnerabilities and Exposures

CVO: Credential Verification Order

CVS: Concurrent Versioning System

CVSS: Common Vulnerability Scoring System

CWA: Communication Workers of America

CWE: Coded With Exceptions

CWE: Common Weakness Enumeration

CWIS: Campus Wide Information System

D2C: Detection to Correction

DA: Data Aggregation

DAC: Discretionary Access Control

DAD: Digital Audio Disk

DAE: Digital Audio Extraction

DAP: Directory Access Protocol

DARPA: Defense Advanced Research Projects Agency

DAS: Direct Attached Storage

DASD: Direct Access Storage Device

DAT: Digital Audio Tap

DAX: Digital Audio Exchange

DB: Data Base

dB: Decibel

DBLC: Data Base Life Cycle

DBM: Data Base Management

dBm: Decibel relative to one milliwatt

DBMMS: Data Base Medical Management System

DBMS: Data Base Management System

DBPSK: Differential Binary Phase Shift Keying

DBT: Digital Business Transformation

DC: Data Condition

DC: Diagnostic Code

DCA: Document Content Architecture

DCC: Data Content Committee

DCC: Designated Content Committee

DCC: Digital Compact Cassette

DCE: Data Circuit-Terminating Equipment

DCE: Distributed Computer Environment

DCG: Diagnostic Code Groups

DCI: Display Control Interface

DCL: Diabetes Care Link

DCN: Document Control Number

D-CODE: HCPS Level II Dental Code

DCOM: Distributed Content Object Model

DCS: Desktop Control Separation

DCS: Distributed Communication System

DD: Data Dictionary

DD: Double Density

DDCC: Designated Data Content Committee

DDE: Direct Data Entry

DDE: Dynamic Data Exchange

DDL: Data Definition Language

DDM: Distributed Data Management

DDN: Defense Data Network

DDNS: Dynamic Domain Name System

DDR: Double Data Rate

DDR2: Double Data Rate

DDS: Dependent Data Suffix

DDS: Digital Data Service (System)

DE: Data Element

DEA: Data Encryption Algorithm

DEA: Data Envelopment Analysis

DEC: Digital Equipment Corporation

DeCC: Dental Content Committee

DEEDS: Data Elements for Emergency Department Systems

DELOS WP5: Network on Excellence on Digital Libraries (EURO); Knowledge Extraction and Semantic Interoperability

DES: Data Encryption Standard

DFASHRM: Distinguished Fellow American Society for Healthcare Risk Management

DFD: Data Flow Diagram

DFS: Distributed File System

DFS: Dynamic Frequency Selection

DHCP: Dynamic Host Configuration Protocol

DHHS: Department of Health and Human Services

DHP: Dynamic Host Protocol

DHS: Department of Homeland Security

DI: Data Integrity

DI: Diagnostic Imaging

DIA: Document Interchange Architecture

DIB: Directory Information Base

DICOM: Digital Imaging and Communications in Medicine

DID: Direct Inward Dialing

DIF: Data Interchange Format

DII: Defense Information Infrastructure

DIMM: Double (Dual) Inline Memory Module

DIP: Dual Inline Package

DIS: Data Interchange Standard

DIS: Dental Information System

DIS: Draft International Standard

DIS: Drug Information System

DISA: Data Information Standards Association

DISA: Data Interchange Standards Association

DISA: Defense Information Systems Agency

DLC: Dynamic Link Control

DLL: Data Link Layer

DLL: Dynamic Link Library

DLS: Data Link Switch

DMA: Direct Memory Access

DMAA: Disease Management Association of America

DMCA: Digital Millennium Copyright Act

DMDS: Dental Minimum Data Set

DME: Durable Medical Equipment

DMERC: Durable Medical Equipment Regional Carrier

DMI: Desktop Management Interface

DMIS: Defense Medical Information System

DMIS: Department of Medical Information Services

DML: Data Manipulation Language

DNS: Digital Nervous System

DNS: Domain Name Server (System)

DNSSEC: Domain Name Server Secured

DOD: Department of Defense

DODIIS: Department of Defense Intelligent Information Systems

DOE: Department of Energy

DOE: Direct Order Entry

DOH: Department of Health

DOI: Date of Incident

DOI: Digital Object Identifier

DOJ: Department of Justice

DOL: Department of Labor

DOM: Document Object Model

DOQ: Doctor's Office Quality

DOQ-IT: Doctor's Office Quality-Information Technology

DOR: Date of Report

DOS: Date of Service

DOS: Denial of Service

DOS: Disk Operating System
DOSA: Denial of Service Attack
DP: Data Processing
DPAHC: Durable Power of Attorney for Health Care
DPH: Department of Public Health
DPI: Deep Packet Inspection
DPI: Dots Per Inch
DPM: Data Protection (Project) Manager
DPSK: Differential Phase Shift Key
DQDB: Distributed Queue Dual Bus
DQPSK: Differential Quadrature Phase Shift Keying
DRAM: Dynamic Random Access Memory
DRDA: Distributed Relation Database Architecture
DRI: Digital Research Inc.
DRM: Digital Rights Management
DRP: Disaster Recovery Plan
DRS: Designated Record Set
DRS: Distributed Resource Scheduler
DRV: Driver
DS: Digital Signal
DSA: Digital Signal Analyzer
DSA: Digital Signature Algorithm
DSA: Digital Storage Architecture
DSA: Directory Server Agent
DSI: Data Scene Investigation
DSL: Digital Subscriber Line
DSLAM: Digital Subscriber Line Access Multiplexor
DSM-IV: *Diagnostic and Statistical Manual of Mental Disorders,* Fourth Edition
DSML: Directory Services Markup Language
DSMMD: Diagnostic and Standard Manual of Mental Disorders—IV
DSMO: Designated Standards Maintenance Organization

DSP: Digital Signal Processor
DSR: Data Set Ready
DSS: Decision Support System
DSS: Digital Signature Standard
DSSS: Direct Sequence Spread Spectrum
DSTU: Draft Standards for Trial Use
DSU: Data (Sharing) Service Unit
DSVD: Digital Simultaneous Voice Data
DTD: Document Type Definition
DTE: Data Terminating Equipment
DTP: Desktop Publishing
DTR: Data Terminal Ready
DTS: Desktop Server
DTS: Digital Termination Service
DTV: Digital TV
DVCR: Digital Video Cassette Recorder
DVD: Digital Video (Versatile) Disc
DVD-R: Digital Video Disc—Recordable
DVD-RAM: Digital Video Disc—Random Access Memory
DVD-ROM: Digital Video Disc—Read Only Memory
DVD+RW: Digital Video Disc—Read Write
DVI: Digital Video Interactive
DWMS: Data Warehouse Management System

EA: Enterprise Architecture
EAI: Enterprise Application Integration
EAP: Extensible Authentication Protocol
EARN: European Academic Research Network
EBB: Eligibility Based Billing
EBCDIC: Extended Binary Code Decimal Information Code

EBM: Evidence Based Medicine

EC: Electronic Claim

EC: Electronic Commerce

ECC: Elliptic Curve Cryptography

ECF: Enhanced Connected Facility

ECHO: Electronic Computer Health Orientated

ECM: Enterprise Content Management

ECMF: Enhanced Connected Medical Facility

ECMQL: Electronic Care Management Qualification Logic

ECN: Electronic Communication Network

ECN: Explicit Congestion Notification

ECP: Explicit Congestion Packet

ED: Encapsulated Data

ED: Evidence Document

EDA: Event Driven Architecture

EDE: Electronic Data Exchange

EDGAR: Electronic Data Gathering, Analysts, and Retrieval

EDI: Electronic Data Interchange

EDIFACT: Electronic Data Interchange for Admission, Commerce, and Trade

EDIS: Electronic Data for Information Systems

EDIS: Electronic Data Interchange Standards

EDLIN: Edit Line

EDM: Electronic Data Management

EDMS: Electronic Document Management System

EDO RAM: Extended Data Output Random Access Memory

EDP: Electronic Data Processing

EDR: Enhanced Data Rate

EDS: Electronic Data Systems

EDS: European Digital Signal

EDU: Education and Training

EDW: External Developer Workstation

EEMR: Enterprise Electronic Medical Record

EEPROM: Electronic Erasable Programmable Read Only Memory

EF: Exposure Factor

EFF: Electronic Frontier Foundation

EFI: Electronic File Interchange

EFIO: Electronic File Interchange Organization

EFM: Electronic Forms Management

EFM: Enterprise Feedback Management

EFT: Electronic Funds Transfer

EGA: Enhanced Graphics Adapter

EGARCH: Exponential Generalized Autoregressive Conditional Heteroskedasticity

EGL: Enterprise Generation Language

EGP: Exterior Gateway Protocol

eHI: Electronic Health Information

eHI: e-Health Initiative

EHCR: Electronic Health Care Record

EHMR: Electronic Health Medical Record

EHNAC: Electronic Healthcare Network Accreditation Commission

EHR: Electronic Health Record

EHRS: Electronic Health Record System

EHRVA: Electronic Health Record Vendor's Association

EIA: Electronic Industries Association

EIDE: Enhanced Integrated Digital Electronics

EIN: Employee Identification Number

EIN: Employer Identification Number

EIN: Enterprise Information Networks

EIP: Electronic Information Portal

EIRP: Equivalent Isotropically Radiated Power

EIS: Enterprise Imaging Sharing

EIS: Enterprise (Executive) Information System

EIS: Executive Information Systems

EISA: Extended Industry Standard Architecture

EITM: Enterprise Information Technology Management

ELOC: Executable Line of Code

EM: Evaluation and Management

EM64T: Extended Memory 64 Technology

EMA: Electronic Mail Association

EMA: Enterprise Management Architecture

E-MAIL: Electronic Mail

EMAR: Electronic Medication Administration Record

EMC: Electronic Media (Medical) Claim

EMDS: Essential Medical Data Set

EMF: Electric and Magnetic Fields

EMI: Electro Magnetic Interface

EMI: Electro Magnetic Interference

EMOP: Emergency Mode Operating Plan

EMPI: Enterprise Master Patient (Person) Index

EMR: Electronic Medical Record

EMS: Emergency Management Service

EMVA©: Economic Medical Value Added©

ENIAC: Electronic Numerical Integrator and Computer

ENS: Enterprise Network Service

EOB: Explanation of Benefits

EOF: End of File

EOL: End of Line

EOM: End of Message

EOMB: Explanation of Medicaid Benefits

EOMB: Explanation of Medical Benefits

EOMB: Explanation of Medicare Benefits

EOMB: Explanation of Member Benefits

EOT: End of Transmission

EOTD: Enhanced Observer Time Difference

EPA: Environmental Protection Agency

EPF: Electronic Patient Folder

EPFT: Electronic Payment Funds Transfer

EPHI: Electronic Protected Health Information

EPIC: Explicitly Parallel Instruction Computing

EPR: Electronic Patient Record

EPSS: Electronic Performance Support System

EPSS: Electronic Preventive Services Selector

ERA: Electronic Remittance Advice

ERD: Emergency Repair Disk

ERD: Entity Relationship Diagram

ERISA: Employment Retirement Income Security Act

ERL: Electronic Receipt Listing

ERM: Electric Records Management

ERM: Enterprise Risk Management

ERMT: Electronic Records Management Technology

ERP: Enterprise Resource Planning

ES: Electronic Signature

ESA: Enterprise Service Architecture

ESB: Enterprise Service Bus

ESD: Electronic Software Distribution
ESDI: Enhanced Small Device Interface
ESF: External Source Format
ESIGN: Electronic Signature in Global National Commerce Act
ESL: Extensible Style sheet Language
ESP: Enhanced Service Provider
ESS: Electronic Switching System
ESS: Executable Support System
ETF: Electronically Traded Funds
ETL: Extraction Transformation Loading
EUA: Enterprise User Authentication
EUHID: Encrypted Universal Healthcare Identifier
EULA: End User License Agreement
EVA: Enterprise Virtual Array
EVDO: Evolution Data Optimized
EVNHID: Encrypted Voluntary National Healthcare Identification
EVRS: Electronic Viral Records System
EWCIS: Enterprise Wide Clinical Information Sharing
Ex-ASCII: Extended American Standard Code for Information Interchange
EXT-2FS: Second Extended File System

4FP: Fourth Framework (Health Telematics) Program
F2F: Face to Face
FAQ: Frequently Asked Questions
FAR: Federal Acquisition Regulation
FASHRM: Fellow American Society for Healthcare Risk Management
FAT: File Allocation Table
FAX: Facsimile Technology
FBCA: Federal Bridge Certification Authority

FCC: Federal Communications Commission
FCFS: First Come, First Served
FCS: Forefront Client Security
FDCPA: Fair Debt Collection Practices Act
FDDI: Fiber Distributed Data Interface
FDI: Foreign Direct Investment
FDM: Frequency Division Multiplex
FEC: Forward Error Correction
FEEA: Facilitated Enrollment by Electronic Application
FeHI: Foundation for e-Health Initiative
FEIN: Federal Employee Identification Number
FERPA: Family Educational Rights and Privacy Act
FF: Forefront
FFS: Fee-For-Service
FFS: Fast File System
FG: First Generation
FG: Fourth Generation
FHA: Federal Health Architecture
FHA: Forensic Health Accountant
FHFMA: Fellow Healthcare Financial Management Association
FHIMSS: Fellow of the Health Information and Management Systems Society
FI: Fiscal Intermediary
FIBRIC: First Boot RPM Installer and Configurator
FIM: Federal Identity Management
FIN: Federal Identification Number
FIP: Fair Information Practices
FIPS: Federal Information Processing Standard
FIX: Financial Information eXchange
FMEA: Failure Mode Effects Analysis
FOAF: Friend of a Friend
FOIA: Freedom of Information Act

FORE: Foundation of Research and Education
FORTRAN: Formula Translator
FPA: Federal Privacy Act
FPGA: Field Program Gate Array
FPMRAM: Fast Page Mode Random Access Memory
FPNW: File and Print Services for Netware
FPO: Facility Privacy Officer
FPS: Frames per Second
FQDN: Fully Qualified Domain Name
FQHC: Federally Qualified Health Center
FR: Federal Register
FRAD: Frame Relay Assemble/Disassemble
FSCSI: Fast Small Computer Systems Interface
FSMA: Financial Services Modernization Act of 1999
FSN: Full Service Network
FSO: Free Space Optics
FTAM: File Transfer, Access, and Management
FTC/A: Federal Trade Commission/Act
FTF: Face To Face
FTP: File Transfer Protocol
FTX: Fault Tolerant UNIX
FUD: Fear Uncertainty Doubt
FYI: For Your Information

<g.>: grin
GALEN: Generalized Architecture for Languages, Encyclopedias, and Nomenclatures
GALENM: Generalized Architecture for Languages, Encyclopedias, and Nomenclatures in Medicine
GAO: General Accounting Office

GARCH: Generalized Autoregressive Conditional Heteroskedasticity
GASSP: Generally Accepted Systems Security Principles
GB: Gigabyte
GBDSS: Graphics Based Decision Support System
GBPS: Gigabytes per Second
GCPR: Government Computer-based Patient Record
GDI: Graphics Device Interchange
GEHR: Good Electronic Health Record
GEHR: Good Electronic Healthcare Record
GEHR: Good European Healthcare Record
GHZ: Gigahertz
GIF: Graphic Interchange Format
GIG: Global Information Grid
GIGO: Garbage In–Garbage Out
GILS: Global Information Locator Service
GLBA: Gramm-Leach-Bliley Act
GMA: Graphics Media Accelerator
GMDN: Global Medical Device Nomenclature
GNU: GNU's Not Unix
GNU/GPL: GNU/General Public License
GOSIP: Government Open Systems Interconnections Profile
GPL: General Public License
GPMC: Group Policy Management Console
GPO: Group Policy Objects
GPRS: General Packet Radio Service
GPS: Global Positioning System
GSA: General Services Administration

GSI: Government Secure Intranet
GSM: Global System of Mobility
GSMC: Global System of Mobile Communications
GSNW: Gateway Services for Netware
GTEPS: General Telephone Electric Processing System
GUI: Graphical User Interface
GWSN: Gate Way Service Network

H: Hexadecimal
HACI: Health Associated Computer Infection
HAEI: Health Associated Electronic Infection
HAI: Health Associated Infection
HAMR: Heat Assisted Magnetic Recording
HAN: Health Alert Network
HBCS: Hospital Billing and Collection Service
HCAHPS: Hospital Consumer Assessment of Health Providers and Systems
HCC: Health Care Clearinghouse
HCCA: Health Care Conference Administrators
HCCMC: Health Care Code Maintenance Committee
HCCSI: Health Care Claims Status Inquiry
HCEA: Healthcare Convention and Exhibitors Association
HCFA: Health Care Financing Administration
HCFA 1500: Health Care Financing Administration Universal Billing Form
HCFA-PSF: Health Care Financing Administration—Provider Specific File

HCFAR: Health Care Financing Administration Ruling
HCII: Health Care Information Infrastructure
HCIN: Health Care Information Network
HCIRC: Health Care Information Resource Center
HCISPP: Health Care Information Standards Planning Panel
HCIT: Health Care Information Technology
HCL: Hardware Compatibility List
HCPCS: Healthcare Common Procedural Coding System
HCPCS: HCFA Common Procedure Coding System
HCQIA: Health Care Quality Improvement Act
HCTA: Health Care Technology Assessment
HCTP: Health Care Technology Package
HCTS: Health Care Technical Service
HDC: Health Data Center
HDC: HCFA Data Center
HDRD: High Dynamic Range Display
HDS©: Health Dictionary Series©
HDSC: Health Data Standards Committee
HDSL: High-Bit-Rate Digital Subscriber Line
HDSS: Healthcare Decision Support System
HDTV: High Definition Television
HDVON: High Definition Video Over Net
HDWA: Healthcare Data Warehousing Association

HEDIC: Healthcare Electronic Data Information Coalition

HEDIS: Health Plan Employer Data Information System

HEDITP: Healthcare Electronic Data Information Trading Partner

HEFM™: Healthcare Enterprise Feedback Management©

HEITM: Health Information Technology Management

HEN: Healthcare EDI Network

HF: High Frequency

HFMA: Healthcare Financial Management Association

HFS: Hierarchical File System

HGC: Hercules Graphics Card

HHCC: Home Health Care Classification

HHIC: Hawaii Health Information Corporation

HHSS: Health and Human Services Survey

HI: Healthcare Informatics

HI: Health Information

HIAA: Health Insurance Association of America

HIAL: Health Information Access Layer

HIBCC: Health Industry Business Communications Council

HIC: Healthcare Industrial Complex

HIC: Health Information Center

HIC: Health Insurance Claim

HIE: Health Information Exchange

HIEDIC: Health Industry Electronic Data Information Corporation

HIF: Healthcare Information Framework

HIM: Health Information Management

HIMA: Health Industry Manufacturers Association

HIMI: Health Information Management Infrastructure

HIMICS: Health Insurance Management Information Control System

HIMS: Health Information Management Systems

HIMSS: Healthcare Information and Management Systems Society

HIN: Health Information Networking

HIN: Health Information Networks

HINA: Health Information Network Australia

HINT: Healthcare Information Networks and Technology

HIPAA: Health Insurance Portability and Accountability Act of 1996

HIPAADD: Health Insurance Portability and Accountability Act Data Dictionary

HIPDB: Healthcare Integrity and Protection Data Bank

HIPPSC: Health Insurance Prospective Payment System Code

HIPS©: Hospital (Healthcare) Investment Policy Statement©

HIPS: Host Intrusion Protection System

HIS: Health (Healthcare) Information System

HIS: Hospital Information System

HISAC: Healthcare Information Sharing and Analysis Center

HISB: Healthcare Informatics Standards Board

HISCC: Health Information Standards Coordinating Committee

HISDG: Health Information Systems Development Guide

HISP: Health Infrastructure Support Program

HISPC: National Health Information Security and Privacy Collaboration

HISPP: Healthcare Informatics Standards Planning Panel

HIT: Health Information Technology

HIT: Hospital Information Technology

HITA: Health Information Technology Auditor

HITPA: Health Information Technology Promotion Act

HITSP: Healthcare Information Technology Standards Panel

HIX: Health Information Exchange

HL7: Health Level 7

HL7: Health Level Seven International

HLC: Healthcare Leadership Council

HLL: High Level Language

HMG: Hospital Medical Group

HMIS: Health (Hospital) Management Information System

HMO: Health Maintenance Organization

HMRI: Hospital Medical Records Institute

HOA: Health Oversight Agency

HOLAP: Hybrid Online Analytic Processing

HON: Health on the Net

HONCode: Health on the Net Code

HONF: Health on the Net Foundation

HOST: Healthcare Open Systems Trial

HPAG: HIPAA Policy Advisory Group

HPCC: High Performance Computing Communications

HPFS: High Performance File System

HPO: Hospital Privacy Officer

HPSA: Health Professional Shortage Area

HR: Health Records

HR: High Rate

HR 4157: Healthcare IT Bill

HRA: Health Risk Assessment

HRDUC: High Resolution Displays Unlimited Colors

HRF: Health Related Facility

HRIMS: Human Resource Information Management System

HRIS: Human Resources Information System

HRSA: Health Resources and Services Administration

HSC: Health System Change

HSPD: Homeland Security Presidential Directive

HSM: Hierarchical Storage Management

HSO: Healthcare Security Officer

HSO: Health Security Officer

HSO: Hospital Security Officer

HSSI: High Speed Serial Interface

HTML: Hyper Text Markup Language

HTTP: Hyper Text Transmission Protocol

HTTPS: Hyper Text Transmission Protocol Secure

HW: Hard Wire

IA: Identification and Authentication

IA: In Area

IAIABC: International Association of Industrial Accident Boards and Commissions

IANA: Internet Assigned Numbers Authority

IAP: Internet Access Provider

IBE: Internet Based Education

IBFS: Interim Billing and Follow-up System

IBG: International Biometric Group

IBIA: International Biometric Industry Association

IBM: International Business Machines, Corp.

IBMT: Internet Based Medical Training

IBT: Internet Based Training

IC: Integrated Circuit

ICANN: Internet Corporation for Assigned Names and Numbers

ICC: Integrated Circuit Chip

ICD: *International Classification of Diseases*

ICD-9-CM: *International Classification of Diseases, Ninth Edition, Clinical Modification*

ICD-10-CM: *International Classification of Diseases, Tenth Edition, Clinical Modification*

ICF: Internet Connection Firewall

ICIDH: International Classification of Impairments, Disability, and Handicaps

ICIDH-2: International Classification of Functioning, Disability, and Health International

ICM: Information Classification Management

ICMP: Internet Control Message Protocol

ICN: International Council of Nurses

ICON: International Council of Nurses

ICPC-2: *International Classification of Primary Care* (2nd Edition)

ICQ: I Seek You

ICR: Intelligent Call Routing

ICR: Intelligent Character Recognition

ICS: Internet Connection Sharing

ICT: Information Communication Technology

ICU: I See You

ICWs: Internet-based Collaborative Workgroups

ID: Identification

IDE: Integrated Development Environment

IDE: Integrative Drive (Device) Electronics

IDHI: Individually Identifiable Health Information

IDM: Image Document Management

IDN: Integrated Delivery Network

IDR: Intelligent Document Recognition

IDS: Intrusion Detection System

IE: Internet Explorer®

IEC: International Electrotechnical Commission

IEEE: Institute of Electrical and Electronics Engineers, Inc.

IETF: Internet Engineering Task Force

IFC: Internet Foundation Class

IFQC: Illinois Foundation for Quality Healthcare

IG: Implementation Guide

IGARCH: Integrated Generalized Autoregressive Conditional Heteroskedasticity

IGES: Initial Graphics Exchange Specifications

IGP: Internet Gateway Protocol

IGRP: Interior Gateway Routing Protocol

IHC: Internet Health Coalition

IHCEBI: Interactive Health Care Eligibility and Benefits Inquiry

IHCEBR: Interactive Health Care Eligibility and Benefits Response

IHDN: Integrated Health Delivery Network

IHE: Integrated Healthcare Enterprise

IHI: Institute for Healthcare Improvement

IHIE: Indian Health Information Exchange

IHO: Integrated Health Organization

IHRBA: Independent Health Record Bank Act

IHS: Indian Health Service

IIA: Information Industry Association

IIA: Information Interchange Architecture

IID: Individually Identifiable Data

IIHI: Individually Identifiable Health Information

IIR: Institute for International Research

IIS: Internet Information Server (Service)

IITF: Information Infrastructure Task Force

IKE: Internet Key Exchange

IKEP: Internet Key Exchange Protocol

ILD: Injection Laser Diode

ILEC: Independent Local Exchange Carrier

ILM: Information Lifecycle Management

IM: Instant Message

IMAP: Internet Message Access Protocol

*i*MBA: Institute of Medical Business Advisors, Inc©

IMCO: In My Considered Opinion

IMD: Internet Management Department

IMHO: In My Humble Opinion

IMIA: International Medical Informatics Association

IMKI: Institute for Medical Knowledge Implementation

IMNSO: In My Not So Humble Opinion

IMO: In My Opinion

IMP: Internet Control Message Protocol

IMP: Internet Message Protocol

IMS: Information Management System

IMS: Integrated Medical System

IMS: IP Multimedium Subsystem

IMSDN: Integrated Medical Systems Digital Network

INCITS: InterNational Committee for Information Technology Standards

INI: Initiation

I/O: Input/Output

IOM: Institute of Medicine

IOS: Internet Operating System

IP: Internet Protocol

IP: Intrusion Protection

IPA: Internet Protocol Address

IPL: Intellectual Property Litigator

IPMI: Intelligent Platform Management Interface

IPN: Internet Planetary Network

IPS: Intrusion Prevention System

IPSEC: Internet Protocol Security

IPX: Internet Packet Exchange

IR: Information Retrieval

IR: Interrupt Request

IRC: Internet Relay Chat

IRD: Information Resource Department

IRDA: Internet Resource Department Architecture

IRL: In Real Life

IRM: Information Resource Management

IRMI: International Risk Management Institute

IRQ: Interrupt ReQuest

IRTF: Internet Research Task Force

IRV: Imaging, Robotics, Virtual Reality

IS: Information Services (Systems)
ISA: Internet (Industry) Security Acceleration
ISA: Internet (Industry) Standard Architecture
iSAC: Information Sharing and Analysis Center
ISCSI: Internet Small Computer System Interface
ISDN: Integrated Services Delivery Network
ISDN: Integrated Services Digital Network
ISHTAE: Implementing Secure Healthcare Telematic Applications in Europe
ISIPP: Institute for Spam and Internet Public Policy
ISM: Industrial, Scientific, and Medical
ISN: Integrated Service Network
ISO: Independent Sales Organization
ISO: International Standards Organization
ISOC: Internet Society
ISO/TC: International Organization for Standardization/Technical Committee for Health Informatics
ISP: Internet Service Provider
ISSA: Information Systems Security Association
ISTM: It Seems To Me
ISTR: I Seem To Recall
ISV: Independent Software Vendor
IT: Information Technology
IT: Internet Telephony
ITAA: Information Technology Association of America
ITAC: Information Technology Association of Canada

ITI: Information Technology Industry
ITIL: Information Technology Infrastructure Library
ITL: Information Technology Laboratory
ITMRA: Information Technology Management Reform Act
ITR: Internet Talk Radio
ITS/CAES: Intermarket Trading System/Computer Assisted Execution System
ITU: International Telecommunications Union
ITUCCT: International Telecommunications Union Consultative Committee for Telecommunications
ITV: Internet TV
ITV: In Transit Visibility
IVD: Interactive Video Disk
IVDS: Interactive Video Data Services
IVR: Interactive Video Response
IVR: Interactive Voice Response
IVT: Interactive Voice Technology
IXC: Interchange Carrier

JAAS: Java Authentication and Authorization Service
JAIM: Journal of Artificial Intelligence in Medicine
JAM: Java Agent-enabled Marketplace
JBOD: Just a Bunch of Disks
JCAHO: Joint Commission on Accreditation of Healthcare Organizations
J-CODE: Higher level II HCPCS code

JDBC: Java Data Base Connectivity
JDK: Java Development Kit
JEIDA: Japanese Electronic Industry Development Association
JFC: Java Foundation Class
JHITA: Joint Healthcare Information Technology Alliance
JMAPI: Java Management Application Program Interface
JMS: Java Message Service
JNI: Java Native Interface
JOE: Java Objects Everywhere
JPEG: Joint Photographic Experts Group
JRE: JAVA Runtime Environment
JSF: Java Server Face
JSR: Java Specific Request
JTC: Joint Technical Committee
JV: Joint Venture
JVM: Java Virtual Machine
JWG: Joint Working Group

K: Kilobytes; KB
KB: Kilobyte, or 1,024 bytes
Kbps: Kilobytes per second
KBS: Knowledge Based System
KHz: Kilohertz; one thousand cycles per second
KIN: Key Image Note
KMS: Key Management Services
KNN: K-Nearest Neighbor
KPI: Key Performance Indicator

L2TP: Layer 2 Tunneling Protocol
L8R: Later
LA: Lightweight Authentication
LAMP: Linux, Apache, MySQL, and PHP/Python/Perl
LAN: Local Area Network
LAP: Link Access Procedure
LAT: Local Area Transport
LBRV: Low Bit Rate Voice

LCA: Labor Condition Application
LCC: Life-Cycle Cost
LCD: Liquid Crystal Display
LCMS: Learning Content Management System
LDAP: Lightweight Directory Access Protocol
LEADERS: Lightweight Epidemiology Advanced Detection and Emergency Response System
LEAP: Lightweight and Efficient Application Protocol
LEC: Local Exchange Carrier
LED: Light Emitting Diode
LEO: Low Earth Orbit
LF: Line Feed
LF: Low Frequency
LFN: Long File Name
LHII: Local Health Information Infrastructure
LIMS: Laboratory Information Management System
LIS: Library Information System
LKG: Last Known Good
LLC: Logic Link Control
LMD: Lab Model Data
LMS: Learning Management System
LOINC: Logical Observations Identifiers, Names, and Codes
LOIS: Limited Order Information System
LOL: Laughing Out Loud
LONI: Laboratory of Neuro Imaging
LPI: Lines per Inch
LPM: Lines per Minute
LQS: Lexicon Query Service
LSD: Least Significant Digit
LSI: Large Scale Integration
LSL: Links Support Layer
LSM: Linux Security Module

LU: Logical Unit
LUA: Limited User Account
LUN: Logical Unit Number
LWF: Laboratory Scheduled Workflow
LWP: Lightweight Protocol

MA: Medicare Advantage
MAC: Mandatory Access Control
MAC: Media Access Control
MAC: Message Authentication Code
MACA: Media Access Control Address
MAE: Macintosh Application Environment
MAE: Metropolitan Area Exchange
MAGE: MicroArray and Gene Expression
MAID: Massive Array of Idle Disks
MAN: Metropolitan (Mobile) Area Network
MAP: Manufacturing Automaton Protocol
MAPD: Medicare Advantage Prescription Drugs
MAPI: Messaging Application Program Interface
MAPS: Mail Abuse Prevention System
MAR: Medical Administration Record
MAS: Medical Archiving System
MASHARE: Massachusetts Health Area Regional Exchange
MATMO: Medical Advanced Technology Management Office
MAU: Multiple Access Units
Mb: Megabit; 1,024 KB; 1,048, 576 bits
MB: Megabyte
MB: Mother Board

MBA©: Medical Business Advisors, Inc©
MBAVN©: Medical Business Advisors Virtual Network©
MBAVU©: Medical Business Advisors Virtual University©
MBDS: Minimum Basic Data Set
Mbps: Megabytes per Second
MBR: Master Boot Record
MBS: Microsoft Business Solutions
MBWA: Management By Walking Around
MCCA: Medicine Coding Council of Australia
MCCIP: Medicare Chronic Care Improvement Program
MCNE: Master Certified Network Engineer
MCP: Microsoft Certified Professional
MCSE: Microsoft Certified Systems Engineer
MCT: Microsoft Certified Trainer
MCU: Micro Controller Unit
MCU: Multipoint Control Unit
MCV: Mobile Command Vehicle
MDA: Model Drive Architecture
MDC: Medical Data Condition
MDDBMS: MultiDimensional Database Management Systems
MDM: Medical Document Management (Message)
MDS: Minimum Data Set
MDSS: Medical Decision Support System
MEC: Medical Education Collaborative
MEDIX: Medical Data Interchange Standard
MEDLARS: Medical Education Literature Analysis and Retrieval System

MEDLINE: Medical Literature and Analysis Retrieval System Online

MEDPAR: Medicare Provider Analysis and Review

MeDRA: Medical Dictionary for Regulatory Activities

MEDS: Minimum Emergency Data Set

MEFM: Medical Enterprise Feedback Management©

MEHUG: Minnesota EDI Healthcare Users Group

MEPS: Medical Expenditure Panel Survey

MeSH: Medical Subject Headings database

MEVA©: Medical Economic Value Added©

MEVA: Medical Enterprise Virtual Array

MFD: MultiFunction Device

MFIPS©: Medical Financial Investment Policy Statement©

MFM: Modified Frequency Modulation

MFS: Medicare Fee Schedule

MFT: Master File Table

MGMA: Medical Group Management Association

MHDC: Massachusetts Health Data Consortium

MHDI: Minnesota Health Data Institute

MHS: Medicare Health Support

MHS: Military Health System

MHS: Medical Health Systems

MHS: Message Handling Service

MHSP: Medical Health Support Program

MHz: Megahertz

MI: Medical Imaging

MIA: Medicare Imaging Act of 2006

MIAME: Minimum Information About a Microarray Experiment

MIB: Management Information Block

MIB: Medical Information Bureau

MIB: Medical Information Bus

MIC: Message Integrity Code

MICM: Medical Information Classification Management

MICR: Magnetic Ink Character Recognition

MID: Management Information Department

MIDI: Musical Instrument Digital Interface

MIIPS©: Medical Institution Investment Policy Statement©

MILM: Medical Information Lifecycle Management

MIME: Multipurpose Internet Mail Extension

MIPS©: Medical Investment Policy Statement©

MIPS: Millions of Instructions Per Second

MIRC: Medical Information Resource Center

MIS: Management Information System

MISB: Medical Information Standards Board

MIT: Master of Information Technology

MLA: Medical Library Association

M-LEARN: Mobile or wireless distance learning

MLM: Medical Logic Model (Mode)

MLP: Medical Language Processing

MMA: Medical Marketing Association

MMA: Medicare Modernization Act of 2003

MMC: Microsoft Management Console

MMDN: Managed Medical Data Network

MMDS: Medical Minimum Data Set

MMSRT: Microsoft Malicious Software Removal Tool

MOBB: Month of Browser Bugs

MODEM: Modulate/Demodulate

MoHCA: Mobile Health Care Alliance

MOLAP: Multidimensional Online Analytical Processing

MOU: Memorandum of Understanding

MP3: MPEG-1 Audio Layer 3

MPEG: Motion Picture Experts Group

MPI: Master Patient Index

MPI: Master Person Index

MPIPS©: Medical Practice Investment Policy Statement©

MPLS: MultipleProtocol Label Switch

MPOA: Multi Protocol Over ATM

MPP: Massive Parallel Processing

MR: Medical Record(s)

MRAM: Magnetic Resistant Access Memory

MRARC: Medicare Remittance Advice Remark Codes

MRI: Magnetic Resonance Image

MRI: Medical Records Institute

MSAU: Multiple Station Access Unit

MSCHAP: Microsoft Challenge Handshake Protocol

MSD: Microsoft Diagnostic

MS-DOS: Microsoft Disk Operating System©

MSH: Medical Subject Heading

MS-HUG: Microsoft Healthcare Users Group©

MSO: Management Services Organization

MSP: Management Service Provider

MSP: Medicare Secondary Payer

MSRT: Malicious Software Removal Tool

MSSP: Managed Security Service Provider

MTBF: Mean Time before Failure

MTBF: Mean Time between Failures

MTS: Medicare Transaction System

MTTD: Mean Time to Diagnose

MTTR: Mean Time to Repair

MTU: Maximum Transition Unit

MUE: Medically Unbelievable Event

MUG: Macintosh User Group

MUMPS: Massachusetts General Hospital Utility Multiprogramming System

MUX: Multiplexer

MVNO: Mobile Virtual Network Operator

MVS: Multiple Virtual Storage

MWS: Medical Warning System

MY: Member Year

MYOB: Mind Your Own Business

NAC: Network Administration (Admission) Control

NACDS: National Association of Chain Drug Stores

NACHA: National Automated Clearinghouse Association

NAHAM: National Association of Healthcare Access Management

NAHDO: National Association of Health Data Organizations

NAHIT: National Alliance for Health Information Technology

NAK: Negative Acknowledgment

NANDA: North American Nursing Diagnoses Association

NAP: Network Access Point
(Protection)

NAR: Nursing Assessment Record

NAS: Networked Attached Storage

NASI: Netware Asynchronous
Service Interface

NASMD: National Association of
State Medicaid Directors

NAT: Network Address Translation

NAU: Network Access Unit

NBS: National Bureau of Standards

NC: Network Computer

NCA: Network Computing
Architecture

NCCA: National Commission for
Certifying Agencies

NCCH: National Center for
Classification in Health

NCCI: National Correct Coding
Initiative

NCEMI: National Center for Emergency Medicine Informatics

NCH: National Claims History

NCHICA: North Carolina Healthcare
Information and Communications
Alliance

NCHIT: National Coordinator for
Health Information Technology

NCHS: National Center for Health
Statistics

NCHSR: National Center for Health
Services Research

NCLSI: National Clinical and
Laboratory Standards Institute

NCP: Network Controlled Program

NCP: Not Copy Protected

NCPA: National Community
Pharmacist Association

NCPDP: National Committee for
Prescription Drug Programs

NCQA: National Committee for
Quality Assurance

NCSA: National Computer Security
Association

NCSC: National Computer Security
Center

NCSC: North Carolina Supercomputing Center

NCSDC: National Community Services Data Committee

NCSDD: National Community
Services Data Dictionary

NCSI: Network Communications
Services Interface

NCSIMG: National Community
Services Information Management Group

NCTA: National Cable and Telecommunications Association

NCVHS: National Committee on
Vital and Health Statistics

NDC: National Drug Code

NDIS: Network Driver Interface
Specifications

NDSS: Nursing Decision Support System

NE: Never Event

NEC: Not Elsewhere Classified

NEDSS: National Electronic Disease
Surveillance System

NEHEN: New England Healthcare
EDI Network

NEMA: National Electrical
Manufacturer's Association

NetBEUI: NetBIOS Extended User
Interface

NetBIOS: Network Basic Input
Output System

NFS: Network File System

NGC: National Guideline
Clearinghouse

NHCAFA: National Health Care
Anti-Fraud Association

NHCSR: National Health Care
Standards Reform

NHDC: National Health Data Committee

NHDD: National Health Data Dictionary

NHDR: National Healthcare Disparities Report

NHI: National Health Index (NZ) New Zealand

NHIA: National Health Information Agreement

NHII: National Health Information Infrastructure

NHIMAC: National Health Information Management Advisory Council

NHIMG: National Health Information Management Group

NHIN: National Health Information Network

NHISAC: National Health Information Standards Advisory Council

NHIT: National Health Information Technology

NHMRCA: National Health and Medical Research Council Australia

NHQR: National Healthcare Quality Report

NHS: National Health Service

NHSC: National Health Service Corps

NHSnet: National Health Service Network

NI: National Identifier

NI: Nursing Informatics

NIAP: National Information Assurance Partnership

NIC: Network Information Center

NIC: Network Interface Card

NIC: Nursing Intervention Classification

NICE: National Institute for Clinical Excellence

NIDSEC: Nursing Information and Data Set Evaluation Center

NIH: National Institute of Health

NII: National Information Infrastructure

NII-HIN: National Information Infrastructure—Health Information Network

NIMH: National Institute of Mental Health

NIS: Network Information Service

NIS: Nursing Information System

NIST: National Institute of Standards and Technology

NITC: National Information Technology Coordinator

NJSHORE: New Jersey Strategic HIPAA/Healthcare Organization and Regional Effort

NLM: National Library of Medicine

NLP: Natural Language Processing

NLSP: Network Layered Security Protocol

NM: Nuclear Medicine

NMI: Nuclear Medicine Integration

NMDS: National Minimum Data Set

NMDS: Nursing Minimum Data Set

NMMDS: Nursing Management Minimum Data Set

NNTP: Network News Transfer Protocol

NOAR: National Organization for Amateur Radio

NOC: Network Operations Center

NOC: Not Otherwise Clarified

NOC: Nursing Outcome Classification

NOI: Notice of Intent

NOS: Network Operating System

NOS: Not Otherwise Specified

NPDB: National Practitioner Data Bank

NPDW: National Patient Data Warehouse

NPEPS: National Plan Enumerator and Provider System

NPF: National Provider File

NPI: National Provider Identification

NPID: National Patient ID

NPID: National Payer ID

NPID: National Provider ID

NPP: Non-Participating Physician/ Provider

NPP: Non-Participating Practitioner

NPP: Non-Professional Provider

NPP: Notice of Privacy Practice

NPPES: National Plan and Provider Enumeration System

NPR: National Provider Registry

NPRM: Notice of Proposed Rulemaking

NPS: National Provider System

NRCNAS: National Research Council of the National Academy of Sciences

NSA: National Security Agency

NSABB: National Science Advisory Board for Biosecurity

NSF: National Standard Format

NSIT: Networking Service Information Technology

NSP: Network Service Provider

NSTL: National Software Testing Laboratory

NT: New Technology

NTFS: Net Technology File System

NTIA: National Telecommunications and Information Administration

NTK: Need to Know

NTM: National Technology Management

NTSC: National Television System Committee

NUBC: National Uniform Billing Committee

NUCC: National Uniform Claim Committee

NUCC: Numbering Uniform Code Council

NUMA: Non-Uniform Memory Architecture

NVD: National Vulnerability Database

NVSS: National Vital Statistics System

NWIP: New Work Item Proposal

NYACH: New York Automated Clearing House

NYCHA: New York Clearing House Association

NZHIS: New Zealand Health Information Service

OA: Open Access

OA: Out of Area

OACIS: Open Architecture Clinical Information System

OAI: Open Application Interface

OASIS: Organization for the Advancement of Structured Information Standards

OASIS: Outcome and Assessment System Information Set

OAV: Object, Attribute, Value

OBRA: Omnibus Budget Reconciliation Act of 1987 and 1989

OCA: Outstanding Claims Account

OCE: Outpatient Code Editor

OCIE: Online Computer Image (Information) Exchange

OCIE: Optical Character Information Exchange

OCMIE: Optical Character Medical Information Exchange

OCR: Office of Civil Rights

OCR: Optical Character Recognition

OCSP: Online Certificate Status Protocol

OD: On Demand

ODA: Open Document Architecture

ODC: On-Demand Computing

ODF: Open Document Format

ODM: Operational Data Model

ODS: Operational Data Store

OEM: Original Equipment Manufacturer

OER: Outcomes and Effectiveness Research

OFCN: Organization for Community Networks

OFDM: Orthogonal Frequency Division Multiplexing

OFNC: Office of National Coordinator

OHCA: Organized Health Care Arrangement

OHIH: Office of Health and Information Highway

OHPA: Ontario Health Providers Association

OIC: Oh, I See

OID: Object Identifier

OIG: Office of Inspector General

OIS: Organization for Internet Safety

OISDAHCPR: Office of Information Systems and Development Agency for Health Care Policy and Research

OLA: Object Linked Embedding

OLAP: Online Analytic Processing

OLE: Object Linked Embedding

OLPC: One Laptop Per Child

OLTP: On Line Transaction Processing

OMB: Office of Management and Budget

OMDS: Optometric Minimum Data Set

OMDS: Osteopathic Minimum Data Set

OMG: Object Management Group

ON: Operations Network

ONA: Open Network Architecture

ONC: Open Network Computer

ONCHIT: Office of National Coordination for Health Information Technology

OOA: Out of Area

OODB: Object Orientated Data Base

OODBMS: Object Orientated Data Base Management System

OOFS: Object Oriented File System

OON: Out of Network

OOP: Object Oriented Programming

OOP: Out of Pocket

OP: On Premise

OPN: Other Physician (Provider) Number

OPSEC: Operational Security

ORB: Object Request Broker

ORBMS: Open Relay Behavior Modification System

ORF: Operating Room of the Future

ORM: Order Message (general)

OS: Operating System

OS/2: Operating System/2

OSHA: Occupational Safety and Health Act

OSI: Open System Interconnection

OSIL: Open System Interface Layer

OSP: Online Service Provider

OSPF: Open Shortest Path First

OSS: Open Source Software

OSS: Open Source Strategy

OSS: Operations Support System

OSS: Order Support System

OTOH: On the Other Hand

OU: Organizational Units

OVAL: Open Vulnerability and Assessment Language

OWASP: Open Web Application Security Project

P2P: Patient to Patient
P2P: Patient to Physician
P2P: Peer to Peer
P2P: Provider to Patient
P2P: Provider to Provider
P2V: Physical to Virtual
P4P: Pay for Performance
PA: Patriot Act
PACS: Picture Archiving and Communication System
PAG: Policy Advisory Group
PAP: Password Authentication Protocol
PAS: Patient Administration System
PATA: Parallel Advanced Technology Attachment
PAYERID: Medicare Pre-HIPAA National Payer ID Initiative
PBCC: Packet Binary Convolution Coding
PBM: Pharmacy Benefits Manager
PBX: Private Branch Exchange
PC: Personal Computer
PC: Professional Component
PCHRI: Personally Controlled Health Records Infrastructure
PCI: Payment Card Industry
PCI: Peripheral Component Interconnect
PCIS: Patient Care Information System
PCM: Pulse Code Modulation
PCMCIA: Personal Computer Memory Card International Association
PCR: Patient Care Record
PCS: Personal Communications Service
PCTS: Patient Care Tracking System
PD: Peripheral Device

PDA: Personal Digital Assistant
PDC: Primary Domain Controller
PDCA CYCLE: Plan-Do-Check-Act Cycle
PDF: Portable Document Format (File)
PDI: Portable Data Imaging
PDN: Packet Data Network
PDP: Prescription Drug Plan
PDP: Programmed Data Processor
PDPSA: Personal Data Privacy and Security Act
PDQ: Patient (Provider/Practitioner) Demographic Query
PDU: Protocol Data Unit
PE: Portable Execution
PEF: Portable Execution File
PEM: Privacy Enhanced Mail
PERL: Practical Extraction and Report Language
PET: Positron Emission Tomography
PFCRA: Program Fraud Civil Remedies Act
PFFS: Private Fee-For-Service
PGP: Presentation of Grouped Procedures
PGP: Pretty Good Privacy
PHI: Protected Health Information
PHI: Public Health Informatics
PHIE: Philadelphia Health Information Exchange
PHIEF: Protected Health Information Electronic Form
PHII: Public Health Informatics Institute
PHIN: Public Health Information Network
PHIPA: Protected Health Information Privacy Act
PHIT: Private Health Information Technology

PHITP: Private Health Information Technology Program
PHP: Personal Home Page
PHR: Personal Health(care) Record
PHR: Protected Health(care) Record
PHS: Public Health Service
PI: Personal Information
PI: Podiatric Imaging
PIC: Patient Information Center
PIC: Physician Information Center
PICS: Patient (Provider) Information Control System
PICS: Physician Information Control System
PID: Patient Identifiable Data
PIDS: Personal (Physician/Practitioner) Identification Service
PIFI: Personally Identifiably Financial Information
PIHI: Personally Identifiable Health Information
PIM: Platform Independent Model
PIN: Personal Identification Number
PING: Packet Internet Grouper
PIP: Periodic Interim Payment
PIR: Patient (Physician/Practitioner) Information Reconciliation
PIRT: Phishing Incident Reporting and Termination
PIS: Pathology (Pharmacy) Information System
PIS: Podiatry Information System
PIT: Pathology (Pharmacy) Information Transfer
PITAC: President's Information Technology Advisory Committee
PIX: Patient (Physician/Practitioner) Identifier Cross-reference profile
PKAF: Public Key Authentication Framework

PKI: Private Key Infrastructure
PKI: Public Key Infrastructure
PKIX: Public Key Infrastructure for X.509 Certificates
PL: Public Law
PLL: Phase Lock Loop
PLM: Product Lifecycle Management
PMDS: Podiatric Minimum Data Set
PMI: Patient Master Index
PMN: Patient Management Network
PMO: Program Management Office
PMP: Project Management Professional
PMS: Practice Management System
PNDS: Peri-operative Nursing Data Set
PNG: Potable Network Graphics
PnP: Plug and Play
POC: Proof of Concept
POCCSP: Point of Care Clinical Support System
POCS: Point of Care System
POD: Ping Of Death
POE: Point of Entry
POL: Physician Office Link
POP: Point of Presence
POP3: Post Office Protocol 3
PORT: Patient Outcomes Research Teams
POS: Palm Operating System
POS: Physician (Provider/Practitioner) Office Systems
POS: Place of Service
POS: Point of Service
POSIX: Portable Open (Operating) Systems Interface
POST: Power On-Self Test
POTS: Plain Old Telephone System
POW: Point of Welcome
PP: Protection Profile

PPP: Point to Point Protocol
PPPoE: Point to Point Protocol Entry
PPS: Prospective Payment System
PPTP: Point to Point Transmission Protocol
PPWF: Post Processing Workflow
PQA: Pharmacy Quality Alliance
PRA: Paperwork Reduction Act
PRAM: Parameter Random Access Memory
PRG: Procedure-Related Group
PRI: Patient Review Instrument
PRIT: Physician Regulatory Issues Team
PRM: Patient (Partner) Relationship Management
PRM: Patient Resource Management
PROM: Programmable Read Only Memory
ProPAC: Prospective Payment Assessment Commission
PROREC: Promotion Strategy for European Electronic Health Care Records
PRRB: Physician (Provider) Reimbursement Review Board
PRS: Patient Record System
PSA: Patient (Physician/Provider/ Practitioner) Synchronized Application
PSI: Payment Status Indicator
PSS: Patient Self-Service
PSS: Physician Self-Service
.PST: MSN Outlook Personal Storage file
PSTN: Public Switched Telephone Network
PSU: Power Supply Unit
PTC: Provider Taxonomy Code
PTL: Program Triage Logic
PTT: Postal, Telegraph, and Telephone

PVC: Peripheral Virtual Circuit
PVR: Personal Video Recorder
PWF: Processing Work Flow
PWP: Personal White Pages
PXE: Preboot Execution Environment

QALY: Quality of Life Years
QDOS: Quick and Dirty Operating System
QIO: Quality Improvement Officer
QIO: Quality Improvement Opinion
QMF: Query Management Facility
QMR: Quick Medical Reference
QOS: Quality of Service
QPSK: Quadrature Phase Shift Keying
QTVR: Quick Time Virtual Reality

RA: Registration Authority
RA: Remittance Advice
RC: Release Candidate
RC: Reasonable and Customary
RAD: Resource Access Decision
RADARS: Research and Data Analysis Reporting System
RADIUS: Remote Authentication Dial-In User Service
RAI: Resident Assessment Instrument
RAID: Redundant (Random) Array of Inexpensive (Independent) Disks (levels 0–5)
RAM: Random Access Memory
RAN: Rural Area Network
RAP: Resident Assessment Protocol
RAPIDS: Real-time Automated Personnel Identification System
RARP: Reverse Address Resolution Protocol
RAS: Remote Access Server

RAT: Remote Access Trojan

RAVEN: Resident Assessment Validation and Entry

RBAC: Role-Based Access Control

RBLEX: Regional Bell Local Exchange Carrier

RC: Rivest Cipher

RCP: Rich Client Platform

RCS: Remote Computer Service

RDBMS: Regional Database Management System

RDF: Resource Description Framework

RDISK: Repair Disk

RDMS: Relational Database Management System

REC: Recommendation

REG: Regional Exchange Carrier

RELMA: Regenstrief LOINC Mapping Assistant

RF: Radio Frequency

RFA: Regulatory Flexible Act

RFC: Request for Capabilities

RFC: Request for Comments

RFI: Radio Frequency Interface

RFI: Request for Information

RFID: Radio Frequency Identification

RFP: Request for Proposal

RHA: Regional Health Administrator

RHEL: Red Hat Enterprise Linux

RHIA: Registered Health Information Administrator

RHIN: Regional Health Information Networks

RHIO: Regional Health Information Organization

RHIT: Registered Health Information Technologist

RHPC: Responsible Health Policy Coalition

RHPM: Red Hat Package Manager

RI: Radiographic Imaging

RICOA: Racketeer Influenced and Corrupt Organization Act

RID: Retrieve Information for Display

RIFF: Resource Interchange File Format

RIM: Reference Information Model

RIM: Research In Motion

RIMS: Radiology Information Management System

RIP: Routing Information Protocol

RIS: Radiology Information System

RISC: Reduced Instruction Set Computer (Computing)

RISS: Reference Information Storage System

RLE: Run Length Encoding

RLEC: Regional Local Exchange Carrier

RM: Risk Management

RM: Risk Monitoring

RMA: Real Media Architecture

RMDS: Remote Medical Diagnosis System

RMI: Remote Method Invocation

RMODP: Reference Model for Open Distributed Processing

RN: Read News

RNM: Remote Network Monitor

RO: Read Only

ROC: Receiver Operating Characteristics

ROFL: Rolling On Floor Laughing

ROI: Release of Information

ROLAP: Relational Outline Analytical Processing

ROM: Read Only Memory

ROR: Ruby On Railes

RPACS: Radiology Picture Archiving Communication System

RPC: Remote Procedure Call

RPM: RedHat Package Manager
RPP: Rich Patient Platform
RPP: Rich Physician Platform
RPS: Revolutions Per Second
RSA: Really Slow Algorithm
RSA: Rivest, Shamir, Adelman
RSAC: Recreational Software Advisory Council
RSN: Real Son Now
RSNA: Radiological Society of North America
RSS: Really Simple Syndication
RSS: Resource Security System
RSSR: Really Simple Syndication Reader
RT: Reference Terminology
RT: Recreational Therapy
RTF: Rich Text Format
RTFM: Read The Friendly Manual
RTM: Real Time Monitoring
RTM: Reference Terminology Model
RTP: Rapid Transit Protocol
RTP: Real-time Transfer Protocol
RTS: Request to Second
RTS: Request to Send
RTSP: Real Time Streaming Protocol
RTT: Round Trip Time
RUG-III: Resource Utilization Group—Version III
RUGS: Resource Utilization Groups
RV: Relative Value
RVU: Relative Value Units
RWF: Reporting Work Flow
RWW: Real World Web

SA: Security Association
SAAS: Software As A Service
SACE: Single Affiliated Covered Entity
SAF: Store and Forward

SALT: Speech Application Language Tag
SAM: Smart Attachment Manager
SAML: Security Assertion Markup Language
SAN: Storage Area Network
SANS: System Administration, Networking, and Security
SARBOX: Sarbanes-Oxley Act
SAS: Serial Attached SCSI
SATA: Serial American Telemedicine Association
SATAN: Security Administration Tool for Analyzing Networks
SBS: Small Business Server
SC: Subcommittee
SCA: Secure Content Architecture
SCA: Service Component Architecture
SCAR: Society for Computer Applications in Radiology
SCI: Scalable Coherent Interface
SCL: Switch Computer Link
SCOM: Systems Center Operations Manager
SCOS: Smart Card Operating System
SCSA: Signal Computing System Architecture
SCSI: Small Computer Systems Interface
SCUI: Smart Card User Interface
SD: Secure Digital
SDBN: Software Defined Broadband Network
SDE: Structured Data Entry
SDF: Standard Data Format
SDH: Synchronous Digital Hierarchy
SDK: Software Development (Developer) Kit
SDL: Security Development Language

SDLC: System Development Life Cycle
SDM: Semantic Data Model
SDM: Shared Decision Making
SDN: Sun Developer Network
SDO: Standards Development Organization
SDRAM: Synchronous Dynamic Random Access Memory
SDS: Smart Document Solution
SDS: Submissions Data Standard
SDTV: Standard Definition Television
SDX: Storage Data Accelerator
SEC: Secure Electronic Conversion
SED: Surface-Conduction Electron-Emitter Display
SEISMED: Secure Environment for Information Systems in Medicine
SEL: Security Enhanced Linux
SEO: Search Engine Optimization
SET: Secure Electronic Transmission
SFM: Services for the Macintosh
SG: Second Generation
SGA: Sustainable Growth Adjustments
SGML: Standard General Markup Language
SGMP: Simple Gateway Monitoring Protocol
SGRAM: Synchronous Graphics Random Access Memory
SHI: Secure Health Information
SHI: Summary Health Information
SHP: Small Health Plan
SHPCC: Sun High Performance Computing Consortium
SHS: Society for Health Systems
SHSE: Society for Health Systems Engineers
SHTTP: Secure Hyper Text Transmission Protocol
SIDF: System Independent Data Format

SIG: Signal Processing
SIG: Special Interest Group
SIMM: Single Inline Memory Module
SINR: Simple Image and Numeric Report
SIP: Session Initiation Protocol
SIPC: Simply Interactive Personal Computer
SIR: Society of Interventional Radiology
SIS: Single Instance Storage
SKE: Senior Knowledge Engineer
SKO: Senior Knowledge Officer
SKU: Stock Keeping Unit
SLA: Service Level Agreement
SLED: SUSE Linux Enterprise Desktop
SLEE: Service Logic Execution Environment
SLES: SUSE Linux Enterprise Server
SLIP: Simple (Serial) Line Internet Protocol
SMB: Service Message Block
SMB: Small Medium Business
SMDA: Safe Medical Devices Act
SME: Subject Matter Expert
SMF: Standard Message Format
SMI: Simple Mail Interface
SMIME: Secure Multipurpose Internet Mail Extension
SMKO: Senior Medical Knowledge Officer
SMP: Symmetric Multiprocessing
SMS: Short Message Service
SMS: Storage Management Software
SMS: System Management Server
SMSBP: Small and Medium Sized Business Partner
SMTP: Simple Mail Transfer Protocol
SNA: Systems Network Architecture
SNF: Semantic Normal Form
SNI: Storage Network Industry

SNIP: Strategic National Implementation Project

SNMP: Simple Network Monitoring Protocol

SNODENT: Systemized Nomenclature of Dentistry

SNOMED: Systemized Nomenclature of Medicine

SNOMED-CT: Systemized Nomenclature of Medicine—Clinical Terminology

SNOMED-RT: Systemized Nomenclature of Medicine—Reference Terminology

SOA: Service Oriented Architecture

SOAP: Simple Object Access Protocol

SOHO: Small Office Home Office

SONET: Synchronous Optical Network

SOP: Standard Operating Procedure

SOW: Statement of Work

SP: Service Pack

SP: Sub Portal

SPA: Software Publishers Association

SPAP: State Pharmacy Assistance Program

SPARC: Scaleable Performance Architecture

SPARCS: Statewide Planning and Research Cooperative System

SPD: Summary Plan Description

SPECT: Single Photon Emission Computed Tomography

SPIN: Standard Prescriber Identification Number

SPL: Structured Product Label for pharmaceutical products

SPOOL: Simultaneous Peripheral Operation On-Line

SPS: Standby Power System

SPX: Secure Packet Exchange

SQL: Structured Query Language

SQM: Software Quality Metrics

SRAM: Static Random Access Memory

SRM: Supplier Relationship Management

SSE: Simple Sharing Extension

SSFDC: Solid State Floppy Disk Card

SSH: Secure Shell

SSI: Service Set Identifier

SSID: Service Set Identifier

SSIS: Social Services Information System

SSL: Secure Sockets Layer

SSL: Standards, Social, or Legal Issues

SSN: Social Security Number

SSO: Signal Sign On

SSO: Standard Setting Organization

STCS: Standard Transaction Code Sets

STEM: Science, Technology, Engineering, and Math

STFCS: Standard Transaction Format Compliance System

STP: Shielded Twisted Pair

SUA: Subsystem Unix-based Applications

SUBC: State Uniform Billing Committee

SunSHINE: Sun Solutions for Healthcare, Information, Networking, and Education

SUSE: Software- und System-Entwicklung

SUT: Server Under Test

SV: Storage Virtualization

SVC: Switched Virtual Circuit

SVGA: Super Video Graphics Array

SVGD: Super Video Graphics Display

SVS: Software Virtual System

SW: Software

SWF: Scheduled Work Flow

SWG: Sub Workgroup
SWI: Secure Windows Initiative
SWIFT: Society for Worldwide Interbank Financial Telecommunication
SWT: Standard Widget Toolkit

T: Number of transactions
t: Time
TA: Technology Assessment
TAC: Technology Advisory Committee
TACACS+: Terminal Access Controller Access Control System +
TAD: Telephone Answering Device
TAG: Technical Advisory Group
TAP: Technology Adoption Program
TAPI: Telephony Application Program Interface
TASC: Telematics Applications Supporting Cognition
TAT: Turn Around Time
TBN: Token Bus Network
TC: Technical Committee
TC: Technical Component
TCO: Total Cost of Ownership
TCP: Transfer Control Protocol
TCP/IP: Transfer Control Protocol/Internet Protocol
TDMA: Time Division Multiple Access
TDMP: Technology Decision Maker Panel
TDR: Time Domain Reflectometer
TDX: Transparent Desktop Extension
TEL: Telemedicine
TELNET: Telecommunications Network
TEPR: Toward an Electronic Patient Record

TFS: Team Foundation Server
TFT: Thin Film Transistor
TFTP: Trivial File Transfer Protocol
TG: Task Group
TG: Third Generation
TG1: Property and Casualty Task Group
TG2: Healthcare Task Group
TG3: Business Transaction Coordination and Modeling Task Group
TG4: Implementation Guide Task Group
TG8: Architecture Task Group
THINC: Taconic Health Information Network and Community
THZ: Terahertz
TIA: Telecommunication Industry Association
TIE: Telemedicine Information Exchange
TIFF: Tag Image File Format
TIN: Tax Identification Number
TKIP: Temporal Key Integrity Protocol
TLD: Top Level Domain
TLS: Thread Local Storage
TLS: Transport LAN Service
TLS: Transport Layer Security
TNC: Trusted Network Connection
TOS: Type of Service
TPA: Third Party Administrator
TPA: Trading Partner Agreement
TPC: Transmitter Power Control
TPM: Trusted Platform Model
TPO: Treatment, Payment, and Operations
TPV: Third Party Vendor
TRILAB: TriService Laboratory
TRIMIS: TriService Medical Information System
TRN: Token Ring Network
TS: Telemedicine Systems

TSR: Terminate and Stay Resident
TTL: Time to Live
TTP: Trusted Third Party
TWAIN: Technology Without an Interesting Name
TXD: Transmitting Data

U: You
UAC: User Account Control
UACDS: Uniform Ambulatory Care Data Set
UART: Universal Asynchronous Receiver Transmitter
UB: Uniform Bill
UB-82: Uniform Billing Code, 1982
UB-92: Uniform Billing Code, 1992
UBE: Unsolicited Bulk E-mail
UBR: Unspecified Bit Rate
UCC: Uniform Code Council
UCC: Uniform Commercial Code
UCE: Unsolicited Commercial E-mail
UCF: Uniform Claim Form
UCR: Usual, Customary, Reasonable
UCTF: Uniform Claim Task Force
UDDI: Universal Description, Discovery, and Integration
UDF: Universal Disk Format
UDF: User Defined Format
UDK: User Defined Key
UDP: User Data (Datagram) Protocol
UDSMR: Uniform Data Set for Medical Rehabilitation
UEFI: Unified Extensible Firmware Interface
UEMR: Use of Electronic Mail Release
UFS: Unix File System
UGS: Unigraphics Solutions Inc.
UHCIA: Uniform Health Care Information Act

UHDDS: Uniform Hospital Discharge Data Set
UHF: Ultra High Frequency
UHI: Unique Health Identifier
UHI: Unique Health Information
UHID: Universal Healthcare Identifier
UHIN: Utah Health Information Network
UIC: Unique Identification Code
UIDL: User Interface Definition Language
UIMA: Unstructured Information Management Architecture
UMDNS: Universal Medical Device Nomenclature System
UMIMA: Unstructured Medical Information Management Architecture
UML: Unified Modeling Language
UMLS: Unified Medical Language System
UMLSI: Unified Medical Language System International
UMPC: Ultra Mobile Personal Computer
UMPS: Utility Multi-Programming System
UMS: Unified Message System
UNC: Universal Naming Convention
UN/CEFACT: United Nations Center for Trade Facilitation and Electronic Business
UN/EDIFACT: United Nations/Rules for Electronic Data Interchange for Administration, Commerce and Transport
UNSM: United Nations Standard Message
UPC: Uniform Practice Code
UPI: Unique Patient (Practitioner) Identifier

UPIN: Unique Patient Identification Number

UPIN: Unique Physician (Provider) Identification Number

UPLC: United Power Line Council

UPN: Universal Product Number

UPS: Uninterruptible Power Supply

UR: Under Review

URI: Uniform Resource Identifier

URL: Uniform Resource Locator

URU: Understandable, Reproducible, and Useful

USB: Universal Serial Bus

USC: United States Code

USMT: User State Migration Tool

USTA: United States Telecommunications Association

UTP: Unshielded Twisted Pair

VA: Department of Veteran's Administration

VAN: Value Added Network

VAR: Value Added Reseller

VAX: Virtual Address Extension

VB: Visual Basic

VBA: Visual Basic Application

VBX: Visual Basic Extension

V-Code: Supplementary Classification of Factors Influencing Health Status and Contact with Health Services (VO1-V82)

VCT: Video Claims Taking

VDM: Virtual DOS Machine

VDT: Video Display Terminal

VESA: Video Electronics Standards Association

VFAT: Virtual File Allocation Table

VGA: Video Graphics Array

VHCI: Virtual Hosted Client Infrastructure

VHF: Very High Frequency

VHLL: Very High Level Language

VI: Vulnerability Index

VIPPS©: Verified Internet Pharmacy Practice Site©

ViPR: Visual Pattern Recognition

VIRT: Vhising Incident Reporting and Termination

VI/VO: Video In/Video Out

VLAN: Virtual Local Area Network

VLOG: Video Blog

VM: Voice Mail

VM: Virtual Machine

VMI: Virtual Machine Interface

VMS: Virtual Memory System

VMT: Virtual Machine Technology

VNHID: Voluntary National Healthcare Identification

VOICEXML: Voice Extensible Markup Language

VOIP: Voice Over Internet Phone

VPN: Virtual Private Network

VRAM: Video Random Access Memory

VRAM: Virtual Random Access Memory

VRML: Virtual Reality Modeling Language

VRU: Voice Response Unit

VSTS: Virtual Studio Team System

VTC: Video Teleconferencing

VTL: Virtual Tape Library

W3: WWW (World Wide Web)

W3C: World Wide Web Consortium

WAA: Wide Area Adaptor

WAIS: Wide Area Information Server

WAN: Wide Area Network

WAP: Wired Access Point

WAP: Wireless Application Protocol

WASP: Wireless Application Service Provider

WATS: Wide Area Telephone Service

WAV: Waveform Audio Format

WBA: Web-Based Application

WBEM: Web-Based Enterprise Management

WBEMM: Web-Based Enterprise Medical Management

WBS: Work Breakdown Structure

WBT: Web-Based Training

WCF: Windows© Communication Foundation

WCS: Wireless Control System

WDD: Windows Distributed Desktop

WebDAV: Web-based Distributed Authoring and Versioning

WECA: Wireless Ethernet Compatibility Association

WEDI: Workgroup for Electronic Data Interchange

WEDI-SNIP: Workgroup for Electronic Data Interchange— Strategic National Implementation Process

WEP: Wired Equivalent Privacy

WFM: Wired for Management

WFMM: Wired for Medical Management

WFO: Workforce Optimization

WG: Work Group

WG1: Healthcare Eligibility Work Group

WG2: Healthcare Claims Work Group

WG3: Healthcare Claim Payments Work Group

WG4: Healthcare Enrollments Work Group

WG5: Healthcare Claims Status Work Group

WG9: Healthcare Patient Information Work Group

WG10: Healthcare Services Review Work Group

WG12: Interactive Healthcare Claims Work Group

WG15: Healthcare Provider Information Work Group

WG19: Healthcare Implementation Coordination Work Group

WH: White Hat

WHITC: World Health Information Technology Congress

WHO: World Health Organization

WIC: Wireless Internet Caucus

Wi-Fi: Wireless Fidelity

WIMP: Windows, Icon, Menu, Pointing device

WIN 16: Windows© NT 16-bit system

WIN 32: Windows© NT 32-bit system

WIN-FS©: Windows File Sharing™

WINS: Windows© Internet Naming Service

WINTEL: Windows/Intel

WISP: Wireless Internet Service Provider

WLAN: Wireless Land Area Network

WLM: Windows© Live Messenger

WMAN: Wireless Metropolitan Area Network

WMF: Windows Meta File

WMIS: Welfare Management Information System

WMM: Windows Movie Maker

WMP: Windows Media Player

WMV: Windows Media Video

WM-W: Wimax Wild

WNC: Wireless Network Connection

WOL: Wake-on-LAN

WONCAAA: World Organization of National Colleges, Academies, and Academic Associations

WORM: Write Once Read Many

WOW: Windows on Windows

WPA: Wi-Fi Protected Access

WPC: Washington Publishing Company

WPS: Washington Publication Company

WRAIR: Walter Reed Army Institute for Research

WSCSI: Wide Small Computer Systems Interface

WSDL: Web Service Description Language

WSI: Web Services Interoperability

WSS: Web Services Security

WSSR: Web Sphere Service Registry

WWAN: Wireless Wide Area Network

WWW: World Wide Web

WWWC: World Wide Web Consortium

WYSIWYG: What You See is What You Get

X12N: ASC designation for health EDI in the insurance industry

X.25: Packet switching network protocol for permanent virtual circuits, switched virtual circuits, and packet assemblers/disassemblers

XAM: Extensible Access Method

XCCDF: Extensible Configuration Checklist Description Format

XECD: Cross Enterprise Clinical Document

XECDS: Crossed Enterprise Clinical Document Sharing

XML: eXtensible Markup Language

XNS: Xerox Networking System

XOR: Exclusive, OR

XSL: Extensible Style sheet Language

XSS: Cross Site Scripting

XST: Cross Site Tracing

XT: Extended Technology

XTP: Express Transfer Protocol

Y2K: Calendar Year 2000

YR: Year

YTD: Year to Date

Z: Zero

ZAK: Zero Administration Kit

ZAW: Zero Administration Windows

ZERT: Zero-day Emergency Response Team

Bibliography

PRINT MEDIA

AHIMA. (2006). *Pocket glossary of health information management and technology.* Chicago, IL: American Health Information Management Association (AHIMA).

Amatayakul, M. (2002, May). 10 ways to keep implementation costs under control. *Journal of American Health Information Management Association (AHIMA).*

Amatayakul, M. (2003, February). HIPAA privacy guidelines. *Journal of American Health Information Management Association (AHIMA).*

Ash, J. S., Stavri, P. Z., & Kuperman, G. J. (2003). A consensus statement on considerations for a successful CPOE implementation. *Journal of American Medical Information Association, 10* (3), 229–234.

Ash, J. S., Gorman, P. N., Lavelle, M., Payne, T. H., Massaro, T. A., & Frantz, G. L., et al. (2003). A cross-site qualitative study of physician order entry. *Journal of American Medical Information Association, 10* (2), 188–200.

ASTM. (1997). *A security framework for healthcare information,* February 11. West Conshohocken, PA: ASTM Committee E-31 on Computerized Systems; Subcommittee E31.20 on Authentication.

Bakker, A., & Pluyter-Wenting, E. (2002). Hospital information systems. In J. Mantar and A. Hasman (Eds.), *Textbook in health informatics.* Fairfax, VA: Hospital Press.

Ball, M. J. (2003). Hospital information systems: Perspectives on problems and prospects, 1979 and 2002. *International Journal of Medical Informatics, 69* (2–3), 83–89.

Ball, M. J., Weaver, C. A., & Kiel, J. M. (2004). *Healthcare information management systems.* New York: Springer Publishing, LLC.

Bates, D. W., Evans, R. S., Murff, H., Stetson, P. D., Pizziferri, L., & Hrpicsak, G. (2003). Detecting adverse events using information technology. *Journal of American Medical Information Association, 10* (2), 115–128.

Beaver, K. (2002). *Healthcare information systems.* Boca Raton, FL: Auerbach Publications.

Blyth, A., & Kovacich, G. L. (2001). *Information assurance: Surviving the information environment.* New York: Springer Publishing, LLC.

Boudrie, E. (2003). *HIPAA facility desk reference.* Reston, VA: Ingenix, Inc.

Breslow, M. J., Rosenfeld, B. A., Doerfler, M., Burke, G., Yates, G., Stone, D. J., et al. (2004). Effect of a multiple-site intensive care unit telemedicine program on clinical and economic outcomes: an alternative paradigm for intensivist staffing. *Critical Care Medicine, 32* (1), 31–38.

Briggs, B. (2003). CPOE: Order from chaos. *Health Data Management, 11* (2), 44–48, 50, 52 passim.

Broyles, R. (2006). *Fundamentals of statistics in health administration.* Sudbury, MA: Jones and Bartlett Publishers.

Burke, D. E., & Menachemi, N. (2004). Opening the black box: Measuring hospital information technology capability. *Health Care Management Review, 29* (3): 210–217.

Chen, H., Fuller, S., Friedman, C., & Hersh, W. (2005). *Medical informatics: Knowledge management and data mining in biomedicine.* New York: Springer Publishing, LLC.

Coile, R. C., Jr. (2003). Technowave 2010: Hospitals compete on high-tech care. *Mich Health Hospital, 39* (6), 12–15.

Committee on Quality of Health Care in America, Institute of Medicine. (2000). *To err is human.* Washington, DC: National Academy Press.

Committee on Quality of Health Care in America, Institute of Medicine. (2001). *Crossing the quality chasm: A new health system for the 21st century.* Washington, DC: National Academy Press.

Computerized Physician Order Entry. (2003). *Costs, benefits, and challenges: A case study approach.* Long Beach, CA: First Consulting Group.

Corey, D. (1996–2006). *Glossary of INFOSEC and INFOSEC related terms.* Pocatello, ID: Center for Decision Support, Idaho State University.

Crume, J. (2001). *Inside internet security.* New York: Addison-Wesley.

Delpierre, C., Cuzin, L., Fillaux, J., Alvarez, M., Massip, P., & Lang, T. (2004). A systematic review of computer-based patient record systems and quality of care: More randomized clinical trials or a broader approach? *International Journal in Health Care, 16* (5), 407–416.

Downing, D. A., Covington, M. A., & Covington, M. M. (2006). *Dictionary of computer and internet terms.* Hauppage, NY: Barron's Educational Series.

Eder, L. B. (2000). *Managing healthcare information systems with web-enabled technologies.* New York: Idea Group Publishing.

Feng, D., & Zhang, H. J. (2003). *Multimedia information retrieval and management.* New York: Springer Publishing, LLC.

Ford, R. M. (2004). Respiratory care management information systems. *Respiratory Care, 49* (4), 367–375.

Freedman A., & Glossbrenner, A. E. (1998). *Internet glossary and quick reference guide.* New York: AMACOM.

Fulcrum Analytics. (2005). *Taking the pulse: Physicians and emerging information technologies.* New York: Deloitte Research.

Ginn, G. O. (2007). The Sarbanes-Oxley and Patriot Acts for hospitals. In D. E. Marcinko (Ed.), *Healthcare organizations: Financial management strategies.* Blaine, WA: Specialty Technical Publishers, Blaine.

Glaser, J. P. (2002). *Strategic application of information technology in healthcare organizations.* New York: Jossey-Bass.

Goldman, J., & Mulligan, D. (1996). *Privacy and health information systems: A guide to protecting patient confidentiality.* Seattle, WA: The Center for Democracy & Technology, Foundation for Health Care Quality.

Gray, M. D., & Felkey, B. G. (2004). Computerized prescribe order-entry systems: Evaluation, selection, and implementation. *American Journal of Health-System Pharmacy, 61* (2), 190–197.

Guchelaar, H. J., & Kalmeijer, M. D. (2003). The potential role of computerization and information technology in improving prescribing in hospitals. *Pharmacy World & Science, 25* (3), 83–87.

Halfhill, T. R. (1994). Transforming the PC: Plug and play. *Byte, 19* (9), 78–94.

HIMSS. (2006). *Dictionary of healthcare information technology, terms, acronyms and organizations*. Chicago, IL: Healthcare Information and Management Systems Society (HIMSS).

HISB. (1997–2006). *Glossary of terms related to information security in health care systems*. London: Healthcare Information Technology Standards Panel (HISB).

Honan, T. M., & Ciotti, V. G. (2000). Information technology: Doing more, spending less. *Healthcare Financial Management, 54* (5), 44–48.

Honan, T., & Ciotti, V. (2002a). Controlling information technology costs. *Michigan Health Hospital, 38* (1), 8–11.

Honan, T., & Ciotti, V. (2002b). Controlling information technology costs, Part 2. *Michigan Health Hospital, 38* (2), 33–35.

Honan, T., & Ciotti, V. (2002c). Controlling information technology costs, Part 3. *Michigan Health Hospital, 38* (3), 38–39.

Jacobs, B. (2005). *Healthcare technology: Electronic health record*. San Francisco, CA: Montgomery Research.

Kaushal, R., Shojania, K. G., & Bates, D. W. (2003). Effects of computerized physician order entry and clinical decision support systems on medication safety: A systematic review. *Archives of Internal Medicine, 163* (12), 1409–1416.

Kiel, J. M. (2000). *Information technology for the practicing physician*. New York: Springer Publishing, LLC.

Kilbridge P., Welebob, E., & Classen, D. (2001). *Overview of the leapfrog group evaluation tool for computerized physician order entry*. Washington, DC: Leapfrog Group and First Consulting Group.

King, L. A., Fisher, J. E., Jacquin, L., & Zeltwanger, P. E. (2003). The digital hospital: Opportunities and challenges. *Journal of Healthcare Information Management, 17* (1), 37–45.

Kiser, K. (October 28–29, 2003). Taming the paper tiger. *Minnesota Medicine*.

Kotecha, H. (2005). *PCs in easy steps*. Southam Warwickshire, UK: Barnes and Nobles Books.

Kuperman, G. J., & Gibson, R. F. (2003). Computer physician order entry: Benefits, costs, and issues. *Annals of Internal Medicine, 139* (1), 31–39.

Land, S. (2004). Surgical information systems. The technology-enhanced surgery department. *Health Management Technology, 25* (1), 20–23.

Lojkine, M. (2005). *The internet in easy steps*. Southam Warwickshire, UK: Barnes and Nobles Books.

Manzo, J., Taylor, R. G., & Cusick, D. (February 2001). Measuring medication related ROI and process improvement after implementing POE. *Healthcare Information and Management Systems Society News.*

Marcinko, D. E. (2000) Management in-formation systems. In D. E. Marcinko (Ed.), *The business of medical practice.* New York: Springer Publishing, LLC.

Marcinko, D. E. (2004). *The advanced business of medical practice* (2nd ed.). New York: Springer Publishing, LLC.

Marcinko, D. E. (Ed.) (2007). *Healthcare organizations: Financial management strategies.* Blaine, WA: Specialty Technical Publishers.

Mata, R., Ramberg, K., & Stuart, W. (2003, February 26). *Loriman presentation: HIPAA implementation in Texas: Beyond the basics.* Overview of HIPAA, HIPAA Security Compliance: Austin, TX.

Mata, R. J. (2007). Information technology and security risks. In D. E. Marcinko (Ed.), *Healthcare organizations: Financial management strategies.* Blaine, WA: Specialty Technical Publisher.

May, E. L. (2003). The case for bar coding: better information, better care and better business. *Managed Healthcare Executive, 18* (5), 8–13.

McDonald, C. J., Overhage, J. M., Mamlin, B. W., Dexter, P. D., & Tierney, W. M. (2004). Physicians, information technology, and health care systems: A journey, not a destination. *Journal of American Medical Information Association, 11* (2), 121–124.

McKinley, B. A., Moore, F. A., Sailors, R. M., Cocanour, C. S., Marquez, A., Wright, R. K., et al. (2001). Computerized decision support for mechanical ventilation of trauma induced ARDS: Results of a randomized clinical trial. *The Journal of Trauma, 50* (3), 415–424; discussion 425.

Metfessel, B. A. (2001). *Technology assessment: Computerized physician order entry.* Bloomington, MN: Institute for Clinical Systems Improvement.

Metfessel, B. (2004a). Processes improvement for physicians and health plans. In D. E. Marcinko (Ed.), *The advanced business of medical practice.* New York: Springer Publishing, LLC.

Metfessel, B. (2004b). Using IT systems to track medical care. In D. E. Marcinko (Ed.), *The advanced business of medical practice.* New York: Springer Publishing, LLC.

Metfessel, B. A. (2007). Financial and clinical features of hospital information systems. In D. E. Marcinko (Ed.), *Healthcare organizations: Financial management strategies.* Blaine, WA: Specialty Technical Publishers.

Miller, S. (2003) *The privacy horizon—How close? How far away?* Arlington, VA: Healthcare Information Management System Society (HIMSS).

Miller, C. S. (2004). Medical information systems and office equipment. In D. E. Marcinko (Ed.), *The advanced business of medical practice.* New York: Springer Publishing, LLC.

Miller, C. S. (2007). Financial and operational impact of the health insurance portability and accountability act on hospital. In D. E. Marcinko (Ed.), *Healthcare organizations: Financial management strategies.* Blaine, WA: Specialty Technical Publishers.

Morgan, C. (1981). The new 16-bit operating systems, or, the search for benützerfreunlichkeit. *Byte, 6* (6), 6.

Morrissey, J. (2004). Show them the money. Healthcare providers say it will take more than vision to turn the government's health IT plans into reality. *Modern Healthcare, 34* (30), 6–7, 10.

Murphy, M. (2003). *Understanding HIPAA.* New York: Author-house Press.

Mutter, M. (2003). One hospital's journey toward reducing medication errors. *Joint Commission Journal on Quality and Safety, 29* (6), 279–288.

Swanson, M., & Guttman, B. (1997, August). *Generally accepted principles and practices for securing information technology systems.* NIST Pub 800–14, National Institute of Standards and Technology.

Oren, E., Shaffer, E. R., & Guglielmo, B. J. (2003). Impact of emerging technologies on medication error and adverse drug reactions. *American Journal of Health-System Pharmacy, 60* (14), 1447–1458.

Osborn, C. (2006). *Statistical applications for health information management.* Sudbury, MA: Jones and Bartlett Publishers.

Peden, A. (2004). *Comparative health information management.* New York: Thomas Delmar Learning.

Pfaffenberger, B. (1992). *Ques's computer user's dictionary* (2nd ed.). Carmel, IN: Que Corporation.

Phillips, J., Rivo, M. L., & Talamonti, W. J. (2004, January). Partnerships between health care organization and medical school in a rapidly changing environment: A view from the delivery system. *Family Medicine, 36.*

Posey, L. M. (2002). Medication errors: Technology coming to the rescue. *Pharmacy Today, 8* (2), 1, 11, 23.

Pountain, D. (1994). The last bastion. *Byte, 19* (9), 47.

Rackley, S. (2005). *Networking in easy steps.* Southam Warwickshire, UK: Barnes and Nobles Books.

Rada, R. (2001a). *HIPAA@IT: Reference guide.* Chicago: Healthcare Information Management Systems Society (HIMSS).

Rada, R. (2001b). *HIPAA security: HIMSS compendium.* Chicago: Healthcare Information Management Systems Society (HIMSS). U.S. Department of Health & Human Services, The Federal Register, Final Security/Privacy Regulations. U.S. Department of Health & Human Services, Office of Civil Rights: www.hhs.gov/ocr; ISO-17799/BS-7799: www.securityauditor.net/iso17799.

Rada, R. (2003a). *HIPAA with information technology essentials.* Land O Lakes, FL: HIPAA-IT, e-Document Press, LLC.

Rada, R. (2003b). *HIPAA privacy cost spreadsheets.* Land O Lakes, FL: HIPAA-IT, e-Document Press, LLC.

Rathbone, A. (1999). *Windows 98 for dummies.* New York: Wiley Publishing, Inc.

Reider, J. (2003). Computerized physician order entry: Has the time come? *Medscape General Medicince, 5* (2), 42.

Rettig, R. A. (1996). *Health care in transition: Technology assessment in the private sector.* Santa Monica, CA: RAND.

Rognehaugh, R. (1999). *The health information technology dictionary.* Gaithersburg, MD: Aspen Publishers.

Rosen, L. D. (1997). *Mental health technology bible.* New York: John Wiley and Sons.

Scalise, D. (2003). MDs + IT: Facilitating physician adoption. *Hospital Health Networks, 77*(4), 41–46.

Snyder-Halpern, R. (1999). Assessing health care setting readiness for point of care computerized clinical decision support system innovations. *Outcomes Management in Nursing Practice, 3* (3), 118–127.

Solovy, A. (2001). The big payback: 2001 survey shows a healthy return on investment for info tech. *Hospitals and Health Networks, 75* (7), 40–50.

Stablein, D., Welebob, E., Johnson, E., Metzger, J., Burgess, R., & Classen, D. C. (2003). Understanding hospital readiness for computerized physician order entry. *Joint Commision Journal on Quality and Safety, 29* (7), 336–344.

Terenziani, P., Montani, S., Bottrighi, A., Torchio, M., Molino, G, &. Correndo, G. (2004). A context-adaptable approach to clinical guidelines. *Medinfo,* 169–173.

Tipton, A. F. (2005). *Information security management handbook.* Boca Raton, FL: Auerbach Publications.

Tjahjono, D., & Kahn, C. E. (1999). Promoting the online use of radiology appropriateness criteria. *RadioGraphics, 19* (6), 1673–1681.

Van der Meijden, M. J., Solen, I., Hasman, A., Troost, J., & Tange, H. J. (2005). Two patient care information systems in the same hospital: Beyond technical aspects. *Methods of Information in Medicine, 42* (4), 423–427.

Varon, J., & Marik, P. E. (2002). Clinical information systems and the electronic medical record in the intensive care unit. *Current Opinion in Critical Care, 8* (6), 616–624.

Wager, K. A., Ornstein, S. M., & Jenkins, R. G. (1997). Perceived value of computer-based patient records among clinician users. *MD Computing, 14* (5), 334–340.

Worthley, J. A., & DiSalvio, P. S. (1995). *Managing computers in health care.* Ann Arbor, MI: Health Administration Press.

HEALTH IT LEGISLATION

June 7, 2006: Draft Special Publication 800–100: *Information Security Handbook: A Guide for Managers.*

This Information Security Handbook provides a broad overview of information security program elements to assist health IT managers in understanding how to establish and implement an information security program. The purpose of this publication is to inform members of the information security management team [agency heads, chief information officers (CIO), senior agency information security officers (SAISO), and security managers] about various aspects of information security that they will be expected to implement and oversee in their respective organizations. This handbook summarizes and augments a number of existing National Institute of Standards and Technology (NIST) standard and guidance documents and provides additional information on related topics.

August 31, 2006: Draft Special Publication 800–45A: *Guidelines on Electronic Mail Security.*

This is a newer version of NIST Special Publication (SP) 800–45, *Guidelines on Electronic Mail Security.*

The draft document, SP 800–45A, is a revision of the 2002 guideline and structured similarly, with new information.

The guide is to aid health care organizations in the installation, configuration, and maintenance of secure mail servers and mail clients. Administrators of electronic mail and other infrastructure services are encouraged to provide feedback on all or part of the document.

ELECTRONIC INTERNET MEDIA

www.4.od.nih.gov/nsabb
www.aamc.org
www.access.digex.net
www.adam.com
www.afehct.org
www.ahima.org
www.amia.org
www.amosweb.com
www.amso.com
www.ansi.org
www.aspe.dhhs.gov
www.astm.org
www.bcm.tmc.edu
www.biosecurityboard.gov
www.cdc.gov/nchs/
www.cio-chime.org
www.comed.com
www.dbmotion.com
www.disa.org
www.ehnac.org

www.emdeon.com
www.fcg.com
www.healthcare-informatics.com
www.healthday.com
www.healthprivacy.org
www.healthwise.com
www.healthy.net
www.hedic.org
www.himss.org
www.hipaaadvisory.com
www.hipaa.org
www.hiww.org
www.hl7.org
www.hp.com
www.imedica.com
www.iom.edu
www.jhita.org
www.mahealthdata.org
www.medrecinst.com
www.meds.com

www.mgma.com
www.midmarkdiagnostics.com
www.midtown.net
www.nahdo.org
www.nchica.org
www.ncpdp.org
www.nlm.nih.gov
www.nubc.org
www.nucc.org

www.pjbpubs.co.uk
www.redmedic.com
www.regenstrief.org
www.spi-bpo.com
www.uhs.bhd.uchicago.edu
www.ushc.com
www.wedi.org
www.wpc-edi.com
www.x12.org

HEALTH INFORMATION TECHNOLOGY TOOLS

According to *eWeek Labs*, September 21st and October 9th, 2006, the following utility tools are vital for any IT worker:

- Audacity
- Azureus BittorrentClient
- Bart's Boot Disk
- Dreamweaver
- FileZilla
- Gaim
- Ghost
- Gimp
- Iometer
- iPerf
- Kismet/NetStumbler
- Knoppix
- LogMein
- Metasploit
- Nagios
- Nero 7
- Nessus
- Net Snippets
- Nmap
- OneNote
- Prime95
- Power meter/data logger
- Putty
- Small GigE switches/routers
- SlickEdit
- Sysinternals
- SystemRescueCD
- Tomboy
- VMware Workstation/Server
- VNC
- X-Lite

HEALTH DATA AND INFORMATION SYSTEMS ORGANIZATIONS

- Association for Electronic Health Care Transactions—an industry group addressing technical and policy issues; http://www.afehct.org.
- Department of Health and Human Services (HHS)—the official government site for HIPAA's Administrative Simplification rules; http://aspe.os.dhhs.gov/admnsimp.
- Electronic Healthcare Network Accreditation Commission—an independent, nonprofit accrediting body; http://www.ehnac.org.

- Government Information Value Exchange for States—a state government agency; http://www.hipaagives.org.
- Hawaii Health Information Corp.—a company that collects, analyzes, and disseminates statewide data to support and improve quality care and cost-efficiency, with pilot policies for HIPAA readiness; http://www.hhic.org/hipaa/pilots.html.
- Joint Healthcare Information Technology Alliance—a coalition of the professional organizations American Health Information Management Association, American Medical Informatics Association, Center for Healthcare Information Management, College of Healthcare Information Management Executives, and Healthcare Information and Management Systems Society; http://www.jhita.org.
- National Association of Health Data Organizations—an expertise broker for health systems and policies; http://www.nahdo.org.
- National Council on Vital and Health Statistics—a public advisory body to the Secretary of HHS in the area of health data and statistics; http://www.ncvhs.hhs.gov.
- National Healthkey Program—a multistate coalition of nonprofit health care organizations; http://healthkey.org.
- Southern HIPAA Administrative Regional Process—a regional public and private partnership forum; http://www.sharpworkgroup.com.
- The North Carolina Healthcare Information and Communications Alliance Inc.—a collaborative group promoting advancement and integration of IT in health care; http://www.nchica.org.
- The SANS (System Administration, Networking, and Security) Institute—a cooperative research and education organization; http://www.sans.org/newlook/home.htm.
- Utah Health Information Network—a coalition of health care insurers, providers, and others, including state government; http://uhin.com.
- Workgroup for Electronic Data Interchange's Strategic National Implementation Process Task Group—an industry-wide collaboration focused on implementation standards, HIPAA readiness assessment and national coordination for compliance; http://www.wedi.org/snip.

HEALTH INFORMATION SECURITY AND BIOMETRIC ASSOCIATIONS AND CORPORATIONS

BERGDATA USA (http://www.bergdata.com)
Biometric Access Corp. (http://www.biometricaccess.com)
Biometric Identification (http://www.biometricid.com)
BioNetrix Systems Corp. (http://www.bionetrix.com)
Cyber SIGN Inc. (http://www.cybersign.com)

DigitalPersona Inc. (http://www.digitalpersona.com)
Identix Inc. (http://www.identix.com)
I/O Software Inc. (http://www.iosoftware.com)
Keyware Technologies (http://www.keyware.com)
NEC Technologies Inc. (http://www.nec.com)
PenOp Inc. (http://www.penop.com)
Phyve (http://www.phyve.com)
Presideo (http://www.presideo.com)
SAFLINK Corp. (http://www.saflink.com)
SecuGen Corp. (http://www.secugen.com)
Silanis Technology Inc. (http://www.silanis.com)
True Touch Technologies Inc. (http://www.truetouch.com)
Who? Vision Systems Inc. (http://www.whovision.com)

HEALTH INFORMATION TECHNOLOGY ASSOCIATIONS

American Academy of Medical
Administrators
248-540-4310
www.aameda.org

American Association of
Healthcare Administrative
Management
202-857-1179
www.aaham.org

American College of Healthcare
Administrators
703-549-5822
www.achca.org

American College of Healthcare
Executives
312-424-2800
www.ache.org

American College of Physician
Executives
813-287-2000
www.acpe.org

American Medical Group
Association
703-838-0033
www.amga.org

Center for Healthcare
Information
734-973-6166
www.chim.org

Institute of Medical Business
Advisors, Inc.
770-448-0769
www.medicalbusinessadvisors.
com
Offers an asynchronous live,
online professional designation
program integrating personal financial planning, health care IT,
and medical practice management for financial advisors and
physicians: Certified Medical
Planner©.

Medical Group Management
Association
303-799-1111
www.mgma.com

National Association of Healthcare Access Management
202-857-1125
www.naham.org

INTERNET HEALTH INFORMATION TECHNOLOGY RESOURCES

American Health Information Management Association
American Medical Informatics Association
Association for Electronic Healthcare Transactions
Association of Telehealth Service Providers
Association of the Medical Directors of Information Systems
Center for Health Information Management
Community Health Information Technology Alliance
Computer-Based Patient Record Institute
Electronic Privacy Information Center: Medical Privacy
Foundation for eHealth Initiative
Healthcare Informatics
Healthcare Information Management Systems Society
Health Level Seven (HL7)
Forum on Privacy & Security in Healthcare
Healthcare Information and Management Systems Society
Healthcare Information Systems Directory
Health Privacy Project Inside Healthcare Computing
Medical Records Institute
National Association of Health Data Organizations
Telemedicine Information Exchange
The Informatics Review
The Joint Healthcare Information Technology Alliance
Workgroup for Electronic Data Interchange

VENDORS OF INFORMATION TECHNOLOGY AND SECURITY SYSTEMS FOR HEALTHCARE

Archive America—record storage and management
AtStaff.inc—has "physician scheduler," enterprise-wide, and nurse scheduling software
Cerner Corp—supplier of health care information technology
Eclipsys—HIM integration with clinical and revenue enhancement workflows
eWebHealth—delivers medical records via the Internet
GE Medical Systems—proprietary doctor practice software
HHS—coding, compliance, and reimbursement solutions
IBM ViaVoice—speech recognition system with medical vocabulary
IMPAC—integrated clinical and administrative management systems for cancer care

LanVision—workflow and document management solutions
McKesson—computer systems
MCOL—managed care software
Medical Manager—financial, clinical, and practice management
Medical Software—medical billing, medical records, and practice management
MediScribe—HIM software
Meditech—information system
MedQuist—speech recognition, document workflow management, and coding
QuadraMed—health care information technology
SDS—health document processor and storage
Siemens—health care information systems (formerly SMS)
SoftMed Systems—health care information systems
SonicWALL—integrated Internet security solutions; comply with HIPAA's Security Rule
TSG—integrated solutions for progressive hospitals
ZixCorp—solutions that protect, manage, and deliver sensitive electronic information

PROFESSIONAL HEALTH INFORMATION TECHNOLOGY AND SECURITY ORGANIZATIONS

American Health Information Management Association
A community of professionals engaged in health information management, providing support to members, and strengthening the industry and profession.
American Medical Informatics Association
A nonprofit membership organization dedicated to developing and using information technologies to improve health care. AMIA was formed in 1990 by the merger of three organizations—the American Association for Medical Systems and Informatics, the American College of Medical Informatics, and the Symposium on Computer Applications in Medical Care.
American Telemedicine Association
A nonprofit that seeks to bring together diverse groups from traditional medicine, academic medical centers, technology and telecommunications companies, e-health, medical societies, government, and others to overcome barriers to the advancement of telemedicine through the professional, ethical, and equitable improvement in health care delivery.
Association of Medical Directors of Information Systems
A professional organization for physicians interested in and responsible for health care information technology.

Center for Health Information and Decision Systems
An academia-led effort at the University of Maryland, with collaboration
from industry and government affiliates that is designed to research,
analyze, and recommend solutions to challenges surrounding the introduction and integration of information and decision technologies into
the health care system.
Center for Health Transformation
A collaboration of public and private sector leaders dedicated to the creation
of a twenty-first-century intelligent health system in which knowledge
saves lives and saves money for every American.
Center for Information Technology Leadership
Uncovers and communicates specific financial and clinical values delivered
by standardized Healthcare Information Exchange and Interoperability.
Certification Commission for Healthcare Information Technology
A voluntary, private-sector initiative to certify health IT products that aims
to accelerate the adoption of robust, interoperable health IT throughout
the U.S. health care system, by creating an efficient, credible, sustainable
mechanism for the certification of HIT products.
College of Healthcare Information Management Executives
Serves the professional development needs of health care CIOs and advocates
the more effective use of information management within health care.
Community Health Information Technology Alliance
A member-driven alliance of health care and technology organizations, both
public and private, that advocates marketplace activities and provides
leadership to help expand and enhance the use of electronic commerce
in the health care industry. Since 1999, it has focused on privacy and security of health data and targets the Pacific Northwest's marketplace.
eHealth Initiative
A nonprofit affiliated organization that drives improvement in the quality,
safety, and efficiency of health care through information and information technology. eHI is focused on engaging multiple and diverse
stakeholders—including hospitals and other health care organizations,
clinician groups, employers and purchasers, health plans, health
care information technology organizations, manufacturers, public
health agencies, academic and research institutions, and public sector
stakeholders—to define and then implement specific actions that will
address the quality, safety, and efficiency challenges of the health care
system through the use of interoperable information technology.
Health Information and Management Systems Society
A membership organization exclusively focused on providing leadership for
the optimal use of health care information technology and management
systems for the betterment of human health. HIMSS frames and leads health
care public policy and industry practices through its advocacy, educational,

and professional development initiatives designed to promote information and management systems' contributions to ensuring quality patient care.

Leapfrog Group

Made up of more than 170 companies and organizations that buy health care that works to trigger giant leaps forward in the safety, quality, and affordability of health care by supporting informed health care decisions by those who use and pay for health care and by promoting high-value health care through incentives and rewards.

National Alliance for Health Information Technology

Created in June 2002 by the American Hospital Association along with 29 other organizations to improve quality and performance through standards-based information systems. It focuses on projects that will contribute to the development of a viable health information infrastructure. Its initial focus has been on standardized bar codes on products used by health care organizations.

National Association for Public Health Statistics and Information Systems

Provides national leadership in advocating, creating, and maintaining comprehensive high-quality public health information systems that integrate vital records registration, public health statistics, and other health information. In collaboration with other organizations, develops standards and principles to effectively administer public health statistics and information systems,

National Health Care Innovations Program

The National Governors Association has called on Congress to establish a National Health Care Innovations program to support state-led demonstrations in health care reform. Some of the demonstration programs would focus on deploying information and communications technology to improve services and improving quality of care. (National Governors Association, Feb. 10, 2005)

Physicians' Electronic Health Record Coalition

A coalition to assist physicians, particularly those in small- and medium-size ambulatory care medical practice, to acquire and use affordable, standards-based electronic health records and other health information technology to improve quality, enhance patient safety, and increase efficiency.

Public Health Data Standards Consortium

A voluntary confederation of federal, state, and local health agencies; national and local professional associations, public and private, with individuals for the overall goal of the confederation is to develop, promote, and implement data standards for population health practice and research.

Public Health Informatics Institute

A program of the Robert Wood Johnson Foundation whose goal is to foster collaboration among public health agencies in the conception, design, acquisition, and deployment of software tools in order to eliminate redundant efforts, speed up development processes, and reduce costs.

Scottsdale Institute

A not-for-profit corporation that focuses on the IT and process improvement components of strategic issues in leading health care systems. It assists members in understanding, deploying, and sharing successes in strategic initiatives involving information management and process improvement.

VistA Software Alliance

A group of companies and individuals committed to promoting and supporting VistA as an electronic health record for health care organizations.

Workgroup for Electronic Data Interchange

Dedicated to improving health care through electronic commerce, WEDI provides a forum for facilitating improvements in information exchange and management including the development of strategies and tactics, definition of standards, the resolution of implementation issues, identification of best practices, and the development and delivery of education and training programs.

STATE HEALTH INFORMATION TECHNOLOGY AND SECURITY ASSOCIATIONS

Alaska

Alaska Federal Health Care Access Network

The AFHCAN project will attempt to bring better health care to Alaskans in rural areas, using telemedicine technologies. The 248 sites mobilized by AFHCAN to participate in the Alaska telemedicine project will include military installations, Alaska Native health facilities, regional hospitals, small village clinics, and state of Alaska public health nursing stations. AFHCAN designed a standard telehealth platform of which nearly 300 have been deployed in Alaska. AFHCAN also developed a robust enterprise-wide software solution that is hosted on 42 connected servers throughout Alaska, built a statewide satellite-based IP network reaching to nearly 200 sites, and developed support and training services to implement and sustain telehealth at the AFHCAN sites.

Arizona

Arizona e-Health Connection Roadmap

The Arizona Health-e Connection steering committee will develop a roadmap for health care IT that will outline directions and goals for care providers, insurers, and consumers. The committee will also identify resources to help with technical standards, including possible funding, and recommend patient privacy and security measures.

Arizona Telemedicine Program

The Arizona Telemedicine Program is a large, multidisciplinary, university-based program that provides telemedicine services, distance learning, informatics training, and telemedicine technology assessment capabilities to communities throughout Arizona. It was funded in 1996 by the Arizona legislature, which mandated that it provide telemedicine services to a broad range of health care service users including geographically isolated communities, Indian tribes, and Department of Corrections rural prisons. Currently the Arizona Telemedicine Program is providing medical services via both real-time and store-and-forward technologies in 20 communities.

Arkansas

University of Arkansas for Medical Sciences Telemedicine Program

Telemedicine technology gives community physicians the ability to instantly share visual and audio information with specialists at the University of Arkansas for Medical Sciences. Using telemedicine, doctors at the affiliate rural hospitals can consult with specialists in maternal-fetal medicine, endocrinology, exchange X-rays, EKGs, heart and lung sounds, and a wealth of information vital to making medical decisions with specialists hundreds of miles away. Forty-one affiliates in the Rural Hospital Program now have this technology and are part of the UAMS Telehealth network.

California

California Regional Health Information Organization

The California Regional Health Information Organization—CalRHIO—is a collaborative, statewide effort to support the use of information technology and the creation of a secure health information data exchange system that will improve the safety, quality, and efficiency of health care for all Californians. It serves as an umbrella organization that brings together health care stakeholders to jointly develop all of the common elements—such as governance, operational processes, technology, and financing—that are required for the formation of one or more RHIOs within the state.

California Telemedicine & eHealth Center

CTEC, formerly known as the California Telehealth and Telemedicine Center (CTTC), has made significant contributions toward increasing the technological expertise of California health care organizations through capacity building, training, education, and regranting. In particular, CTEC has emerged as the primary source for hospitals and clinics in promoting the use of telemedicine and eHealth within underserved communities.

Northern Sierra Rural Health Network

NSRHN serves health care professionals, organizations, and agencies covering more than 30,000 square miles of northeastern California. Major services and activities of NSRHN since its inception in 1996 include managed care for isolated communities, telemedicine, videoconferencing, and development of regional technology services.

Santa Barbara County Care Data Exchange

The Santa Barbara County Care Data Exchange (SBCCDE) operates as a public utility and allows patient-specific clinical information to be securely and readily accessible to any authorized person, including the patient. It serves the County of Santa Barbara as a peer-to-peer health information exchange, including the sharing of reports, results, and personal health information.

Colorado

Colorado Health Information Exchange

The Colorado Health Information Exchange (COHIE) project involves four major health centers in the development of a technical prototype for statewide health information exchange. In addition, throughout the state, several local projects are underway to implement health information exchange among a variety of local providers, hospitals, and agencies.

Denver Health Telemedicine

Since its inception in 1995, Denver Health Telemedicine specialists have been providing consultations to inmates at several jails and prisons throughout Colorado. Denver Health is the first and only Colorado program to furnish ongoing EMS/trauma consultations.

High Plains Rural Health Network

High Plains Rural Health Network was established in 1989 to provide economies of scale for rural hospitals in frontier and medically underserved areas of Northeast Colorado. In 1994, the Network expanded into Western Kansas and the Panhandle of Western Nebraska. After receiving a three-year grant from the Office of Rural Health Policy (ORHP) in 1995, the Network transitioned into a Telemedicine Network utilizing two-way interactive video conferencing technology to deliver specialty medical care, continuing medical education, and administrative business services to member hospital facilities throughout the region. HPRHN is now a totally member-supported Telemedicine Network.

Delaware

Delaware Health Information Network

The Delaware Health Information Network (DHIN) was created by an act of the General Assembly and signed into law in 1997 as a public instrumentality of the state to advance the creation of a statewide health information and electronic data interchange network for public and private use. The DHIN organization falls under the purview of the Delaware Health Care Commission. The development of a clinical information sharing utility is the primary focus of DHIN at this time.

Florida

Florida Telehealth Work Group

The mission of the Department of Health Telehealth Work Group is to lead and provide strategic direction for the department and apostle efforts as it relates to telehealth and telemedicine. The group works collegially to facilitate the use of advanced telecommunications technology in the enhancement of the mission, goals, and objectives of the department by assuring coordinated, educated, and comprehensive deployment of services and resources.

Georgia

Medical College of Georgia Center for Telehealth

The Center for Telehealth at the Medical College of Georgia is involved in a variety of different projects and services. The Patient Data Management System (PDMS) simplifies and organizes the collection of all consult-related information, tracking administrative details, such as the time of the consult, the patient and providers & payers; names and the names of the sites involved. Patient images and heart and lung sounds associated with telemedicine consultations can be captured and added to the patient & payers; electronic record.

Hawaii

Hawaii Health Information Corporation

Hawaii Health Information Corporation is Hawaii & payers leading health care information organization that collects, analyzes, and disseminates statewide health information to support efforts to improve the quality and cost-efficiency of Hawaii & payers; health care services. It maintains one of Hawaii & payers largest health care databases, which contains nearly one million inpatient discharge records collected from Hawaii & payers 22 acute care hospitals for each year since 1993.

Indiana

Indiana Health Information Exchange

The Indiana Health Information Exchange (IHIE) is a nonprofit venture backed by a unique collaboration of Indiana health care institutions. The strategy for achieving this vision is to "wire" health care—first in Central Indiana and eventually across the entire state—by creating a common, secure, electronic infrastructure that expands communication and information-sharing among participating providers, hospitals, public health organizations, and other health care entities. Ultimately, the system will give providers better information for treatment purposes at the point-of-care, and it will give researchers a richer pool of data to guide more far-reaching treatment improvements over the longer run.

Kansas

University of Kansas Center for Telemedicine and Telehealth
Beginning in 1991 with a single connection to a community in western Kansas, the Kansas telehealth network has grown to more than 60 sites across the state. One of the functions of the KUCTT is to research telemedicine and telehealth applications, comparing the effectiveness of telemedicine to traditional health care delivery.

Kentucky

Kentucky e-Health Network
The Kentucky e-Health Network was created to help develop a secure state-wide electronic network through which patients, physicians, and other health care providers can access and transfer medical information.
Kentucky Health Care Infrastructure Authority
Senate Bill 2 (SB 2) calls for the development of a statewide program to reduce medical costs and improve health care by establishing the Kentucky Health Care Infrastructure Authority, a joint venture between the University of Kentucky and the University of Louisville. The program would investigate ways to use information technology and other means to improve health care. The authority is also aimed at implementing pilot projects to improve patient care and control costs.
Kentucky Telehealth Network
The Kentucky Telehealth Network & payers goal is to provide quality health care to individuals in rural areas without regard to time or distance. It is overseen by a nine-member Board of Directors and includes all three medical schools in the state and nearly 70 rural health care facilities.

Louisiana

Louisiana Rural Health Information Technology Partnership
The Louisiana Rural Health Information Technology Partnership developed a project to implement an electronic medical record system in the

emergency departments of 10 critical access hospitals. The grant will also allow electronic information to be shared with other community-based health care providers such as federally qualified health centers and rural health clinics. As a partner in the project, the Louisiana Department of Health and Hospitals—Bureau of Primary Care and Rural Health will assist in the implementation of the project.

Maine

Maine Health Data Organization
The mission of the Maine Health Data Organization is to create and maintain a useful, objective, reliable, and comprehensive health information database that is used to improve the health of Maine citizens and that will be publicly accessible.
Maine Health Information Network
The Maine Health Information Network Technology (MHINT) Steering Committee has begun the Phase II Planning and Development process necessary to establish a statewide interconnected clinical information sharing system for Maine. Phase II plans call for quickly assembling key clinical and IT leaders to address the many technical issues that need to be resolved. The leadership of consumer groups also convened early in Phase III. In mid-June 2006 a group of stakeholders from across the state met at the Hanley Leadership Forum for the second time at Bowdoin College to begin the process of developing an implementation plan and discuss system governance, financing, consumer engagement, and other important elements of the MHINT project.
Maine Telemedicine Services
Maine Telemedicine Services is a statewide professional and technical service of the Regional Medical Center at Lubec that supports health care, mental health, social service, education, government, and industry to increase access throughout Maine to high quality services delivered through interactive video-conferencing and other electronic systems. MTS provides this support to about 100 sites throughout the State greatly through its sponsored telemedicine networks (as well as through consultation services). It currently supports participants in three telemedicine networks: DownEast Telemedicine Network, Maine Telehealth Network, and the Northeast Maine Telemedicine Network.

Maryland

Maryland/D.C. Collaborative for Healthcare Information Technology
The Collaborative & payers long-term goal is to implement and "operationalize" a secure, HIPAA-compliant, regional health care information

organization (RHIO) for the State of Maryland and Washington, D.C. region. The RHIO will ultimately link all the components in the Maryland/D.C. health care delivery chain.

Massachusetts

Massachusetts eHealth Collaborative

The mission of the Collaborative, formed in 2004, is to improve the safety, cost effectiveness, and quality of health care in Massachusetts through the promotion of widespread implementation and use of secure and confidential electronic clinical information systems, including electronic health records, medical decision support, and clinical data exchange capabilities. The Collaborative will also evaluate and promote reimbursement and other financial mechanisms to facilitate widespread adoption and continued use of electronic clinical information systems technology by all health care professionals and provider organizations.

Massachusetts Health Data Consortium

The Massachusetts Health Data Consortium was founded in 1978 by the state and payer's major public and private health care organizations to be a neutral "honest broker," independent of special interests, to collect, analyze, and disseminate health care information. The Consortium offers information on products, services, and special projects that support health policy development, technology planning and implementation, and improved decision making in the allocation and financing of health care. It recently launched MedsInfo-ED, an electronic health information exchange that uses the internet to make patient prescription history information more accurate and accessible to health care providers in hospital emergency departments.

Michigan

Michigan Electronic Medical Record Initiative

MEMRI's goal is to build an EMR from the data generated from standard health care transactions. Aggregated and de-identified to protect patient privacy, the database of all EMRs will also allow purchasers, providers, and patients to make more meaningful comparisons among providers and health plans in terms of cost, quality, value, and availability of health care services. It would also enable government, academic, and public health research institutions to track diseases and infections and monitor, on a real-time, ongoing basis, and thereby be in a position to derive more timely and effective policies and interventions.

Upper Peninsular Telehealth Network

What started in 1994 as a small effort to provide distance learning to physicians among five initial sites has led to a sophisticated 38-site network that provides over 6,000 annual connections to nine critical access hospitals, four community hospitals, a regional referral center, a tribal health center, a summer camp for handicap children, behavioral health clinics, and several medical clinics.

Minnesota

Fairview University of Minnesota Telemedicine Network

Fairview University of Minnesota Telemedicine Network (FUMTN) has evolved from a small telemedicine network originally started by the University of Minnesota in 1994 to a network consisting of the University, which supplies the majority of specialty physicians, Fairview Health Services, owner of Fairview University Medical Center, the primary teaching hospital for the University, community hospitals, and the Ne-Ia-Shing clinic on Mille Lacs Reservation near Onamia, Minnesota. Available specialty services include dermatology, child and adolescent psychiatry, adult psychiatry, asthma and allergy, gastroenterology, neurology, orthopedics, and wound care. FUMTN operations are funded by network members, patient fees, and a major grant from the Federal Office for the Advancement of Telehealth, a division of the U.S. Public Health Service.

Minnesota e-Health Initiative

The Minnesota e-Health Initiative is a public-private collaborative effort to improve health care quality, increase patient safety, reduce health care costs and enable individuals and communities to make the best possible health decisions by accelerating the adoption and use of health information technology.

Minnesota Community Health Information Collaborative

The mission of the Community Health Information Collaborative (CHIC) is to plan and develop a shared information network linking hospitals, medical clinics, academic health programs, public health agencies, and other appropriate organizations that will build connectivity between health care providers in the region in order to improve the quality of, and access to, health care for citizens and to reduce costs for health care providers and consumers.

Mississippi

Mississippi TelEmergency

In response to a lack of emergency care and physicians in many rural areas of Mississippi, the University of Mississippi Medical Center has developed and will direct the operation of a rural health telemedicine initiative called TelEmergency, using nurse practitioners as the health care providers. The program is also linked to the Mississippi Department of Health, which has funded access to electronic medical records generated by the nurse practitioners. This allows them to survey the state and rural areas and Jackson for potential trends in public health or bioterror.

Missouri

Missouri Telehealth Network
The targets of the Missouri Telehealth Network are rural communities in mid-Missouri, with a goal to provide high quality specialty care in participating rural communities through the use of digital telecommunications technology, and to evaluate the clinical utility and cost impact of telemedicine. Three of the project counties are designated as Primary Care Health Professional Shortage Areas, but all of them lack specialty resources of the kind provided by MTN.

Montana

Eastern Montana Telemedicine Network
Eastern Montana Telemedicine Network is a consortium of not-for-profit medical and mental health facilities linking health care providers and their patients throughout Montana and Wyoming.
Montana Healthcare Telecommunications Alliance
The Montana Healthcare Telecommunications Alliance was formed in 1997 by individuals from health care organizations across Montana to share common interests and expertise and to promote advancements in telecommunications through video-teleconferencing and telemedicine. Its goals include cost reduction for the operation of telemedicine networks, promoting Interoperability among and between systems by exploring the use of a state-wide network, promoting services, the pursuit of legislative activities, and the development of a reasonable approach for evaluation and research of telemedicine systems.
Montana Public Health Informatics
Public Health Informatics was formed as a work unit within the Public Health System Improvement and Preparedness Bureau during the Department of Public Health and Human Services' 2004 reorganization of State-level public health. The change was necessary due to the increasing number of systems Montana's public health community was being required to support at both the State and local levels. The need for

these changes became apparent during the public health visioning process where it was concluded that Montana's public health programs had no unifying strategy for the creation of systems to support the public health "enterprise."

Nebraska

Nebraska Statewide Telehealth Network

The Nebraska Statewide Telehealth Network (NSTN) will provide the opportunity for all hospitals and public health departments in the state to connect, provide access to consultations with medical specialists, continuing medical education, transmission of digital clinical information, bioterrorism alerts, and training for homeland security and other emergency issues. Connections between hub hospitals and connecting rural hospitals were initiated in August 2004, and all Nebraska hospitals and health departments are to be connected to the NSTN by 2007.

New Jersey

New Jersey Electronic Medical Records Network

The New Jersey Department of Banking and Insurance will develop a more efficient way of providing medical services through development of electronic health records system statewide, in the process also putting downward pressure on health insurance rates (May 11, 2005 statement).

New Mexico

New Mexico Center for Telehealth

The goal of the Center for Telehealth based at the University of New Mexico, is to help improve the health of all New Mexicans through development of a highly visible and sustainable telehealth network, foster and develop telehealth alliances and collaborative activities, provide support to users, and conduct research, evaluation, and analysis of telehealth technologies and programs, and their impact on health outcomes.

New Mexico Telehealth Alliance

The New Mexico Telehealth Alliance will provide a forum for individuals and organizations to improve the health of New Mexicans through the collaboration and sharing of health resources statewide. The Alliance seeks to enable the development and delivery of technology assisted programs that promote access, utilization, and affordability of telehealth services.

New York

State University of New York Telemedicine Project

The SUNY Telemedicine Program was launched in 1994 with the first ever remote telepathology consult in Central New York and has successfully grown over the years providing a multitude of telemedicine services and specialty care to the rural communities.

Taconic Health Information Network and Community

The goal of Taconic Health Information Network and Community is to provide connectivity for the physician community in the Hudson Valley area of New York State and, longer term, to move physicians toward a community-based electronic health record.

North Carolina

East Carolina University Telemedicine Center

Telemedicine at East Carolina University (ECU) began with the first consults with Central Prison (Raleigh) in 1992. Over the subsequent 11 years, services and infrastructure grew and evolved through the support of the University, University Health Systems, rural health facilities, and several grants and contracts.

North Carolina Healthcare Information and Communications Alliance

NCHICA was created in 1994 as a nonprofit consortium by then Gov. James B. Hunt's executive order to improve health care through information technology and secure communications. Over 235 organizations in the state, including leading providers, payers, corporate partners, professional associations, and state and local government agencies, have joined together to direct pilot projects and other programs. Projects include the Community Medication Management Project, Provider Access to Immunization Registry Securely, the North Carolina Emergency Department Database, and various projects on electronic health records.

Oregon

Oregon Community Health Information Network

The Oregon Community Health Information Network is a collaborative project of stakeholders, safety net health care providers, and CareOregon. The first phase of the OCHIN project is to design and implement a statewide data infrastructure that will offer practice management software to safety net project partners. The second phase of the project is the rollout of medical record software facilitating continuity of care for uninsured Oregonians. The final stage is the activation of a data warehouse on the health demographics of the populations served by the health safety net.

Oregon Health Information Infrastructure
A multistakeholder collaboration to demonstrate the application of health care information and communication technology to improve the quality, safety, cost-effectiveness, and accessibility of health care for all Oregonians.

Pennsylvania

Pennsylvania e-Health Technology Consortium
A consortium of 28 health care organizations plan to build the Pennsylvania electronic patient data network that will be tied into a national system so that patients and their doctors can securely access medical records from any part of the country. The consortium started meeting in March 2005 with a statewide summit in Harrisburg in July 2006 to move the project another step forward. Details such as standardizing software and ensuring data security are important concerns for the group.

Rhode Island

Rhode Island HIT Development Fund
Rhode Island Gov. Cacieri in 2004 signed into law an act aimed at setting up a Health Care Information Technology and Infrastructure Development Fund. The program seeks to jumpstart the health care industry's use of IT by creating a fund that could accept private, federal, and state allocations to pay for health IT in the state.

Tennessee

Tennessee Volunteer eHealth Initiative
The Volunteer eHealth Initiative will begin by providing a framework for hospitals, physicians, clinics, health plans, and other health care stakeholders in Shelby, Fayette, and Tipton counties to work together to establish regional data sharing agreements. Although TennCare is a catalyst for this work, the effort is designed to improve the health care of all Tennesseans. The Volunteer eHealth Initiative is managed by the State of Tennessee in partnership with Vanderbilt University Medical Center.

Utah

Utah Health Information Network
The Utah Health Information Network is a broad-based coalition of health insurers, providers, and other interested parties, including state

government, who have joined together to reduce health care administrative costs through data standardization of administrative health data and electronic commerce.

Utah Telehealth Network

The Utah Telehealth Network consists of a hub at the University of Utah Health Sciences Center directly connected to numerous sites throughout Utah, and is used to provide patient care, continuing education for health professionals and patients, and connections to facilitate business and administrative meetings. UTN can also link with most other videoconferencing sites across the country and internationally.

Virginia

Virginia Task Force on Information Technology in Health Care

The Task Force, created in January 2005, is responsible for developing and implementing a state health information system that better uses technology and electronic health record (EHR) systems to improve the quality and cost-effectiveness of health care in Virginia. It delivered a preliminary report to the Governor and the General Assembly on November 1, 2005.

Virginia Telehealth Network

The VTN presently has a membership of over 50 individuals representing 35 public and private agencies/organizations. During 2003—2004, the VTN Infrastructure Work Group assessed the current telehealth capacity and the anticipated future needs in the Commonwealth and identified weaknesses in the existing infrastructure, developing a white paper that recommends the development of a statewide integrated telehealth network.

MedVirginia

The goal of MedVirginia, established in 2000, is to organize, coordinate, and serve provider interests in health care information technology by providing a system for community-wide clinical data and information exchange that enables and supports improved business and clinical transactions.

Washington

PeaceHealth

PeaceHealth is a nonprofit, integrated health care system headquartered in Bellevue, WA, that operates five hospitals, medical groups, a chemical dependency program, health care joint ventures, and other services in Washington, Oregon, and Alaska. It is recognized nationally for its use of health care information technology, including a fully integrated electronic medical records network, and is considered a possible precursor for a regional health care information organization (RHIO).

Washington State Public Health Information Technology Committee

The Public Health Information Technology Committee provides a forum for coordination of IT planning across many separate public health entities so that communications and data transfer systems are compatible, reliable, secure, and cost-effective. It is a part of the Public Health Improvement Partnership, which guides the development and implementation of a plan for collaborative action to bring about improved health in all the communities of Washington State.

Inland Northwest Health Services

INHS is a nonprofit corporation formed in 1994 with the intent and purpose of bringing high quality, cost effective health care to Spokane and the region through innovative and successful collaborations of health care services, including through the use of its Northwest Telehealth network.

West Virginia

West Virginia Health Task Force

Gov. Joe Manchin appointed Dr. Julian E. Bailes, Professor and Chairman of the Department of Neurosurgery at West Virginia University School of Medicine, to oversee a statewide working group studying implementation of electronic medical records technology.

Wisconsin

Wisconsin Health Information Exchange

The Wisconsin Health Information Exchange, established in 2004, is a nonprofit collaborative that includes public and private organizations whose goal is to provide timely and accurate access to information to improve the quality, safety, efficiency, and accessibility of health care and public health. Its first phase is a three-year start-up of the organizational and technical framework for information exchange between members with electronic health information systems.

Wyoming

Wyoming Healthcare Commission

The State of Wyoming is working toward the development of a long-term, sustainable plan for supporting the effective, efficient, and secure exchange of health information across the spectrum of health care stakeholders. The Wyoming Healthcare Commission, created in 2003, is charged with examining a wide range of health care issues and drafting specific recommendations designed to improve access to, and quality of, health care in Wyoming communities.

MULTINATIONAL HEALTH INFORMATION TECHNOLOGY ASSOCIATIONS

Africa Telehealth Project

The Africa TeleHealth Project provides a staged introduction to telehealth programs in the African market, focusing on geographic coverage and service issues. Initially, the services are being introduced in cooperation with a variety of international development agencies, including private sector participation with Mediastats leading and academic institutions.

ArabMedicine.com

Web portal for health care professionals serving the Arab world.

EU eHealth

eHealth is an eEurope 2005 policy priority, setting targets for both the European Commission and Member States to meet in areas such as promoting a European electronic health card, developing Health Information Networks, and putting health services online.

European Health Telematics Association

EHTEL, as a membership driven European association, offers a platform to all stakeholders of eHealth in order to exchange information, to identify problems, and find solutions for the implementation of the above goals. This is realized through networking between the stakeholders, the organization of conferences, workshops, and specific task forces.

European Health Telematics Observatory

EHTO provides a Web-integrated and innovative approach to dissemination of information on IT and on RTD results to the specific audiences of professionals involved in health telematics. The objective is to create an efficient IT-health telematics market by overcoming the high fragmentation of decisional structures of the health sector. The target is to facilitate and to enhance the relations between users of technologies at all levels (health professionals, decision and policymakers, and hospital administrators) and providers of IT equipment and services (including telecom operators).

Health Metrics Network

The World Health Assembly has launched a new global partnership called the Health Metrics Network (HMN) that will work to improve public health decision making by having better health information systems available. HMN, a partnership comprised of countries, multilateral and bilateral development agencies, foundations, global health initiatives, and technical experts will increase the use of timely, reliable health information by catalyzing the funding and development of core health information systems in developing countries. HMN will help countries gather vital health information and bring together health and statistical constituencies.

World Health Organization's E-Health Development Plan

The World Health Organization (WHO) Regional Office for the Eastern Mediterranean (EMRO) organized the meeting of Health and Medical Informatics Focal Points in EMR in Cairo, Egypt, in May 2001. The meeting made a number of recommendations addressed to WHO and to member states. Based on these recommendations a plan of action was developed, including capacity building and applications.

Australia

Australia E-health Standards

E-health standards selected by national body working on health informatics.

Australian Health Information Council

AHIC was established by Australian state and territory health ministers to provide independent advice on effective use of information management and information communications technology in the health sector.

Foundations for the Future

Australian Health Information Council national e-health strategy plan including priorities for health informatics standardization in Australia, 2005–2008.

HealthConnect

The HealthConnect Web site reflects new partnership arrangements between the Australian, State, and Territory governments to implement HealthConnect as an overarching national change management strategy to improve safety and quality in health care by establishing and maintaining a range of standardized electronic health information products and services for health care providers and consumers.

Health Connect Business Architecture

The strategy and plan for Australia's HealthConnect—a network of electronic health records that aims to improve the flow of information across the Australian health sector. It involves the electronic collection, storage, and exchange of consumer health information via a secure network and within strict privacy safeguards.

HealthConnect Strategy Plan
Five phase plan to deploy electronic health care systems by regions and states released in June 2005.

Lesson Learned from the MediConnect Field Test and HealthConnect Trials
The Tasmanian HealthConnect trial centered on Hobart and focused on diabetes management involving a broad range of health care providers. The MediConnect Field Test involved the sharing of medicines information for over 3,000 consumers in two areas, Ballarat and Launceston. The North Queensland trial involved the sharing of information around an episode of elective surgery at the Townsville Hospital and the secure exchange of information with GPs.

Lions Eye Institute Center for e-Health
The Lions Eye Institute telemedicine project was developed to bring about the use of modern electronics and telecommunications facilities to allow on-line analysis of eye images taken in the field anywhere in the world, initially trialing in Western Australia and Indonesia.

National e-Health Transition Authority
Established by the national government to work jointly with the states to develop an e-health architecture and supply the HealthConnect infrastructure.

New South Wales

Information Management and Technology Strategy for General Practitioners
Includes guidelines for HL7 discharge referral messaging standard (NSW Clinical Information Access Program).

New Way of Delivering Information Management and Technology Services
Details patient information system and infrastructure plans to provide a consistent standard of IM&T coverage for all health areas (New South Wales Department of Health, May 2005).

New South Wales Health Connect Trial
The trial's objectives are to develop, test, and evaluate the core components of HealthConnect and NSW Health e-Link, including business and technical architecture, security and consent, communication and implementation of standards. It focuses on chronic disease management system and child information network.

Queensland

North Queensland HealthConnect Trial
Focused on the exchange information between doctors and patients in rural areas needing surgery and hospital in Townsville. Primary care

providers will generate an EHR and send it to hospital in Townsville, with all care providers agreed to by patient able to share record.

Brisbane Health Connect Trial

The Brisbane Southside HealthConnect trial will focus on adults with diabetes who often need to visit a range of different health care providers to meet their health care needs and will use an EHR system to provide interchange of patient information between those providers. Trial will test use of a Web-based open EHR.

South Australia

Rural and Remote Mental Health Service of South Australia Telepyschiatry

Uses two-way video teleconferencing systems to connect psychiatrists in Adelaide with remote patients. Currently 83 videoconferencing units can be accessed by 67 South Australian rural and remote communities.

Tasmania HealthConnect Diabetes Patient Trial

Designed to provide electronic exchange of information among health care providers for diabetes patients.

Tasmania Medical Smartcards

Tasmania is the first state in Australia to use medical smart cards.

Finland

Finnish Society of Telemedicine

The Finnish Society of Telemedicine aims to promote the health of the population through telecommunication and to disperse the expert knowledge within health care.

Hong Kong

Hong Kong Society of Medical Informatics

The society promotes the establishment of information infrastructure, applications, and information technology in medicine.

India

Framework for Information Technology Infrastructure for Health in India

The primary objective of building an Information Technology Infrastructure for Health (ITIH) is to address all information needs of different stakeholders (government, hospitals, insurance companies, patients, vendors, and others) in the health care industry and to streamline health care activities across the country (Ministry of Communications and Information Technology).

IT Infrastructure for Health & Telemedicine Standardization

The Department of Information Technology (DIT) is responsible for defining the standards for telemedicine systems in India and for defining the framework for IT Infrastructure for Health (ITIH) to efficiently address information needs of different stakeholders in the health care sector.

Narayana Hrudayalaya Telemedicine Project

This project is a "Non-Profitable" project sponsored by Rabindranath Tagore International Institute of Cardiac Sciences, Calcutta; Narayana Hrudayalaya, Bangalore; Hewlett Packard; Indian Space Research Organisation; and state governments of the seven northeastern states of India.

Recommended Guidelines & Standards for Practice of Telemedicine in India (Ministry of Communications and Information Technology, May 2003)

Kenya

Mosoriot Medical Record System

An electronic medical record system supporting a primary care health center in rural Kenya. During initial project phases, the system was used as the sole means to capture clinical data in the Mosoriot Rural Health Center run by the Kenyan Ministry of Health, which provides primary health services to 40,000 patients annually.

AMPATH Medical Record System

The Academic Model for the Prevention and Treatment of HIV/AIDS (AMPATH) is the next generation EMR and is focused primarily on supporting the prevention and treatment of HIV/AIDS in Kenya.

Norway

KITH—Norwegian Centre for Informatics in Health and Social Care

KITH was formed to contribute to coordinated and cost-efficient applications of information technology in the health and social care sector. KITH focuses on codes and terminology, electronic Information exchange, information security, electronic health record systems, and digital imaging systems/radiology.

Norwegian Centre for Telemedicine

The Norwegian Centre for Telemedicine (NST) is a research and development center that aims to gather, produce, and provide knowledge about telemedicine and ehealth both nationally and internationally. The NST works actively to ensure that telemedicine and ehealth services are integrated into health service provision.

Teamwork 2007: Electronic Interaction in the Health and Social Sector

Norway's eHealth strategy has two main priorities: improving the flow of information in the sector and including new actors in electronic interaction in the sector.

South Africa

Health Technology Assessment

South Africa is in the process of developing a Health Technology Assessment mechanism as part of a broader regulatory framework.

National Health Information System

A nationally coordinated effort to support the effective delivery of services at all levels of the health system.

Strategic Priorities for the National Health System, 2004–2009

The Department of Health conducted a review of the period 1999–2005 to determine what work is outstanding and what new work is needed to provide the necessary stewardship of the South African health system. This process resulted in the adoption of a new set of priorities for the next 5 years (Ministry of Health, July 2006).

United Kingdom

Care Record Development Board

CRDB brings together patients and service users, the public, and social and health care professionals in a single forum that will set the new model for care. It will work with the NHS National Programme for IT to enable sharing of information, scheduling, and processes.

National Health Service Programme for IT

UK Department of Health Agency's Connecting for Health is a 10-year project to provide 50 million NHS patients in England with electronic health records accessible by 30,000 doctors with an award of $11 billion in contracts in late 2003 and early 2004.

NHS Health Informatics Community

This site aims to facilitate the exchange of knowledge in support of health informatics through peer to peer exchange, collective intelligence, networking, debate, sharing, learning, and discussion in support of the individual and the organization. Users include health informatics professionals, doctors, nurses, midwives, consultants, suppliers, academics, librarians, and students.

NHS Health Technology Assessment Programme
HTA's mission is to ensure high-quality research information on the costs, effectiveness, and broader impact of health technologies is produced in the most effective way for those who use, manage, and provide care in the NHS.

Northern Ireland

Information and Communications Technologies Strategic Plan
High-level plans and policies for the deployment of an electronic health record system in Northern Ireland (Health and Personal Social Services Agency, March 2005).

Scotland

A National Framework for Service Change in the NHS in Scotland
An expert group, led by international cancer specialist Professor David Kerr, has produced a detailed set of recommendations on how the health service could be shaped over the coming decades. It represents the culmination of 14 months of investigation (Kerr Group, May 26, 2005).
Building a Health Service Fit for the Future
Strategy document calls for Scotland-wide EHR and Telehealth system to improve and speed patient care (National Framework for Service Change in the NHS Scotland Report May 2005).
National Ehealth/Information Management and Technology Strategy Plan, 2004–2008
Detailed planning document for deployment of electronic health care systems in Scotland (NHS Scotland, April 2004).

Wales

Designed for Life: Creating World Class Health and Social Care in Wales In The 21st Century
High level planning document, which includes ehealth and telehealth strategies (NHS Wales, May 2005).
Modernizing Diagnostic Imaging Services in Wales
Details plans for regional collaboration and networked systems to maximize use of diagnostic imaging systems in Wales and reduce patient time patients need to wait for an appointment (Wales Pathology Modernization Project Report, May 9, 2005).

HEALTH INFORMATION AND TECHNOLOGY STANDARDS ASSOCIATIONS

American Health Information Community

AHIC is the public-private entity that will develop standards and work to develop a national approach to interoperability. The committee will include HHS officials and representatives of key agencies including DOD and VA.

American Society for Testing and Materials

A component of the American National Standards Institute (ANSI) that has a subcommittee (E31) for general health care informatics. This E31 Subcommittee on Healthcare Informatics develops standards related to the architecture, content, storage, security, confidentiality, functionality, and communication of information used within health care and health care decision making, including patient-specific information and knowledge.

Certification Commission for Health Care Information Technology

The purpose of the Commission is to create an efficient, credible, sustainable mechanism for the certification of health care information technology products. The Commission will focus its initial efforts on HIT market sectors expected to enjoy the greatest potential acceleration of adoption from Product Certification. The consensus has emerged, supported by Dr. Brailer's report, that EHRs and related clinical HIT products marketed to the physician office practice represent the most appropriate place to start. The Commission will have the goal of having its initial certification requirements and processes in place for testing in spring or summer 2007.

The Clinical Informatics Wiki—Clinfowiki

Wiki technology applied to the growing content of informatics terminology.

Clinical Data Interchange Standards Consortium

The Clinical Data Interchange Standards Consortium (CDISC) is committed to the development of standards to support the electronic acquisition, exchange, submission, and archiving of clinical trials data and metadata for medical and biopharmaceutical product development. Microsoft serves on the organization's Industry Advisory Board.

Connecting for Health

Connecting for Health is a public–private collaborative designed to address the barriers to development of an interconnected health information infrastructure. Connecting for Health organized several working groups focusing on understanding the business and organizational issues of community-based information exchange, sharing electronic information with patients, and several aspects of technical interoperability.

Consolidated Health Informatics

CHI is a collaborative effort to adopt health information interoperability standards, particularly health vocabulary and messaging standards, for implementation in federal government systems.

EHR Collaborative

The EHR Collaborative is a group of organizations representing key stakeholders in health care, including practicing clinicians, payers, purchasers, researchers, health care providers, IT suppliers, information and technology managers, accrediting groups, public health organizations, manufacturers, and public sector partners. The goal of the EHR Collaborative is to facilitate rapid input from the health care community in this and other development initiatives that advance the adoption of information standards for health care.

Electronic Healthcare Network Accreditation Commission

EHNAC works to set standards for electronic health care industry participants to facilitate the electronic transmission of bills and payments in a manner consistent with all federal laws and regulations.

Federal Health Architecture

The FHA will create a consistent federal framework to facilitate communication and collaboration among all health care entities to improve citizen access to health-related information and high-quality services. It will link health business processes to their enabling technology solutions and standards to demonstrate how these solutions achieve improved health performance outcomes.

Health Information Standards Board (HISB)

HISB provides an open, public forum for the voluntary coordination of health care informatics standards among all U.S. standard developing organizations. Every major developer of health care informatics standards in the United States participates in ANSI HISB. The ANSI HISB has 27 voting members and more than 100 participants, including ANSI-accredited and other standards developing organizations, professional societies, trade associations, private companies, federal agencies, and others.

HHS Data Council

The HHS Data Council coordinates all health and human services data collection and analysis activities of the Department of Health and Human Services, including an integrated data collection strategy, coordination of health data standards, and health information and privacy policy activities.

HL7

Health Level Seven is an accredited ANSI standard organization that produces the HL7 messaging standard. It is the accepted messaging standard for communicating clinical data. It is supported by every major medical informatics system vendor in the United States. The HL7 mission is to provide a comprehensive framework and related standards for the exchange, integration, sharing, and retrieval of electronic health information that supports clinical practice and the management, delivery, and evaluation of health services. Specifically, to create flexible, cost effective standards, guidelines, and methodologies to enable health care information system interoperability and sharing of electronic health records. The HL7 Reference Information Model (RIM) is an object model with a large pictorial representation of the clinical data (domains) and identifies the life cycle of events that a message or groups of related messages will carry.

HL7 Electronic Health Record Technical Committee's Home Page

This site is a gateway for information related to the ongoing HL7's Electronic Health Record Systems standards development work. You will find information describing the Technical Committee's work, how to get involved in a project, how to contribute to the current EHR-S Draft Standard for Trial use and future ballots, and information about other organizations that continue to support this critical initiative.

Institute of Electrical and Electronics Engineers's Standards Association

The Institute of Electrical and Electronics Engineers Standards Association (IEEE-SA) is the leading developer of global industry standards in a broad-range of industries, including biomedical and health care, information technology, and information assurance.

MedBiquitous

MedBiquitous is the ANSI-accredited developer of information technology standards for health care education and competence assessment. Their XML and Web Services Standards enable communications among diverse entities in professional medicine and provide opportunities to seamlessly support the clinician learner. MedBiquitous has developed standards for health care learning objects (HLOs), discrete units of online instruction that may be used at the time of need, as well as standards for communicating clinician profile information, education, and certification activities, journal information, and educational metrics. These standards will facilitate collaboration across organizations and make it easier to track licensure, certification, and educational changes or activities.

National Committee on Vital and Health Statistics

The National Committee on Vital and Health Statistics was established by Congress to serve as an advisory body to the Department of Health and Human Services on health data, statistics, and national health information policy. It fulfills important review and advisory functions relative to health data and statistical problems of national and international interest, stimulates or conducts studies of such problems, and makes proposals for improvement of the Nation's health statistics and information systems. In 1996, the Committee was restructured to meet expanded responsibilities under the Health Insurance Portability and Accountability Act of 1996 (HIPAA).

Public Health Data Standards Consortium (PHDSC)

The Public Health Data Standards Consortium is an important vehicle for promoting standardization of information on health and health care. Members of the Consortium serve as health data collectors and data users who actively support the overall goals of developing, promoting, and implementing data standards for population health practice and research.

ACTUAL HEALTH INFORMATION TECHNOLOGY STANDARDS

Alliance Standards Directory

The Standards Directory is part of the National Alliance for Health Information Technology's drive to accelerate the implementation of world-class, standards-based IT. The directory contains organizations that participate in the definition or spread of health IT standards and the standards publications of those organizations. For each standards publication, the directory provides key summary information and reference links.

Continuity of Care Record (CCR)

Continuity of Care Record (CCR) is being developed in response to the need to organize and make transportable a set of basic information about a patient's health care that is accessible to clinicians and patients.

Current Procedural Terminology (CPT)

CPT Current Procedural Terminology was developed by the American Medical Association in 1966. These codes are used for the billing of medical procedures. Each year, an annual publication is prepared that makes changes corresponding with significant updates in medical technology and practice. The most recent version of CPT, CPT 2003, contains 8,107 codes and descriptors.

Digital Imaging and Communications in Medicine (DICOM)

The Digital Imaging and Communications in Medicine (DICOM) Standard was developed for the transmission of images and is used internationally for Picture Archiving and Communication Systems (PACS). This standard was developed by the joint committee of the ACR (the American College of Radiology) and NEMA (the National Electrical Manufacturers Association) to meet the needs of manufacturers and users of medical imaging equipment for interconnection of devices on standard networks.

EHR-Lab Interoperability and Connectivity Standards

ELINCS will develop a national standard for the delivery of real-time laboratory results from a lab's information system to an electronic health record. Typically this process can be a fractured one in which lab results are sent to the ordering doctor's office via fax or mail. The results must be filed in the patient's paper chart or manually entered into the physician's EHR.

E-Prescribing Standards (Second Set of Recommendations)

The National Committee on Vital and Health Statistics (NCVHS) has been called upon by the Medicare Prescription Drug, Improvement, and Modernization Act of 2003 (MMA) to develop recommendations for uniform standards to enable electronic prescribing (eprescribing) in ambulatory care. This letter is the second set of recommendations on eprescribing and sets forth recommendations relating to electronic signatures and other important issues (National Committee on Vital and Health Statistics, March 4, 2005).

E-Prescribing Standards (First Set of Recommendations)

The first set of recommendations, sent September 2, 2004, addressed message format standards that provide communication protocols and data content requirements, terminologies to ensure data comparability and interoperability, identifiers for all relevant entities within the e-prescribing process, and important related issues for e-prescribing (National Committee on Vital and Health Statistics, Sept. 2, 2004).

HL7 Reference Information Model

The HL7 Version 3 RIM is designed to provide a unified framework for, and to serve as a comprehensive source of, all information used by an HL7 Specification. The RIM specifically and unambiguously articulates both the explicit definitions of health care concepts—the "things of interest" to the world of health care information systems—and the relationships (aka "associations") between these concepts-of-interest.

HL7 Clinical Document Architecture

Provides an exchange model for clinical documents (such as discharge summaries and progress notes) and brings the health care industry closer to the realization of an electronic medical record.

Infoway Reference Implementation Suite

IRIS (Infoway Reference Implementation Suite) is a demonstration of Electronic Health Record (EHR) interoperability messaging created by Canada Health Infoway. The project demonstrates and proves Patient Registry interoperability messaging using HL7 v3.

International Classification of Diseases (ICD-9CM)

The International Classification of Diseases, Ninth Revision, Clinical Modification (ICD-9-CM) was developed in the United States to provide a way to classify morbidity data for indexing of medical records, medical case reviews, and ambulatory and other medical care programs, as well as for basic health statistics. It is based on the World Health Organization (WHO) international ICD-9. A version based on ICD-10 (ICD-10-CM) is in preparation.

International Classification of Diseases (ICD-10)

The ICD has become the international standard diagnostic classification for all general epidemiological and many health management purposes. These include the analysis of the general health situation of population groups and monitoring of the incidence and prevalence of diseases and other health problems in relation to other variables such as the characteristics and circumstances of the individuals affected.

Logical Observations: Identifiers, Names, Codes (LOINC)

Coding system for the electronic exchange of laboratory test results and other observations. LOINC development involved a public–private partnership comprised of several federal agencies, academia, and the vendor community. This model can be applied to other standards setting domains.

National Drug File Reference Terminology (NDF-RT) and RxNorm

The NDF-RT and the RxNorm projects are focused on improving interoperability of drug terminology. The area of clinical drugs is seen as important in the growing issues of patient safety. The National Drug File, Reference Terminology is being developed for the Veterans Administration as a reference standard for medications to support a variety of clinical, administrative, and analytical purposes. The RxNorm Project is a developing project of the NLM where new concepts are being added to the UMLS for clinical drug representations.

National Provider Identifier (NPI)

HIPAA-covered entities must use NPIs to identify health care providers in standard transactions. These transactions include claims, eligibility inquiries and responses, claim status inquiries and responses, referrals, and remittance advices.

Systematized Nomenclature of Medicine

SNOMED-CT (Clinical Terminology) has been created from the combination of SNOMED-RT (Reference Terminology) and Read codes. NLM and others are working to bring coding systems such as this SNOMED-CT (clinical terms) into the public domain.

X12N

X12N is the standard for electronic data interchange (EDI) used in administrative and financial health care transactions (excluding retail pharmacy transactions) in compliance with the Health Insurance Portability and Accountability Act of 1996. Used for external financial transactions, financial coverage verification, and insurance transactions and claims.

INTERGOVERNMENTAL HEALTH INFORMATION TECHNOLOGY ASSOCIATIONS

Consolidated Health Informatics

An essential initiative that adopts a portfolio of existing health information interoperability standards (health vocabulary and messaging) enabling all agencies in the federal health enterprise to communicate based on common enterprise-wide business and information technology architectures. About 20 department/agencies including HHS, VA, DOD, SSA, GSA, and NIST are active in the CHI governance process. Through the CHI governance process, all federal agencies will incorporate the adopted standards into their individual agency health data enterprise architecture used to build all new systems or modify existing ones. There is a Consolidated Health Informatics Council to lead the work.

American Health Information Community

AHIC is the public–private entity that will develop standards and work to develop a national approach to interoperability. The committee will include HHS officials and representatives of key agencies including DOD and VA.

National Electronic Disease Surveillance System

NEDSS is an initiative that promotes the use of data and information system standards to advance the development of efficient, integrated, and interoperable surveillance systems at federal, state, and local levels.

Public Health Information Network

PHIN is CDC's vision for advancing fully capable and interoperable information systems in the many organizations that participate in public health. PHIN is a national initiative to implement a multiorganizational business and technical architecture for public health information systems.

HIPAA Information Tracking System

CMS has launched a database to track HIPAA violation complaints. The database will store information from the Office of E-Health Standards and Services, which is responsible for enforcing HIPAA's administrative simplification rules. The database includes search capability and workflow and reporting tools (Federal Register, July 6, 2005).

Health Resources and Services Administration

The Health Resources and Services Administration envisions optimal health for all, supported by a health care system that assures access to comprehensive, culturally competent, quality care. It focuses on uninsured, underserved, and special needs populations.

Electronic Medical Record Resources

During 2001–2003, the Bureau of Primary Health Care sponsored two pilot projects for electronic health records. These pilot projects were the result of the Health Center Information Systems Workgroup's recommendations to provide community health centers with information on Electronic Medical Records (EMR) and Disease Management (DM) to assist with the implementation of systems that support clinical data management.

Shared Integrated Management Information System

The SIMIS initiative began in 1998, in an effort to assist community health centers to approach economies of scale means to implementing practice management technology through either State or marketplace health center networks.

Integrated Services Development Initiative

The program supports integration efforts in five areas, one of which is information management.

Office for the Advancement of Telehealth

Office for the Advancement of Telehealth serves as a leader in telehealth, a focal point for HRSA's telehealth activities, and as a catalyst for the wider adoption of advanced technologies in the provision of health care services and education.

IHS Electronic Health Record

The site is designed primarily for IHS, Tribal, and Urban (I/T/U) Indian health care facilities that are actively involved in implementation of IHS-EHR, or are contemplating doing so in the near future. It provides a variety of information about the EHR product, as well as links to a number of helpful documents.

The National Data Warehouse

The NDW project is upgrading the IHS national data repository, the National Patient Information Reporting System (NPIRS), to a new, state-of-the-art, enterprise-wide data warehouse environment. It is a collaborative project between Headquarters' Office of Information Technology and the Indian Health Performance Evaluation System, a Phoenix Area program.

Resource and Patient Management System

RPMS is an integrated solution for the management of clinical and administrative information in health care facilities of various sizes and orientations. Flexible hardware configurations, over 35 software applications, and network communication components combine to provide a comprehensive clinical, financial, and administrative solution.

Standard Code Book
The Indian Health Service Standard Codebook is a uniform listing of
    descriptive terms and identifying codes for recording and reporting med-
    ical information collected during the provision of health care services.
National Committee on Vital and Health Statistics
The committee serves as an advisory body to the Department of Health and
    Human Services on health data, statistics, and national health informa-
    tion policy.
National Health Information Infrastructure
The National Health Information Infrastructure (NHII) is a comprehensive
    knowledge-based network of interoperable systems of clinical, public health,
    and personal health information that would improve decision-making by
    making health information available when and where it is needed and the
    set of technologies, standards, applications, systems, values, and laws that
    support all facets of individual health, health care, and public health.
Office of the National Coordinator for Health Information Technology
ONCHIT implements the President's vision for widespread adoption of
    interoperable electronic health records. It serves as the senior advisor
    to the Secretary HHS and the President on all HIT programs and initia-
    tives; it develops and maintains a strategic plan to guide the nationwide
    implementation of interoperable EHRs; it coordinates the spending for
    HIT programs and initiatives across the federal enterprise; it coordi-
    nates all outreach activities to private industry and serve as the catalyst
    for health care industry change.
Office of the National Coordinator for Health Information Technology
    Organization, Functions, and Delegations of Authority
The HHS formalization of the organization, functions, and delegations of
    authority for the Office of the National Coordinator for Health Informa-
    tion Technology (August 2005).

HOMELAND SECURITY ASSOCIATIONS

National Biosurveillance Integration System
NBIS will combine health data from CDC, agricultural data from the
    USDA, food data from a combination of USDA and HHS, and environ-
    mental monitoring from BioWatch to improve detection and response.

Joint Defense Department and Veterans
Affairs Programs

Clinical Data Repository/Health Data Repository
The CHDR initiative seeks to ensure the interoperability of the DOD Clini-
    cal Data Repository (CDR) with the VA Health Data Repository (HDR)

by FY 2006. Under CHDR, the DOD and VA are developing the software component that will permit the Composite Health Care System (CHCS II) CDR and the HealtheVet HDR to exchange clinical data so that both TRICARE and HealtheVet beneficiaries receive seamless care.

Consolidated Health Informatics

The purpose of CHI is to adopt a portfolio of existing health information interoperability standards (health vocabulary and messaging). This project will enable all agencies in the Federal health enterprise to "speak the same language" based on common enterprise-wide business and information technology architectures.

DOD/VA Bidirectional Health Information Exchange

BHIE leverages existing joint DOD/VA infrastructure, IT investments, VA/DOD test facilities, and personnel resources to quickly support a real-time, bidirectional interface. BHIE also enables DOD Military Treatment Facilities and VA medical centers to exchange clinical data, capable of computational actions, when a shared patient presents for care.

Federal Health Information Exchange

This milestone accomplishment was led by the FHIE Program Office and now permits the Departments to share electronic medical information by providing historical data on separated and retired military personnel from DOD's Composite Health Care System to the FHIE Data Repository for use in VA clinical encounters and potential future use for aggregate analysis.

Laboratory Data Sharing and Interoperability Project

The LDSI project focuses on sharing real-time chemistry laboratory order entry and laboratory results retrieval between DOD, VA, and commercial reference laboratories. LDSI provides laboratory order portability between local DOD/VA sites that have a local sharing agreement for laboratory services.

National Defense Authorization Act IM/IT Demonstration Sites

Three information management and technology sites are evaluating health information technology projects as potential national health information technology solutions: bi-directional exchange of data, integrated credentialing functionality, and enhancement of the BHIE HL7 data exchange with the HL7 Clinical Document Architecture.

VA/DOD Health IT Sharing Program

Facilitates and supports the development of mutually beneficial health information technology sharing agreements between VHA and the Military Health System.

VA/DOD Joint Electronic Health Records Interoperability (JEHRI) Program

This overarching initiative guides activities and deliverables of VA and DOD sharing and will result in a "virtual" health record accessible by authorized users within DOD and VA.

DEFENSE DEPARTMENT

Advanced Technology Innovation Center

Executive-Level Briefing and Demonstration Facility, Technology Assessment and Technology Insertion, Computer Training Facility, Joint Medical Testing Center—The ATIC provides a full range of technical and technical support services, ranging from a state-of-the-art demonstration facility and conference room to a computer laboratory where the latest health care applications are tested in a secure environment.

Clinical Information System

The CIS is a commercial off-the-shelf-product that supports health care providers in the delivery of inpatient clinical and selected outpatient care. CIS improves productivity by eliminating many clerical and information processing activities. The core of CIS is automated clinical documentation, freeing users to attend to direct patient care. It provides point-of-care data capture at the patient's bedside for physiological monitors, fetal/uterine monitors, ventilators, and other patient care machines.

Clinical Information Technology Program Office

CITPO is an acquisition office for centrally managed Military Health System (MHS) clinical information technology systems that support the delivery of health services throughout the MHS.

Composite Health Care System

CHCS is one of the largest medical systems in the world and the primary automated medical information system for the Department of Defense. CHCS provides essential, automated information support to Military Health System (MHS) providers, enabling improved quality of care for 8.9 million MHS beneficiaries at more than 700 DOD hospitals and clinics worldwide.

Composite Health Care System II

The CHCS II is a medical and dental clinical information system that will generate and maintain a comprehensive, lifelong, computer-based patient record (CPR) for each Military Health System (MHS) beneficiary.

Executive Information and Decision Support

The Executive Information and Decision Support (EI/DS) Program Office provides decision support information and tools used by Military Health System (MHS) managers, clinicians, and analysts to manage the business of health care within the MHS. To facilitate providing complete, accurate information upon which to make decisions, EI/DS manages the receipt, processing, and storage of tremendous volumes of data that characterize MHS operations and performance. The data, which include beneficiary, provider, financial, and health care use, are processed to improve data quality and then are integrated and made available to MHS users through a variety of EI/DS products and specialized data sets developed to meet business requirements.

Information Management, Technology and Reengineering

Applies the principles of DOD information and technology management by developing and implementing policies, procedures, programs, and technical standards necessary to acquire, manage, integrate, and secure information technology systems and capabilities that support the delivery of high quality, cost effective health care services across the operational continuum.

Joint Medical Information Systems

The Department of Defense (DOD) Military Health System (MHS) operates TRICARE as the worldwide, integrated health care delivery system for accessible, high quality, and cost effective health care services to 8.9 million beneficiaries. In support of TRICARE, the Information Management and Information Technology (IM/IT) Program oversees the identification of system requirements and the acquisition and worldwide deployment of software/hardware systems to meet DOD/MHS requirements.

Military Health System

The Military Health System ensures the nation has available at all times a healthy fighting force supported by a combat ready health care system; and it provides a cost effective, quality health benefit to active duty members, retirees, survivors, and their families.

Resources Information Technology Program Office

RITPO develops, operates, and maintains automated information systems to support the TRICARE Management Activity, TRICARE Regional Lead Agent offices, and Service Surgeon General offices in managing the resources of the more than $20 billion annual Defense Health Program.

Telemedicine and Advanced Technology Research Center

The Telemedicine and Advanced Technology Research Center (TATRC), a subordinate element of the U.S. Army Research and Materiel Command (USAMRMC), is charged with managing core Research Development Test and Evaluation (RDT&E) and congressionally mandated projects in telemedicine and advanced medical technologies.

Theater Medical Information Program

TMIP's other prime purpose is as a major technology enabler of the Department of Defense's (DOD's) Force Health Protection (FHP) initiative. FHP is a comprehensive management strategy, including wellness and preventative initiatives, to preserve, maintain, and improve individual and collective health.

NASA Electronic Health Records System Task Force

Currently, the EHRS project is a major initiative of the Office of the Chief Health and Medical Officer (OCHMO). An Agency Task Force, comprised of individuals from each of NASA's fourteen centers and facilities and crosscutting many professional disciplines, is focusing its current efforts on the generation of technical and functional requirements necessary for such a system to operate successfully in NASA's environment. Results from this endeavor will drive the development of an Agency-wide system capable of standardizing an improved level of health care for all employees. Interested individuals can check this page regularly to track the progress of this project.

VETERANS AFFAIRS

Decision Support System
The Decision Support System (DSS) is a set of programs that uses relational databases to provide information needed by managers and clinicians, including the cost of specific patient care encounters. DSS has been implemented throughout the U.S. Department of Veterans Affairs (VA) health care systems. All medical centers should have DSS financial data on health care services provided after October 1, 1998.

HealtheVet
Through My HealtheVet, veterans can now begin to build their own Personal Health Record by self-entering information on medications, medical visits, medical events, and military health history. And, they can also enter health readings such as blood pressure, blood sugar, cholesterol, body weight, and pain and track results over time.

VHA Telehealth
Although VHA has engaged in telehealth in 32 different clinical areas, the organization's main emphases in implementing telehealth is in the following major areas: home telehealth, teledermatology, telemental health, telepathology, telerehabilitation, and telesurgery.

Veterans Health Information Systems and Technology Architecture
VISTA is a suite of health care information software that is in the public domain and being used by many public and private sector organizations. VISTA is built on a client-server architecture, which ties together workstations and personal computers with graphical user interfaces at Veterans Health Administration (VHA) facilities, as well as software developed by local medical facility staff. VISTA also includes the links that allow commercial off-the-shelf software and products to be used with existing and future technologies. The Decision Support System (DSS) and other national databases that might be derived from locally generated data lie outside the scope of VISTA.

VistA Monograph Collection
A collection of monographs has been developed as an introduction to VHA developed software that comprises a large part of our integrated hospital information systems.